Multivariate Statistics and Machine Learning in R For Beginners

Andreas Tilevik

Multivariate Statistics and Machine Learning in R For Beginners

With Applications in Biology and Medicine

Springer

Andreas Tilevik
University of Skövde
Skövde, Sweden

ISBN 978-3-032-01850-2 ISBN 978-3-032-01851-9 (eBook)
https://doi.org/10.1007/978-3-032-01851-9

This Springer imprint is published by the registered company Springer Nature Switzerland AG
The registered company address is: Gewerbestrasse 11, 6330 Cham, Switzerland

Preface

In an era where data-driven insights shape every field, mastering multivariate statistics and machine learning techniques has never been more essential. *This book is more than just a book—it is a full course* designed as an interactive guide for beginners in multivariate analysis. Combining theoretical videos with practical examples in R, this book offers readers a unique blend of theory, practice, and application. This book covers a comprehensive range of essential topics in multivariate statistics and machine learning, including fundamentals of matrix operations, multivariate plotting, and correlation, as well as methods for multivariate data analysis such as multivariate analysis of variance (MANOVA), principal component analysis (PCA), clustering, partial least squares (PLS), and canonical correlation analysis (CCA). By integrating videos with practical coding examples, *this book* makes complex topics accessible for beginners. The interactive learning approach ensures that readers not only grasp the statistical theories and machine learning concepts but also gain the confidence to apply them in real-world scenarios.

Skövde, Sweden Andreas Tilevik

Competing Interests The author has no competing interests to declare that are relevant to the content of this manuscript.

About this book

This book is designed to guide you through the concepts of machine learning and multivariate statistics, starting with some basic matrix operations that you need to know before we cover multivariate methods. Although it assumes that you have some basic knowledge of statistics, such as simple linear regression, correlation, and how to interpret p-values, the examples and codes are presented at a basic level. On my homepage, www.tilestats.com, I have plenty of videos about basic statistics that can be used as a complement to the more advanced statistics in this book. Each chapter links directly to videos at www.tilestats.com/ml/, where I explain the theory behind each method. Some of the videos are optional, which means that they usually cover a lot of math, which is good to know, but not essential to understand the concepts in this book. Following each video, you will find R codes that replicate most of the analyses presented in the videos, which will allow you to get a hands-on understanding. You may either type in the code manually into R or use the source code files that you can download from www.tilestats.com/ml/. At the end of each subchapter, you will find several exercises, which will allow you to test your knowledge of each concept through hands-on practice. The suggested answers to these exercises are presented at the end of this book. I have chosen to explain the multivariate methods with simple R code, using small datasets, in order to facilitate the understanding of how the methods work before applying them to larger datasets. I have also consistently used the same example datasets in the exercises so that you are familiar with the data when learning a new method. In the final chapter, you will find case studies that show how you can apply several of the methods covered in this book by reproducing the plots and analyses in two scientific papers.

If you identify possible errors in this book, please leave a comment below the video in the corresponding section.

To learn about multivariate statistics and machine learning, we will first start with some basic matrix operations and see how to plot multivariate data. Then we will discuss principal component analysis (PCA), which is the most fundamental method in multivariate analysis. Understanding the concept of PCA is therefore essential before learning more advanced multivariate techniques like partial least squares regression and canonical correlation analysis. We will also go through several different supervised machine learning methods that can be used to make predictions based on some training data.

Contents

Chapter 1
A Brief Introduction to Machine Learning and Multivariate Statistics

1.1 What Are Machine Learning and Multivariate Statistics?

The fields of machine learning (ML) and multivariate statistics have now become important tools to analyze large data in order to uncover patterns and make predictions. These methods have been developed to handle the complexity of high-dimensional data, where relationships among several variables are difficult to analyze with traditional univariate techniques. ML can be divided into two main categories: supervised and unsupervised learning. In supervised learning, models are trained on labeled data. For example, supervised learning can be used to train a model to predict if a person has diabetes. The model is trained on a dataset where the input features include information, such as age, glucose levels, BMI, and family history, as well as labels that indicate whether the person has diabetes (e.g., "Yes" or "No"), which the model learns to predict based on the input features. Once the model has been trained, it can be used to predict the probability of diabetes for new patients based on their input data. Building a model with several input features usually performs way much better than traditional methods. Supervised ML models are usually validated to estimate their true performance, which is commonly done by training the model on training data and then testing the model on a test dataset to estimate its true performance. Conversely, unsupervised learning deals with unlabeled data. For example, suppose that we have data from patients with diabetes but no data on healthy individuals. The model can therefore not be used to predict whether the patient has diabetes (e.g., "Yes" or "No") because we have no data on healthy individuals. Instead, we can use unsupervised ML to identify, for example, groups of patients that might deviate from the other patients. Patients in a certain group might, for example, respond differently to different treatments or may explain why they experience side effects from a certain drug treatment. ML can be seen as the engine of artificial intelligence (AI) since it is the core component that drives much of the "intelligence" in modern AI. While AI is a broader field concerned with

A. Tilevik, *Multivariate Statistics and Machine Learning in R For Beginners*,
https://doi.org/10.1007/978-3-032-01851-9_1

creating systems that can simulate human intelligence, ML provides the mechanism in AI for learning from data. By using ML methods, AI systems can be trained to detect patterns, make predictions, and support decision-making in complex domains like healthcare. Multivariate statistics and ML share common grounds and are therefore not mutually exclusive. The branch of multivariate statistics that involves hypothesis testing is, however, commonly not associated with ML. For example, MANOVA, which can be seen as the multivariate version of ANOVA, involves hypothesis testing and the computation of p-values. With MANOVA, we can test if there is a significant difference between two or more groups based on several variables. What makes ML and multivariate statistics particularly powerful is their synergy. While ML often focuses on prediction, multivariate statistics is more focused on explaining the underlying relationships in the multivariate data.

It is important to understand the difference between multivariate analysis and multivariable analysis. Multivariate analysis involves analyzing multiple dependent (response) variables, whereas multivariable analysis involves just one dependent variable and multiple independent variables (explanatory or predictor variables). Multivariable analyses are usually associated with multivariable regression, also known as multiple regression, where one wants to predict one dependent variable based on several independent variables. In comparison, in multivariate regression, one wants to predict two or more dependent variables based on one or more independent variables. For example, suppose that we want to predict the systolic blood pressure (SBP) based on the body mass index (BMI) and Age. Then we can use a multivariable regression model such as:

1.1.1 Multiple/Multivariable Regression

$$SBP = BMI + Age$$

Suppose that we instead like to create a model that can predict both the SBP and the diastolic blood pressure (DBP) based on BMI and Age. Such a model is then referred to as a multivariate regression model:

1.1.2 Multivariate Regression

$$SBP + DBP = BMI + Age$$

Thus, if we have two or more variables on the left-hand side of the equation, we will perform multivariate regression, and if we have just one variable on the left-hand side but two or more variables on the right-hand side, we will perform multiple or multivariable regression.

To get an overview of most of the multivariate statistical and ML methods that will be covered in this book, have a look at this video:

1.1.3 Video

https://youtu.be/wJEUgilH-TA
www.tilestats.com/ml/

1.2 An Introduction to R

If you need an introduction to R, I recommend that you first watch this video where I show how to install R and RStudio and then how to get started with the basics.

1.2.1 Video

https://youtu.be/xm1td1kwmBU
www.tilestats.com/ml/

This book involves the use of several R packages. As explained in the video, to use a package in R, we first need to load that package in order to use it. To load a package in R, we use the function "library" and the name of the package:

```
library(NAME OF THE PACKAGE YOU WANT TO LOAD)
```

For example, we will here first load the package **dplyr** by:

```
library(dplyr)
```

If you run this line, you might get a warning that says that the package was built under another R-version than you use. If so, don't worry since the package usually works fine even if it was built on another R-version. However, if you get the following error message:

```
Error in library(dplyr) : there is no package called 'dplyr'
```

that means that you have not yet installed the package. You then need to install it by running:

```
install.packages("dplyr")
```

If you have problems installing or loading the packages, the best way is usually to copy the error message and search on the web or simply paste the code and the error message into AI tools, such as ChatGPT. In most cases, you will find a solution to why the installation of the package has failed. However, the safest way to make sure that a package can be installed without any problems is to use the latest R-version. If you download a new version of R and use RStudio, make sure that you change to that R-version. In RStudio, go to Tools - > Global Options - > General, change to the newly installed R-version and restart RStudio.

Once you have successfully installed the package, you no longer need to install the package again unless you change to a newer version of R. However, you still need to load the package every time you open a new session in R or RStudio.

Chapter 2
Matrix Algebra

Understanding matrix operations and how to compute eigenvectors is essential for learning multivariate statistics and ML. In multivariate statistics, data is often represented as matrices, where rows and columns correspond to observations and variables, respectively. Matrix algebra allows you to manipulate such data in order to perform operations like data transformation and dimensionality reduction. In addition, knowing how eigenvectors and eigenvalues are computed is important to fully understand how PCA works, which is one of the most fundamental methods in multivariate statistics and ML. This chapter therefore provides you with the basics that you need to know before we start learning about multivariate methods.

2.1 Basic Matrix Operations

We will here learn how to create matrices and how to perform some simple matrix operations. Watch the video below to get a basic understanding of matrices and matrix operations.

2.1.1 Video

https://youtu.be/BOas4cXZ4jY
www.tilestats.com/ml/

A. Tilevik, *Multivariate Statistics and Machine Learning in R For Beginners*,
https://doi.org/10.1007/978-3-032-01851-9_2

2.1.2 Create a Matrix

Let's say that we like to create the following matrix in R:

$$A = \begin{bmatrix} 3 & 1 & 0 \\ 5 & 3 & 8 \end{bmatrix}$$

Note that the matrix has two rows and three columns. We can create this matrix in R like this:

```
A=matrix(c(3,5,1,3,0,8),nrow=2,ncol=3)
```

The first argument in the function "matrix" is here c(3,5,1,3,0,8), which is simply a vector with the numbers from the above matrix, where the order of the numbers is entered based on the columns of the matrix. The second and third arguments (nrow = 2,ncol = 3) tell how many rows and columns that we want for our matrix. Since the above matrix has two rows and three columns, we set "nrow" to 2 and "ncol" to 3.

Usually, one places only numbers for the second and third arguments like this,

```
A=matrix(c(3,5,1,3,0,8),2,3)
A
       [,1]  [,2]  [,3]
[1,]     3     1     0
[2,]     5     3     8
```

To create the following matrix:

$$A = \begin{bmatrix} 3 & 1 \\ 0 & 2 \\ 4 & 3 \end{bmatrix}$$

we define that we like to create a matrix with three rows and two columns:

```
A=matrix(c(3,0,4,1,2,3),3,2)
A
      [,1]  [,2]
[1,]     3     1
[2,]     0     2
[3,]     4     3
```

If we set the argument "byrow" to true, we can instead fill in the numbers based on the order of the rows:

```
A=matrix(c(3,1,0,2,4,3),3,2,byrow = TRUE)
A
     [,1] [,2]
[1,]    3    1
[2,]    0    2
[3,]    4    3
```

2.1.3 Extract Rows and Columns of a Matrix

We will now practice how to extract certain elements of the following matrix:

$$A = \begin{bmatrix} 67 & 170 & 120 \\ 77 & 173 & 123 \\ 89 & 179 & 130 \end{bmatrix}$$

```
A=matrix(c(67,77,89,170,173,179,120,123,130),3,3)
```

To print the element in the first row, third column, we type:

```
A[1,3]
[1] 120
```

To print the element in the third row, second column, we type:

```
A[3,2]
[1] 179
```

To print all elements of the first row, we can type:

```
A[1,1:3]
[1]  67 170 120
```

where 1:3 means that we like to print the columns 1–3. Another option is to simply leave the column index blank, such as:

```
 A[1,]
[1]  67 170 120
```

If we like to print the values in columns 1 and 3 on the first row, we can use the function “c” to specify the column indexes:

```
A[1,c(1,3)]
[1]  67 120
```

Suppose that we like to store the last two columns in a new matrix, then we simply extract these two columns and save them in another object that we, for example, here call G:

```
G=A[,2:3]
G
      [,1]  [,2]
[1,]  170   120
[2,]  173   123
[3,]  179   130
```

Note that we here extract all rows, because we leave the row index blank.

2.1.4 Exclude Rows and Columns of a Matrix

Instead of extracting the second and third columns as we did above, we can exclude the first column by using a negative index. For example, in the following code:

```
A[,-1]
     [,1]   [,2]
[1,]  170   120
[2,]  173   123
[3,]  179   130
```

we exclude column 1 from the matrix, which will give the same output as if we use A[,2:3]. To, for example, exclude the second row and the third column, we can type:

```
A[-2,-3]
      [,1]   [,2]
[1,]    67    170
[2,]    89    179
```

The same can be achieved if we instead extract rows 1 and 3 and columns 1–2:

```
A[c(1,3),1:2]
      [,1]   [,2]
[1,]    67    170
[2,]    89    179
```

2.1.5 Create Vectors

To store the following column vector in R:

$$v = \begin{bmatrix} 2 \\ 3 \\ 5 \\ 1 \end{bmatrix}$$

we set the number of rows to 4 and the number of columns to 1:

```
v=matrix(c(2,3,5,1),4,1)
v
     [,1]
[1,]    2
[2,]    3
[3,]    5
[4,]    1
```

To store the following row vector:

$$v = \begin{bmatrix} 2 & 3 & 5 & 1 \end{bmatrix}$$

we instead set the number of rows to 1 and the number of columns to 4:

```
v=matrix(c(2,3,5,1),1,4)
v
      [,1] [,2] [,3] [,4]
[1,]    2    3    5    1
```

2.1.6 Zero Matrix

To create the following square zero matrix:

$$A = \begin{bmatrix} 0 & 0 & 0 \\ 0 & 0 & 0 \\ 0 & 0 & 0 \end{bmatrix}$$

we can type:

```
A=matrix(c(0,0,0,0,0,0,0,0,0),3,3)
A
     [,1] [,2] [,3]
[1,]    0    0    0
[2,]    0    0    0
[3,]    0    0    0
```

However, it is tedious to enter all nine zeros manually like this. To fill a matrix with zeros, or any other number, we can simply just type:

```
A=matrix(0,3,3)
A
     [,1] [,2] [,3]
[1,]    0    0    0
[2,]    0    0    0
[3,]    0    0    0
```

2.1.7 The Identity Matrix

To create, for example, a three-by-three identity matrix, we can use the function "diag":

```
I=diag(3)
I
     [,1] [,2] [,3]
[1,]    1    0    0
[2,]    0    1    0
[3,]    0    0    1
```

which consists of ones in the main diagonal and zeros elsewhere.

2.1.8 Transpose a Matrix

To transpose a matrix in R, we can use the function "t". Suppose that we would like to transpose the following matrix:

$$A = \begin{bmatrix} 1 & 3 & 5 \\ 2 & 4 & 6 \end{bmatrix}$$

```
A=matrix(c(1,2,3,4,5,6),2,3)
A
      [,1]  [,2] [,3]
[1,]     1     3    5
[2,]     2     4    6
```

then we type:

```
t(A)
     [,1] [,2]
[1,]    1    2
[2,]    3    4
[3,]    5    6
```

Note that the rows of the original matrix now correspond to the columns of the transposed matrix.

2.1.9 Symmetric Matrices

From the video, we know the definition of a symmetric matrix. To see if the following square matrix:

$$A = \begin{bmatrix} 1 & 2 & 4 \\ 2 & 1 & 3 \\ 4 & 3 & 1 \end{bmatrix}$$

is symmetric, we can check if the elements in matrix A are equal to the elements of its transpose:

```
A=matrix(c(1,2,4,2,1,3,4,3,1),3,3)
t(A)
A==t(A)
    [,1]  [,2]  [,3]
[1,] TRUE TRUE TRUE
[2,] TRUE TRUE TRUE
[3,] TRUE TRUE TRUE
```

We see that all elements are “TRUE”, which means that all elements in A are equal to the elements of the transpose of A. Thus, matrix A is a symmetric matrix.

A simpler way to check if a square matrix is symmetric is to use the function “isSymmetric”:

```
isSymmetric(A)
[1] TRUE
```

2.1.10 Matrix Addition and Subtraction

We will now practice how to add and subtract two matrices. For example, if we like to add these two matrices in R:

$$A = \begin{bmatrix} 1 & 2 \\ 3 & 4 \end{bmatrix}, B = \begin{bmatrix} 2 & 2 \\ 2 & 2 \end{bmatrix}$$

we first create them and simply type: $A + B$:

```
A=matrix(c(1,3,2,4),2,2)
B=matrix(2,2,2) # Fill a 2 by 2 matrix with twos
A+B
     [,1] [,2]
[1,]    3    4
[2,]    5    6
```

and if we like to subtract B from A, we type:

```
A-B
     [,1] [,2]
[1,]   -1    0
[2,]    1    2
```

2.1.11 Matrix Multiplication

We will now practice how to multiply a matrix by a number (scalar multiplication) and how to multiply two matrices. For example, let's say that we like to compute three times matrix A, then we type:

```
A=matrix(c(1,3,2,4),2,2)
3*A
     [,1] [,2]
[1,]    3    6
[2,]    9   12
```

However, when we like to multiply two matrices in R, we do not just use the symbol "*". Instead, we use these three symbols: "%*%". For example, let's say that we like to multiply matrix A by the column vector v:

$$A \cdot v = \begin{bmatrix} 1 & 2 \\ 3 & 4 \end{bmatrix} \cdot \begin{bmatrix} 3 \\ 4 \end{bmatrix}.$$

We then type:

```
A=matrix(c(1,3,2,4),2,2)
v=matrix(c(3,4),2,1)
A%*%v
     [,1]
[1,]   11
[2,]   25
```

If you would try and multiply these two matrices by using just "*", you will get the following error message:

```
A*v
Error in A * v : non-conformable arrays
```

because if you use only "*", R will multiply the corresponding elements together, and since the two matrices, A and v, do not have the same number of elements, we cannot perform such an operation. Basically, use only "%*%" in R if you like to multiply two matrices. Note that we will get the same error message if we try to add the two matrices:

```
A+v
Error in A + v : non-conformable arrays
```

since adding two matrices requires that they have the same number of rows and columns. Remember from the video that multiplying two matrices requires that the number of columns of the first matrix must be equal to the number of rows of the second matrix. Since matrix A has two columns and matrix v has two rows, we can compute their product by:

```
A%*%v
```

However, if we try to multiply matrix v by A, we will get the following error message:

```
v%*%A
Error in v %*% A : non-conformable arguments
```

because the first matrix, v, has one column, whereas the second matrix, A, has two rows. However, if we transpose vector v, it will have the same number of columns as rows of the second matrix. Then we can compute their product by:

```
t(v)%*%A
        [,1]     [,2]
[1,]      15       22
```

Remember from the video that $A \times B$ does, usually, not result in the same matrix as if we compute $B \times A$. Have a look at this example:

```
A=matrix(c(1,3,2,1),2,2)
B=matrix(c(2,2,2,1),2,2)
A%*%B
      [,1] [,2]
[1,]     6    4
[2,]     8    7

B%*%A
      [,1] [,2]
[1,]     8    6
[2,]     5    5
```

Note that the two resulting matrices are different, which tells us that the order we multiply two matrices matters.

Also, remember that, if we multiply a matrix by the identity matrix, the resulting matrix will be the same as the original matrix. For example, if we multiply the identity matrix by the following column vector v:

```
I=diag(2) # A two-by-two identity matrix
v=matrix(c(3,4),2,1)
v
      [,1]
[1,]     3
[2,]     4
I%*%v
      [,1]
[1,]     3
[2,]     4
```

we see that the product will be identical to vector v.

2.2 Exercises

1. Create the following matrix in R and print only its second column.

$$A = \begin{bmatrix} 4 & 1 \\ 1 & 5 \\ 0 & 9 \end{bmatrix}$$

2. Create the following matrix in R. Once you have created this matrix, extract only the last two columns and the last row (the values 3 and 1) and save these in a vector with the name V.

$$A = \begin{bmatrix} 5 & 2 & 4 \\ 6 & 3 & 1 \end{bmatrix}$$

3. Create a four-by-four identity matrix and print its transpose.
4. Check if matrix A is a symmetric matrix.

$$A = \begin{bmatrix} 3 & 2 & 4 \\ 2 & 1 & 3 \\ 4 & 3 & 2 \end{bmatrix}$$

5. Compute $A - B$.

$$A = \begin{bmatrix} 3 & 2 \\ 1 & 2 \end{bmatrix}$$

$$B = \begin{bmatrix} 4 & 3 \\ 2 & 2 \end{bmatrix}$$

6. Compute $A \times v$.

$$A = \begin{bmatrix} 3 & 2 & 4 \\ 2 & 1 & 3 \\ 4 & 3 & 2 \end{bmatrix}$$

$$v = \begin{bmatrix} 2 \\ 1 \\ 3 \end{bmatrix}$$

7. Is it possible to compute $v \times A$? Explain why, or why not.
8. Multiply matrix A with an identity matrix of appropriate size.

$$A = \begin{bmatrix} 2 & 3 \\ 2 & 3 \\ 1 & 3 \end{bmatrix}$$

2.3 Determinant and Inverse of a Matrix

In this second part of matrices and matrix operations, we will see how to compute the determinant and the inverse of a matrix. We will also learn how to solve a system of equations in R. Watch the video below to get an understanding of how to compute these matrices by hand:

2.3.1 Video

https://youtu.be/DeqqXHJnvyE
www.tilestats.com/ml/

2.3.2 The Determinant of a Matrix

From the video, we know that it is very time-consuming to calculate the determinant and the inverse of a matrix by hand. However, this is easy in R. We compute the determinant of a square matrix by the function "det". For example, to compute the determinant of matrix A:

$$A = \begin{bmatrix} 3 & 2 \\ 2 & 4 \end{bmatrix}$$

we first create the matrix and use the function "det":

```
A=matrix(c(3,2,2,4),2,2).
det(A)
8
```

Similarly, we can compute the determinant of the following matrix:

$$A = \begin{bmatrix} 1 & 2 & 3 \\ 4 & 5 & 5 \\ 3 & 2 & 3 \end{bmatrix}$$

by

```
A=matrix(c(1,4,3,2,5,2,3,5,3),3,3)
det(A)
-10
```

2.3.3 The Inverse of a Matrix

The inverse of a matrix can be computed with the function "solve". For example, to compute the inverse of the following matrix:

$$A = \begin{bmatrix} 3 & 1 \\ 4 & 2 \end{bmatrix}$$

we type:

```
A=matrix(c(3,4,1,2),2,2)
solve(A)
        [,1]  [,2]
[1,]      1   -0.5
[2,]     -2    1.5
```

From the video, we know that we cannot compute the inverse of a matrix when its determinant is equal to zero. For example, we will get the following error message if we try to compute the inverse of the following matrix:

```
B=matrix(c(3,3,2,2),2,2)
det(B)
0
solve(B)
Error in solve.default(B) :
  Lapack routine dgesv: system is exactly singular:
  U[2,2] = 0
```

Remember from the video that if we multiply a matrix by its inverse, we will obtain the identity matrix:

$$AA^{-1} = I$$

Let's test this in R based on the following matrix:

$$A = \begin{bmatrix} 3 & 1 \\ 4 & 2 \end{bmatrix}$$

```
A=matrix(c(3,4,1,2),2,2)
A%*%solve(A)
      [,1]  [,2]
[1,]    1     0
[2,]    0     1
```

We see, as expected, that this computation results in the identity matrix.

2.3.4 Solving a System of Linear Equations

Suppose that we like to solve the following system as shown in the video:

$$3a + 1b = 4$$
$$4a + 2b = 6$$

First, we write the system in matrix form. Let matrix A be our coefficient matrix:

$$A = \begin{bmatrix} 3 & 1 \\ 4 & 2 \end{bmatrix}$$

This matrix stores the coefficients on the left-hand side of the equation. B is our constant column matrix (vector) which stores the numbers on the right-hand side:

$$B = \begin{bmatrix} 4 \\ 6 \end{bmatrix}$$

We can now solve this system by using the function "solve":

```
A=matrix(c(3,4,1,2),2,2)
B= matrix(c(4,6),2,1)
solve(A,B) # solve(A)%*%B   also works
     [,1]
[1,]    1
[2,]    1
```

From the output, we can see that a is equal to 1 and that b is also equal to 1. Try and plug in these numbers by hand in the system above, and make sure that the left-hand side is equal to the right-hand side when you set a and b to 1.

2.4 Exercises

1. Compute the inverse and the determinant of the following matrix.

$$A = \begin{bmatrix} 5 & 2 & 3 \\ 5 & 5 & 5 \\ 3 & 2 & 3 \end{bmatrix}$$

2. Explain why it is not possible to compute the inverse of the following matrix.

$$A = \begin{bmatrix} 4 & 2 \\ 8 & 4 \end{bmatrix}$$

3. Solve the following system of equations.

$$2x + 3y - 2z = 10$$
$$3x - 2y + 2z = 20$$
$$4x + 4y + 3z = 30$$

2.5 Eigenvectors and Eigenvalues

Eigenvectors are special vectors that are often used in multivariate statistical methods, such as in PCA and in linear discriminant analysis. We will first learn how to represent a vector in a plot and then see how to compute eigenvectors and eigenvalues. Watch the first video to get an understanding of eigenvectors and eigenvalues. You may also watch the optional second video that shows how eigenvectors and eigenvalues are calculated by hand.

2.5.1 Videos

https://youtu.be/v6OMIjmixdo
https://youtu.be/YxfxiWrGamI
www.tilestats.com/ml/

2.5.2 Draw a Vector in a Graph

To understand eigenvectors, we will first learn how to draw vectors in R. Let's draw the following vector:

$$v = \begin{bmatrix} 3 \\ 3 \end{bmatrix}$$

in a graph (Fig. 2.1):

```
v=matrix(c(3,3),2,1) # Vector to be drawn
# Coordinates of the starting point of the vector
origin=c(0,0)
plot(NULL,NULL,xlim=c(0,5),ylim=c(0,5),las=1,xlab="x",
ylab="y") # Create an empty plot
grid() # Add a grid
# Add an arrow that represents the vector
arrows(origin[1],origin[2],v[1],v[2],length = 0.15)
```

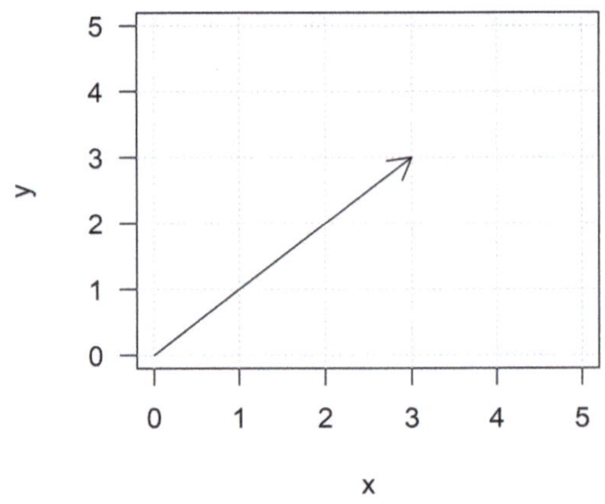

Fig. 2.1 A vector in the Cartesian plane starting at the origin (0,0) and ending at the point (3,3)

We can calculate the length of this vector by:

$$L = \sqrt{x^2 + y^2}$$

```
sqrt(sum(v^2))
[1] 4.242641
```

2.5.3 *Eigenvectors*

From the video, we know that an eigenvector, v, is a non-zero vector that satisfies the following equation:

$$Av = \lambda v$$

Let's test if the following vector:

$$v = \begin{bmatrix} 2 \\ 2 \end{bmatrix}$$

is an eigenvector of matrix A.

$$A = \begin{bmatrix} 1 & 2 \\ 1 & 0 \end{bmatrix}$$

Vector v can be represented in space like this (Fig. 2.2):

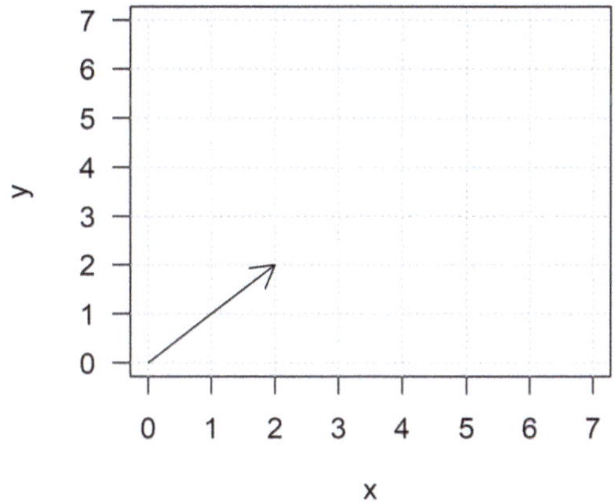

Fig. 2.2 A vector in the Cartesian plane starting at the origin (0,0) and ending at the point (2,2)

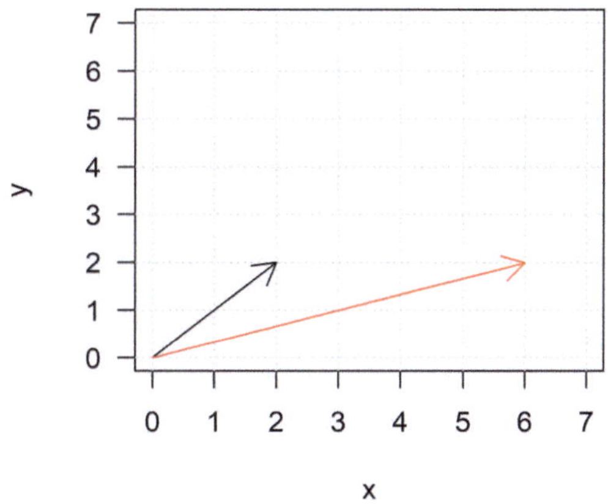

Fig. 2.3 Two vectors in the Cartesian plane starting at the origin (0,0). The black vector points to the coordinates (2,2), while the red vector extends further to (6,2)

```
v=matrix(c(2,2),2,1) # Vector to be drawn
# Coordinates of the starting point of the vector
origin=c(0,0)
plot(NULL,NULL,xlim=c(0,7),ylim=c(0,7),las=1,xlab="x",
ylab="y") # Create an empty plot
grid() # Add a grid
# Add an arrow that represents the vector
arrows(origin[1],origin[2],v[1],v[2],length = 0.15)
```

If we multiply matrix A by vector v, we get:

$$Av = \begin{bmatrix} 1 & 2 \\ 1 & 0 \end{bmatrix} \cdot \begin{bmatrix} 2 \\ 2 \end{bmatrix} = \begin{bmatrix} 6 \\ 2 \end{bmatrix}$$

If we now plot this new vector (Fig. 2.3), Av, by:

```
A=matrix(c(1,1,2,0),2,2)
Av=A%*%v # Calculate new vector
arrows(origin[1],origin[2],Av[1],Av[2],length =
0.15,col="red")
```

we see that the two vectors do not have the same direction (they are not on the same line). Vector v is therefore not an eigenvector of matrix A. Let's see if the following vector is an eigenvector of the same matrix (Fig. 2.4):

$$v = \begin{bmatrix} 2 \\ 1 \end{bmatrix}$$

```
v=matrix(c(2,1),2,1) # Vector to be drawn
# Coordinates of the starting point of the vector
origin=c(0,0)
plot(NULL,NULL,xlim=c(0,7),ylim=c(0,7),las=1,xlab="x",
ylab="y") # Create an empty plot
grid() # Add a grid
A=matrix(c(1,1,2,0),2,2)
Av=A%*%v # Calculate new vector
# Add an arrow that represents vector v
arrows(origin[1],origin[2],v[1],v[2],length = 0.15)
arrows(origin[1],origin[2],Av[1],Av[2],length =
0.15,col="red") # Add an arrow for Av
```

We see that the two vectors, v and Av, now have the same direction. Thus, vector v is therefore an eigenvector of matrix A. Since vector Av has the same direction as vector v, vector Av is also an eigenvector of matrix A.

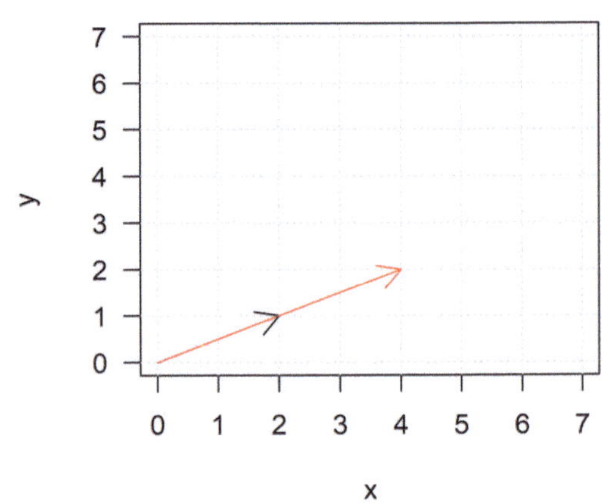

Fig. 2.4 Two vectors in the Cartesian plane starting at the origin (0,0). The black vector points to the coordinates (2,1), while the red vector extends further to (4,2). Since the red vector points in the same direction as the original vector (black), the original vector is therefore an eigenvector of matrix A

2.5.4 Eigenvalue

The eigenvalue tells us how much the eigenvector changes in size when multiplied by the matrix. If we calculate the lengths of the two vectors we previously created:

```
sqrt(sum(v^2))
[1] 2.236068
sqrt(sum(Av^2))
[1] 4.472136
```

and then calculate the ratio of these:

```
sqrt(sum(Av^2))/sqrt(sum(v^2))
[1] 2
```

we see that vector *Av* is twice as long as vector *v*. Our eigenvalue, λ, is therefore equal to two. We therefore satisfy the following equation:

$$Av = \lambda v$$

because *Av* results in a vector with the same direction as vector *v*. When we multiply matrix *A* by vector *v*, we get a new vector, *Av* or λv, with the same direction, but which is two times longer because λ is here equal to two.

2.5.5 Unit Length

Usually, one normalizes eigenvectors to unit length, which means that its length should be equal to one. Let's normalize our eigenvector:

$$v = \begin{bmatrix} 2 \\ 1 \end{bmatrix}$$

to unit length by dividing by its length:

```
v=matrix(c(2,1),2,1)
v / sqrt(sum(v^2))
          [,1]
[1,] 0.8944272
[2,] 0.4472136
```

$$v = \begin{bmatrix} 0.8944272 \\ 0.4472136 \end{bmatrix}$$

The eigenvector has now a length of one.

2.5.6 Compute Eigenvectors and Eigenvalues

From the second video about eigenvectors, we know that it is complicated to calculate eigenvectors and eigenvalues by hand. However, this is easy in R where we simply use the function "eigen". For example, to compute the eigenvector of our previous matrix:

$$A = \begin{bmatrix} 1 & 2 \\ 1 & 0 \end{bmatrix}$$

we simply run the following code:

```
A=matrix(c(1,1,2,0),2,2)
eigen(A)
eigen() decomposition
$values
[1]  2 -1

$vectors
          [,1]         [,2]
[1,] 0.8944272   -0.7071068
[2,] 0.4472136    0.7071068
```

Note that the eigenvector [0.8944272 0.4472136] corresponds to the exact same eigenvector with unit length that we calculated previously. Since matrix A is a two-by-two matrix, there will be two different eigenvectors and two eigenvalues. The first eigenvector [0.8944272 0.4472136] is shown in the first column in the above output, whereas the second eigenvector [−0.7071068 0.7071068] is shown in the second column. The associated eigenvalues, 2 and −1, to the two eigenvectors, are shown at the beginning of the output.

We can extract the eigenvectors and eigenvalues like this:

```
Eig=eigen(A) # Save output from the function eigen
Eig$vectors # Extract and print the eigenvectors
          [,1]          [,2]
[1,] 0.8944272    -0.7071068
[2,] 0.4472136     0.7071068
Eig$values # Extract and print the eigenvalues
[1]  2 -1
```

Note that we store the output from the function "eigen" in an object that we call Eig. If we type:

```
names(Eig)
[1] "values"   "vectors"
```

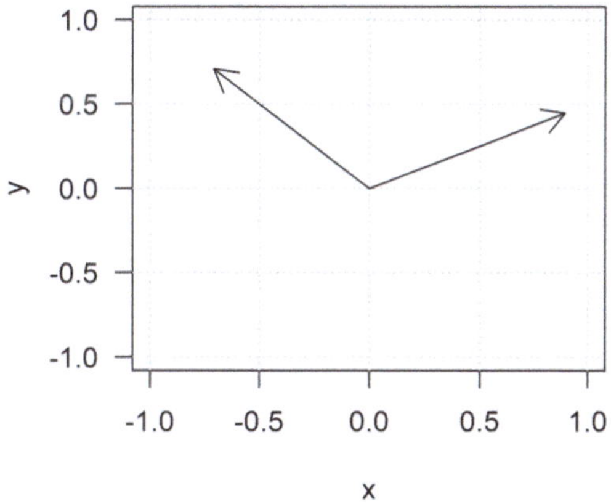

Fig. 2.5 Two eigenvectors in the Cartesian plane

we see that we can extract the eigenvalues with “values” and the eigenvectors with “vectors” by using the $ sign after the name of the object.

Let’s plot the two eigenvectors in a graph (Fig. 2.5):

```
Eig=eigen(A) # Save output from the function eigen
origin=c(0,0) # Coordinates of the start point of the vector
plot(NULL,NULL,xlim=c(-1,1),
ylim=c(-1,1),las=1,xlab="x",ylab="y") # Create an empty plot
grid() # Add a grid
arrows(origin[1],origin[2],Eig$vectors[1,1],
Eig$vectors[2,1],length = 0.15)
arrows(origin[1],origin[2],Eig$vectors[1,2],
Eig$vectors[2,2],length = 0.15)
```

2.6 Exercises

1. Draw the following vector in a plot and compute its length.

$$v = \begin{bmatrix} 4 \\ 3 \end{bmatrix}$$

2. Check if the above vector is an eigenvector of the following matrix.

$$A = \begin{bmatrix} 1 & 2 \\ 1 & 0 \end{bmatrix}$$

Use a plot to illustrate if vector v is an eigenvector of matrix A.

3. Use the function "eigen" in R to compute the eigenvectors, and eigenvalues, of the following matrix:

$$A = \begin{bmatrix} 5 & 2 & 3 \\ 5 & 5 & 5 \\ 3 & 2 & 3 \end{bmatrix}$$

Print the first eigenvector and eigenvalue on the screen after you have extracted them from the output.

Chapter 3
Managing Data in R

The first step in multivariate analysis is to set up multivariate data in R. The second step usually involves plotting the data. In this chapter, we will learn how to create data frames and how to compute some basic descriptive statistics. We will then get to know the classic Iris dataset and the Crab dataset, which are two multivariate datasets that we will work with throughout this book.

3.1 Working with Data Frames

The data that we will use in R for multivariate statistics is in most cases stored as data frames or tibbles. These are usually the type of objects that are created when we read data from, for example, a data file. In the last chapter with case studies, you will learn how to read in data from an Excel file and a CSV file. Data frames or tibbles are the types of objects that most functions in R accept as inputs. The main advantage of a data frame, over a matrix, is that a data frame can store information based on different data types, for example, both numbers and characters, whereas a matrix can only store one data type. We will here introduce some important functions that we will use later on. Start by entering the following code into an empty R script (remember that you can also download the R scripts from www.tilestats.com/ml/ if you do not want to enter the data manually):

```
Gender=factor(c("M","F","F","F","M","M","F"))
Weight=c(80,58,65,70,90,100,50)
Height=c(190,171,175,169,182,183,165)
Temp=c(37.5,38.3,37.0,37.9,38.6,40.1,36.7)
df=data.frame(Gender,Weight,Height,Temp)
```


A. Tilevik, *Multivariate Statistics and Machine Learning in R For Beginners*,
https://doi.org/10.1007/978-3-032-01851-9_3

Let's print the data frame:

```
df
   Gender  Weight   Height    Temp
1    M       80      190      37.5
2    F       58      171      38.3
3    F       65      175      37.0
4    F       70      169      37.9
5    M       90      182      38.6
6    M      100      183      40.1
7    F       50      165      36.7
```

This data frame holds information about the gender, weight (kg), height (cm), and body temperature (°C) of seven individuals. Note that the data frame stores both numbers and characters.

3.1.1 *Trick to Print*

In the above code, we printed the data frame by typing and running its name "df" (we can also use "print(df)"). However, a convenient way to both print and create an object in one line of code is to place parentheses "()" around the entire line of code:

```
(df=data.frame(Gender,Weight,Height,Temp))
   Gender  Weight  Height  Temp
1    M       80     190    37.5
2    F       58     171    38.3
3    F       65     175    37.0
4    F       70     169    37.9
5    M       90     182    38.6
6    M      100     183    40.1
7    F       50     165    36.7
```

3.1.2 *The Pipe Operator*

To first create and then print the data frame, we can, for example, use:

```
df=data.frame(Gender,Weight,Height,Temp)
print(df)
```

However, it is also possible to do this stepwise on a single line by using a pipe (% > %), which can be used if we first load the package **dplyr**:

```
library(dplyr)
df=data.frame(Gender,Weight,Height,Temp) %>% print()
```

The pipe operator feeds the results of the code from the left-hand side of the pipe into the operation to the right-hand side of the pipe.

3.1.3 *str*

To show the internal structure of the data frame, we can use the function called "str".

```
str(df)
'data.frame':   7 obs. of  4 variables:
 $ Gender: Factor w/ 2 levels "F","M": 2 1 1 1 2 2 1
 $ Weight: num  80 58 65 70 90 100 50
 $ Height: num  190 171 175 169 182 183 165
 $ Temp  : num  37.5 38.3 37 37.9 38.6 40.1 36.7
```

This function tells us that "df" is a data frame with seven observations and four variables. One variable is a factor of two levels (Female "F" and Male "M"), whereas the other three variables are numeric.

3.1.4 *tibble*

A tibble is a modern type of data frame. In comparison to data frames, a tibble makes fewer assumptions about the data. For example, a tibble never changes the names of the variables or set row names when we read in data from a file. To create a tibble, we first need to load the package **tibble**. Remember that you first need to install this package, if you have not already done that, by:

```
install.packages("tibble")
```

Note that packages such as **tibble**, **readr**, **dplyr**, and **ggplot2** which we will use later on in this book can also be loaded with the package **tidyverse**, which is a collection of R packages designed for data science. To install all those packages at once, we can instead run:

```
install.packages("tidyverse")
```

One problem when installing the **tidyverse** package is that it installs several packages, and if one of those packages cannot be installed correctly, you will not be able to load the **tidyverse** package. From my experience, the more packages a package depends on, the more likely it is that it will cause problems in the installation. This is the reason why this book does not rely completely on the **tidyverse** package because if a user fails to install this package properly, the user will still be able to work with most examples in this book.

Once you have installed the **tibble** package, or the **tidyverse** package, you can load it like this:

```
library(tibble)   # or library(tidyverse)
```

We can use the function "as_tibble" in the **tibble** package to convert our previous data frame into a tibble:

```
tib=as_tibble(df)
tib
# A tibble: 7 x 4
     Gender   Weight   Height  Temp
     <fct>    <dbl>    <dbl>   <dbl>
1      M        80       19    37.5
2      F        58       17    38.3
3      F        65       175   37
4      F        70       169   37.9
5      M        90       182   38.6
6      M        100      183   40.1
7      F        50       165   36.7
```

In comparison to a data frame, a tibble shows the data type of each column when it is printed. "fct" tells us that the variable Gender is a factor, whereas the other variables are numeric ("dbl" = double).

3.1.5 *summary*

By using the "summary" function, we can compute a range of statistics for each numeric variable: the minimum value (min), first quartile (1st Qu.), median, mean, third quartile (3rd Qu.), and the maximum value (max). For variables on a categorical scale, the function computes the frequency of each category:

```
summary(df)
Gender        Weight             Height             Temp
F:4       Min.   : 50.00    Min.   :165.0    Min.   :36.70
M:3       1st Qu.: 61.50    1st Qu.:170.0    1st Qu.:37.25
          Median : 70.00    Median :175.0    Median :37.90
          Mean   : 73.29    Mean   :176.4    Mean   :38.01
          3rd Qu.: 85.00    3rd Qu.:182.5    3rd Qu.:38.45
          Max.   :100.00    Max.   :190.0    Max.   :40.10
```

We see that we have four females and three males in the dataset. The shortest person in the dataset has a height of 165 cm, whereas the tallest person has a height of 190 cm. The average height of the seven individuals is 176.4 cm.

3.1.6 *subset*

From the "summary" function, we get the statistics for each variable. However, if we, for example, would like to show the statistics for the men and women separately, we can use the function "subset" to extract a certain category from the data frame. For example, let's extract the females (F) from the data frame:

```
Women=subset(df,Gender=="F")
Women # Print
  Gender   Weight   Height   Temp
2   F        58       171    38.3
3   F        65       175    37.0
4   F        70       169    37.9
7   F        50       165    36.7
```

We could now generate, for example, the summary statistics on just the women by "summary(Women)". We can also extract the females by the "manual way", where we extract only the rows that are equal to "F" in the column Gender:

```
df[df$Gender=="F",]
```

3.1.7 *AND and OR Operators*

Suppose that we like to extract only the women with a body weight greater than 60 kg. Then we can use the "&" operator, which is used when several conditions need to be true, such as:

```
Women_weight=subset(df,Gender=="F" & Weight>60)
Women_weight
  Gender   Weight   Height   Temp
3   F        65       175    37.0
4   F        70       169    37.9
```

Note that we now have extracted only the women with a weight larger than 60 kg. Thus, we will extract the rows only when both these conditions are true.

If we instead use the OR operator "|":

```
Women_weight=subset(df,Gender=="F" | Weight>60)
Women_weight
```

we will extract all women, independent of the weight, and all individuals with a weight larger than 60 kg. Thus, we will extract the rows that fulfill either of these two conditions. Try and change the above code so that you extract all women and all individuals with a weight larger than 95 kg. Note that only one man will then be extracted.

3.1.8 *filter*

Another common function to extract a subset of a data frame is the function "filter" in the **dplyr** package:

```
library(dplyr)
Women=filter(df, Gender=="F")
Women
  Gender   Weight   Height   Temp
2   F        58      171     38.3
3   F        65      175     37.0
4   F        70      169     37.9
7   F        50      165     36.7
```

The function "filter" has a lot of options. For example, suppose that we like to extract only women with a weight larger than 60 kg, then we type:

```
# or filter(df, Gender == "F" & Weight > 60)
filter(df, Gender == "F", Weight > 60)
     Gender  Weight  Height   Temp
1      F       65     175     37.0
2      F       70     169     37.9
```

3.1.9 *Select*

When we have a large dataset, we might want to reduce it to include only relevant variables that we will analyze. For example, suppose that we like to select only the variables Weight and Height, we can then extract columns 2 and 3 and save these into a new data frame:

```
df_select=df[,c(2,3)]
```

However, it is very hard to keep track of the column number in a large dataset. A better way is to instead use the names of the columns:

```
df_select=df[,c("Weight","Height")]
```

We can also use the function "select" in the **dplyr** package:

```
library(dplyr)
df_select=select(df, Weight, Height)
```

It is common to also combine the select function with the filter function. Suppose that we like to extract the men and that we like to store only the weight and height of these men. We can then first extract the men and store these in a new data frame with the name Men:

```
Men=filter(df, Gender=="M")
```

Then we select that we like to extract the variables Weight and Height from the data frame Men:

```
df_select=select(Men, Weight, Height)
df_select
   Weight   Height
1    80       190
2    90       182
3    100      183
```

By using piping, we can do this in one step:

```
df_select = df %>% filter(Gender=="M") %>% select (Weight,
Height)
df_select
   Weight    Height
1    80        190
2    90        182
3    100       183
```

Note that, in the functions "filter" and "select" we now do not include the data frames as arguments because the pipe operator (%>%) passes the data frames into the first argument of the function to the right-hand side of the pipe operator.

3.1.10 lapply and apply

Let's say that we want to calculate the mean of the numerical variables in our data frame. We could use a variety of functions to do this. We could do it manually for each variable by:

```
mean(df$Weight)
mean(df$Height)
mean(df$Temp)
```

We could also do this by a for-loop where "i" is a counter that starts at 2 and ends at 4. The reason why we here start at 2, and not 1, is because the first column in the data frame does not hold numeric values.

```
for (i in 2:4){
    print(mean(df[,i]))
}
73.28571
176.4286
38.01429
```

However, the easiest way, and recommended way, is to avoid using for-loops and instead use the apply functions family. The "lapply" function works like the for-loop. Note that we here only apply the function on the columns 2–4 (df[,2:4]) because the first column does not include numeric data:

```
lapply(df[,2:4],mean)
$Weight
[1] 73.28571
$Height
[1] 176.4286
$Temp
[1] 38.01429
```

The "apply" function works in a similar way but it can be used to compute, for example, the mean of either the rows or the columns:

```
apply(df[,2:4],2,mean)
  Weight      Height     Temp
 73.28571  176.42857  38.01429
```

The "2" here tells the apply function to compute the means based on the columns. Try and change the value from "2" to "1" and note that the mean will be computed over the rows instead. We can, for example, calculate the sample standard deviation of the numeric variables if we change "mean" to "sd":

```
apply(df[,2:4],2,sd)
  Weight     Height     Temp
17.764330  8.904253  1.140802
```

3.1.11 colMeans and rowMeans

The functions "colMeans" and "rowMeans" are simple functions to remember if we like to compute the means of numeric columns or rows. For example, to calculate the means of the numeric variables, we can type:

```
colMeans(df[,2:4])
  Weight       Height       Temp
 73.28571    176.42857    38.01429
```

3.1.12 tapply

tapply works similarly to the "lapply" function, but tapply can be used to apply a function on given categories. If we want to generate mean values for men and women separately, the "tapply" function is handy. To calculate the mean weight of men and women we type:

```
tapply(df$Weight,df$Gender,mean)
    F          M
  60.75      90.00
```

3.1.13 Aggregate and Summarize

In contrast to the "tapply" function, which can only be used on one column at a time, the "aggregate" function can be used to calculate the mean values for men and women on all numeric columns:

```
aggregate(.~Gender,df,FUN="mean")
    Gender   Weight     Height    Temp
1     F       60.75      170      37.47
2     M       90.00      185      38.73
```

If we like, we can specify in the "aggregate" function which columns (variables) that we want to compute for. For example, calculating only the mean of the variables Weight and Height can be done by:

```
aggregate(cbind(Weight, Height) ~ Gender, df, FUN = mean)
  Gender  Weight   Height
1   F      60.75    170
2   M      90.00    185
```

The package **dplyr** has a similar function called "summarize" that can be combined with the function "group_by" to compute the same thing as above:

```
library(dplyr)
df %>%
  group_by(Gender) %>%
  summarize(across(c(Weight, Height), mean),
  .groups = "drop")
  Gender Weight Height
   <fct>     <dbl>     <dbl>
1     F        60.8        170
2     M         90         185
```

Note that the output here comes as a tibble, whereas the function "aggregate" generates a data frame.

3.1.14 Your Own Functions

We have previously used the function "mean" which is included in R. However, sometimes we want to compute certain things that are not included as inbuilt functions in R. We can then create our own function. Let's say that we want to create a function that calculates the area of a circle:

```
CircleArea=function(r) {
    area=r^2*pi
    return(area)
}
```

A function consists of the general terms that are required:

1. The name of the function. We have named our function "CircleArea".
2. The word "function" tells R that this is a function.
3. Input to the function (input). In our example, we will use the radius "(r)" as input.
4. The curly braces { } represent the beginning and end of the function.
5. Code that should be run within the function. In our example, the code is: "area=r^2*pi".
6. The function will return the calculated area of the circle by "return(area)".

To use this function, we first need to run all the above code to store the function in the working memory. I recommend that you write the code in a script and then run the code. When you run this code, you should see the following output in the console:

```
> CircleArea=function(r) {
+ area=r^2*pi
+ return(area)
+ }
```

Note that R just reads and stores the function in the workspace. Hence, it is enough to run this code only once because R will remember this function as long as we do not clear the memory. To use this function, we just type the name of the function and include some value. Let's calculate the area of a circle with a radius of 4:

```
CircleArea(4)
50.26548
```

The function will return the value 50.26, which is the area of the circle.

3.1.15 *Applying your Function*

When we have created our function, we might want to apply it to a data frame. Let's say that we want to normalize the values in each column by dividing them by the maximum value in each column. We first create a function that takes a vector (a column from the data frame) and divides all its values by its maximum value:

```
normalize=function(x){
    norm_val=x/max(x)
    return(norm_val)
}
```

Let's test the function before we use it on the data frame. For example, a vector with the values 10, 4, and 3 should be normalized to 1, 0.4, and 0.3:

```
v=c(10,4,3)
normalize(v)
[1] 1.0 0.4 0.3
```

We see that our function works! Now, let's try this function on our data frame and apply it to each column that holds numeric data:

```
lapply(df[,2:4],normalize)
$Weight
[1] 0.80 0.58 0.65 0.70 0.90 1.00 0.50
$Height
[1] 1.0000000 0.9000000 0.9210526 0.8894737 0.9578947
0.9631579 0.8684211
$Temp
[1] 0.9351621 0.9551122 0.9226933 0.9451372 0.9625935
1.0000000 0.9152120
```

It seems like each variable has been normalized. However, lapply returns a list and we commonly want a data frame. We can then use the function "data.frame" to convert the list to a data frame:

```
data.frame(lapply(df[,2:4],normalize))
    Weight          Height          Temp
1   0.80            1.0000000       0.9351621
2   0.58            0.9000000       0.9551122
3   0.65            0.9210526       0.9226933
4   0.70            0.8894737       0.9451372
5   0.90            0.9578947       0.9625935
6   1.00            0.9631579       1.0000000
7   0.50            0.8684211       0.9152120
```

We can also write simple functions in just one line of code by:

```
data.frame(lapply(df[,2:4],function(x) x/max(x)))
   Weight      Height        Temp
1   0.80       1.0000000     0.9351621
2   0.58       0.9000000     0.9551122
3   0.65       0.9210526     0.9226933
4   0.70       0.8894737     0.9451372
5   0.90       0.9578947     0.9625935
6   1.00       0.9631579     1.0000000
7   0.50       0.8684211     0.9152120
```

3.2 Generate Random Data

In this book, we will generate random data that will be used in several examples. Later on, we will use random data during the validation of ML models. We will here only cover the basics of how to generate random data in R. Let's start to generate four random numbers from a normal distribution with a mean of zero and a standard deviation of one:

```
rnorm(4,0,1)
```

The first argument specifies how many random numbers that we want to generate. The second argument sets the mean of the normal distribution that we sample from, whereas the last argument specifies the standard deviation of the normal distribution. Try and run the code. When I ran the code, I got the following random numbers:

```
0.64806912    0.22057142   -0.71928584    0.09141874
```

Your values will, of course, be different from my values because the numbers are randomly generated. Try and run the code many times and observe that you will get different numbers every time.

3.2.1 Set a Seed

Sometimes we would like to generate the same random numbers over and over again because we might want to be able to reproduce the results. For example, when you work with this book, it would be nice if you get the same random numbers as I got when creating this book so that you get the same results as shown in the examples. To generate the same random numbers, we can use the function "set.seed". For example:

```
set.seed(12)
rnorm(4,0,1)
-1.4805676    1.5771695   -0.9567445   -0.9200052
```

Here I have set the seed number arbitrarily to 12, but we could have selected another integer. If you run the above code (the two lines including set.seed(12)), you should get the same random numbers as the ones above. If you get different numbers, you might use a different R-version where they have updated some functions that are used for random numbers. When I created this book, I used R-version 4.4.2.

Try and run the two lines above many times and note that you will get the same random numbers every time.

Note, if you do not get the same random numbers as the ones above, although you use the same seed, it means that you will not get the exact same results as shown in this book when random numbers are used.

If we change the seed number to 100, we will get different random numbers compared to when we used the seed number 12:

```
set.seed(100)
rnorm(4,0,1)
-0.50219235   0.13153117  -0.07891709   0.88678481
```

3.2.2 Simulated Data

One nice thing with random numbers is that we can simulate an experiment. Let's say that we would like to generate a sample dataset of the height of 40 men from a certain population. We know that the mean body height is normally distributed, with a mean of 175 cm and a standard deviation of 7 cm in this population. We could simulate such a dataset by drawing, for example, 40 random data points from a normal distribution with a mean of 175 and a standard deviation of 7:

```
set.seed(107) #For reproducibility
sim_data=rnorm(40,175,7)
```

Since the data comes from a normal distribution, we expect that our sample should follow a normal distribution. Let's make a histogram of the data:

```
hist(sim_data)
```

We see that the distribution of our sample data seems to follow a normal distribution (Fig. 3.1). Since the mean of the distribution is 175, we expect that the mean of our sample is also about 175:

```
mean(sim_data)
175.3087
```

We see that the mean of our sample is close to 175. Try to change the previous code so that you generate one million random numbers instead. Create a histogram of the data (hist(sim_data,100)) and calculate the mean of the data points. Note that the more data we generate, the closer we will get to the true mean (175), and that our histogram will more or less be identical to a bell-shaped curve.

To draw random numbers between zero and one from a uniform distribution, we can instead use the function "runif":

```
sim_data=runif(100000)
hist(sim_data)
```

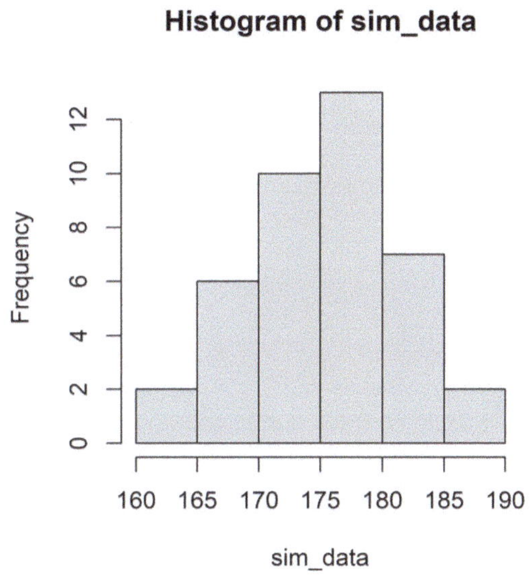

Fig. 3.1 A histogram of 40 random values drawn from a normal distribution with a mean of 175 and a standard deviation of seven

3.3 Missing Data and Imputation

There are several reasons why we may have missing data in our dataset. One common reason is that the data was not collected due to problems with a machine failing to read the sample, or that the data could not be collected because it was simply not possible or due to mistakes. R represents missing values as NA. Let's create a dataset with some missing values:

```
Gender=factor(c("M","F","M","F",NA))
Weight=c(80,58,65,70,NA)
Height=c(190,NA,165,179,182)
Temp=c(37.5,NA,NA,NA,NA)
(df=data.frame(Gender,Weight,Height,Temp))
  Gender   Weight   Height   Temp
1   M        80       190     37.5
2   F        58       NA      NA
3   M        65       165     NA
4   F        70       179     NA
5  <NA>      NA       182     NA
```

One simple way to check the amount of missing data in a data frame is to run the following code, which sums the number of NAs in each column:

```
colSums(is.na(df))
Gender Weight Height   Temp
  1       1      1       4
```

We see that we have, for example, four missing values in the variable Temp.

One problem with missing data is that we might get strange outputs, or errors, in R if we try to use a function on data, including NAs. Suppose that we like to compute the mean of the variable Height by:

```
mean(df$Height)
NA
```

then we just get an output that says NA. If we type:

```
?mean
```

we can read the documentation about the function, which says that its argument na.rm. can be set to TRUE in order to remove missing values before the computation proceeds, such as:

```
mean(df$Height, na.rm=TRUE)
179
```

By setting the argument na.rm. to TRUE, we now remove the missing value before the mean is computed. If you have missing values in your dataset, make sure to read the documentation to see how the R function that you like to use deals with missing data.

Some functions in R might not include arguments for how to deal with missing data. We must therefore remove missing data before using such a function. This can be done with the function "na.omit":

```
cleaned_data = na.omit(df)
cleaned_data
  Gender Weight Height Temp
1   M      80     190   37.5
```

However, note that the "na.omit" removes all rows that have at least one column with NA, which means that we only have the first person left in the dataset. This is something that we do not want to do because we lose a lot of data. To use this function, it is a good idea to first remove columns with a lot of missing data, such as column number four:

```
df2=df[,-4] # Remove the fourth column
cleaned_data = na.omit(df2)
cleaned_data
  Gender    Weight       Height
1   M          80          190
3   M          65          165
4   F          70          179
```

By removing the fourth column before using the "na.omit" function, we rescue the data for person numbers 3 and 4. However, we still lose the data for person number 2 and 5. Another strategy is to replace the NAs with plausible values. This is called imputation. There are a range of different methods to do imputation but I will here show a simple method that is based on the k-nearest neighbors (KNN) technique. The method fills in missing values in a dataset by relying on the values of similar (neighboring) data points. Below, we use the values from the three closest persons ($k = 3$) to predict a reasonable value for replacing the NA with:

```
library(VIM)
imputed_data = kNN(df2, k = 3)
imputed_data
  Gender  Weight  Height  Gender_imp  Weight_imp  Height_imp
1   M       80     190      FALSE       FALSE       FALSE
2   F       58     179      FALSE       FALSE       TRUE
3   M       65     165      FALSE       FALSE       FALSE
4   F       70     179      FALSE       FALSE       FALSE
5   M       70     182      TRUE        TRUE        FALSE
```

Make sure you remove variables (columns) that have a large amount of missing data before you use imputation. Generally, remove columns that have more than 50% of missing data. The value of k is usually set to 3 or 5. To extract our dataset with imputed values we can simply select the first three columns by:

```
imputed_data = imputed_data[,1:3]
```

3.4 Datasets Used in This Book

Most datasets used in this book are in silico data, which means that they have been randomly generated. Hence, results from analyses in this book should not be seen as "true" results. Also, note that most datasets are small in order to help the reader to get a quick overview of the data. Hence, if you design your own study, you should not use the examples in this book as a guide to determine the sample size of your experiments. The more data you have, the more reliable model you will create. In addition to the in silico data, we will also use the Iris dataset and the Crab dataset. At the end of this book, we will also use datasets from two scientific papers.

3.4.1 The Iris Dataset

The Iris dataset is a classic dataset when it comes to multivariate analysis and ML. If you want to learn more about multivariate statistical methods, you will for sure encounter the Iris dataset. The Iris data was collected by Edgar Anderson (Anderson,

1935) and was later used by Ronald Fisher (Fisher, 1936) to show the application of linear discriminant analysis.

The Iris dataset is an inbuilt multivariate dataset in R, which is stored as a data frame with the name iris:

```
iris
```

After you have run this line of code, you should see the dataset, which includes sepal length, sepal width, petal length, and petal width in centimeters of the 150 Iris flowers. The measurements are illustrated in Fig. 3.2. Fifty flowers from three different species (Setosa, Versicolor, and Virginica) have been measured.

If we print the head of the Iris data frame (the first six rows):

```
head(iris)
  Sepal.Length  Sepal.Width  Petal.Length Petal.Width  Species
1    5.1           3.5           1.4          0.2       setosa
2    4.9           3.0           1.4          0.2       setosa
3    4.7           3.2           1.3          0.2       setosa
4    4.6           3.1           1.5          0.2       setosa
5    5.0           3.6           1.4          0.2       setosa
6    5.4           3.9           1.7          0.4       setosa
```

we see that the data frame “iris” includes five variables, where the variable “Species” defines which species the flower belongs to: Setosa, Versicolor, or Virginica.

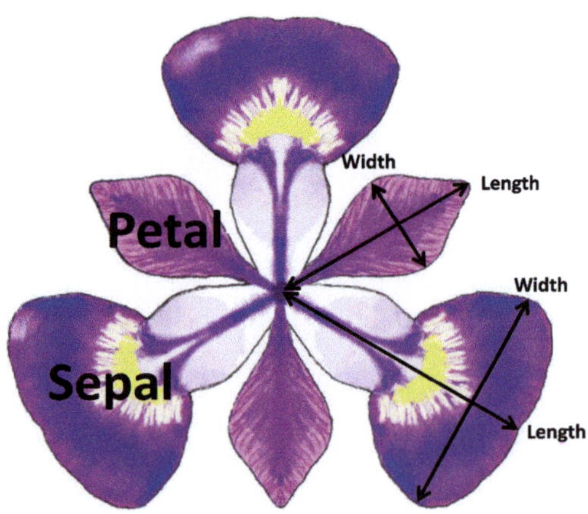

Fig. 3.2 An illustration of the measurements in the Iris dataset

Let's print the average values for each variable for the three different species:

```
aggregate(.~ Species, iris, FUN="mean")
   Species    Sepal.Length  Sepal.Width Petal.Length Petal.Width
1  setosa        5.006         3.428        1.462        0.246
2  versicolor    5.936         2.770        4.260        1.326
3  virginica     6.588         2.974        5.552        2.026
```

We see that the Setosa flowers have, for example, the shortest mean sepal length but the longest sepal width.

3.4.2 *The Crab Dataset*

The Crab dataset comes from the study by Campbell and Mahon (1974). The dataset is stored in the **MASS** package, so to access it, we first need to load this package:

```
library(MASS) # Remember that you might need to install it
# first by: install.packages("MASS")
head(crabs)
   sp sex  index    FL      RW     CL     CW    BD
1  B   M     1      8.1     6.7    16.1   19.0  7.0
2  B   M     2      8.8     7.7    18.1   20.8  7.4
3  B   M     3      9.2     7.8    19.0   22.4  7.7
4  B   M     4      9.6     7.9    20.1   23.1  8.2
5  B   M     5      9.8     8.0    20.3   23.0  8.2
6  B   M     6      10.8    9.0    23.0   26.5  9.8
```

The dataset consists of measurements of 200 blue and orange-form species of rock crabs. The different measurements are illustrated in Fig. 3.3. The columns show the two color forms of this crab species (*sp*): B = blue, O = orange, *sex*: M = Male, F = Female, *index*: 1:50 for each group (sex and sp), *FL*: frontal lobe size (mm), *RW*: rear width (mm), *CL*: carapace length (mm), *CW*: carapace width (mm), and *BD*: body depth (mm).

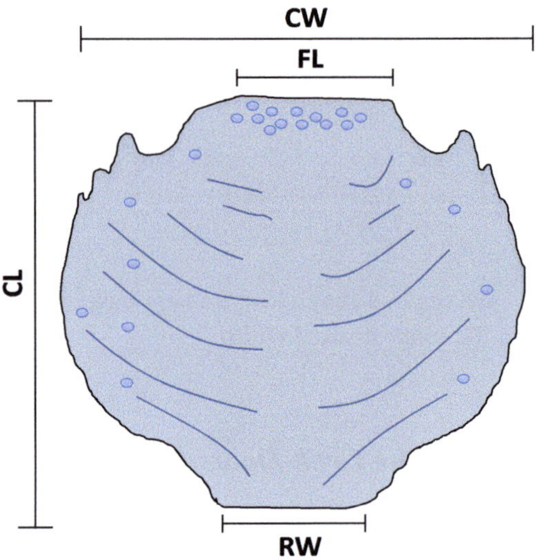

Fig. 3.3 An illustration of the measurements used in the Crab dataset

3.5 Exercises

1. Use the "str" function on the data frame "crabs" and tell which variables are on a categorical or a numerical scale.
2. Save the data frame "crabs" as a tibble with the name crab_tibble. Print this tibble and note that the output essentially gives the same information as using the function "str".
3. Calculate the mean value for all numerical variables in the Crab dataset, separated by sex.
4. Extract only the Setosa flowers in the Iris dataset.
5. Extract only Versicolors and Virginicas from the Iris dataset, which have a sepal length larger than 6.8. Tip: use the OR operator "|" to select both Versicolors and Virginicas and the AND operator "&" to select only flowers that have a sepal length larger than 6.8.

References

Anderson, E. (1935). The irises of the Gaspé Peninsula. Bulletin of the American Iris Society. 59: 2–5.

Campbell, N. A., & Mahon, R. J. (1974). A multivariate study of variation in two species of rock crab of the genus Leptograpsus. *Australian Journal of Zoology, 22*(3), 417–425.

Fisher, R. A. (1936). The use of multiple measurements in taxonomic problems. *Annals of Eugenics, 7*(2), 179–188.

Chapter 4
Graphical Illustration of Multivariate Data

Before we start to analyze a multivariate dataset, we should always start with some graphical illustrations. Besides helping us to understand the data distribution and identify any patterns, the graphical illustration may help us to detect outliers. We will here illustrate a range of different plotting techniques by using the Iris dataset. We will first see how to use the inbuilt plotting functions in R and then see how to make the same plots by using the **ggplot2** package. **ggplot2** is a powerful data visualization package in R, designed for creating plots that look nicer compared to the inbuilt plot function in R. Also, **ggplot2** includes a lot more functions compared to the basic plots in R.

4.1 Scatter Plots

We will first start with a simple scatter plot, using the function "plot". We will here plot the petal width versus the petal length in the Iris dataset:

```
plot(iris$Petal.Width,iris$Petal.Length,xlab="Petal width (cm)",
ylab="Petal Length (cm)")
```

From the plot (Fig. 4.1), we can see that there is a positive linear relationship between the two variables. A flower with a long petal length is likely also to have a long petal width. In the plot, we can also see that there seems to be a distinct cluster of flowers with short petal length and width. Since the dataset includes three different species of flowers, the cluster that we see might come from one class. A simple way to identify different categories in the data is to use different colors in the scatter plot. The argument "col" can be used to change the color of the points. For example, the following code:

A. Tilevik, *Multivariate Statistics and Machine Learning in R For Beginners*,
https://doi.org/10.1007/978-3-032-01851-9_4

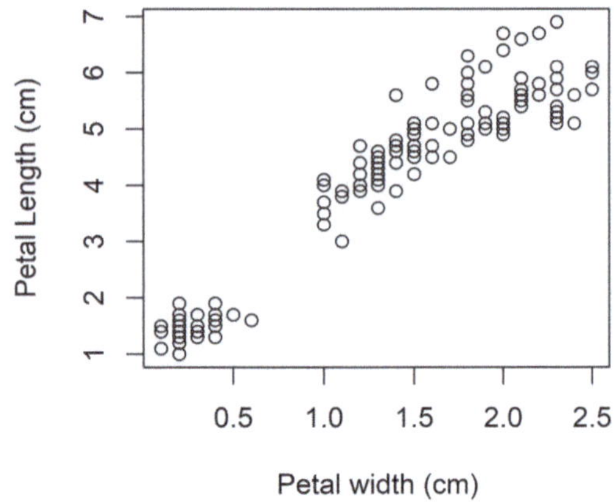

Fig. 4.1 A scatter plot of the petal length and width of the Iris dataset

```
plot(iris$Petal.Width,iris$Petal.Length,col=2)
```

will generate a plot with red points because we set col = 2 (we can also type: col="#DF536B", which will give the corresponding red color). To see which color that corresponds to an integer, we can type:

```
palette()
"black"    "#DF536B" "#61D04F" "#2297E6" "#28E2E5" "#CD0BBC"
"#F5C710" "gray62"
```

For example, 1 = "black", 2 = "#DF536B" (red), 3 = "#61D04F" (green), and so forth. To see all the colors that you can set as a text string, type "colors()". For example, to use blue color, we can type:

```
plot(iris$Petal.Width,iris$Petal.Length,col= "blue")
```

If we now set "col" equal to the class of each flower, we will generate a plot with a unique color for each class: Setosa = 1 (black color), Versicolor = 2 (red color), and Virginica = 3 (green color). The order of the class is defined per default according to the alphabetic order. To check the order, we can type:

```
levels(iris$Species)
"setosa"  "versicolor"   "virginica"
```

Let's generate a scatter plot where we plot each class with a unique color:

```
plot(iris$Petal.Width,iris$Petal.Length,col=iris$Species)
```

With this plot (Fig. 4.2), it is now easy to see that the distinct cluster with small petal width and length consists of Setosa flowers (black points).

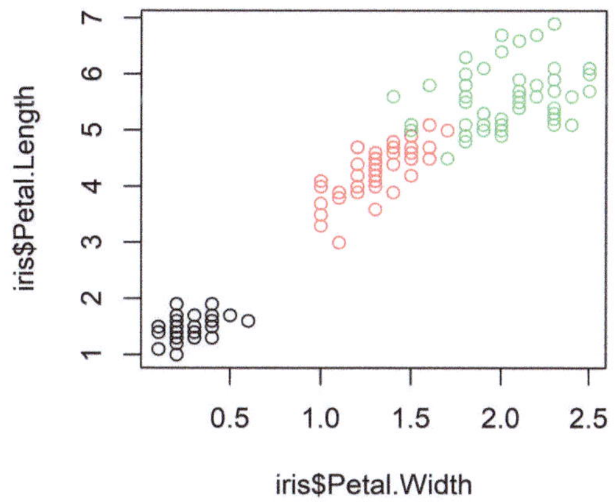

Fig. 4.2 A scatter plot of the petal length and width of the Iris dataset. The different species are represented by different colors: black (Setosa), red (Versicolor) and green (Virginica)

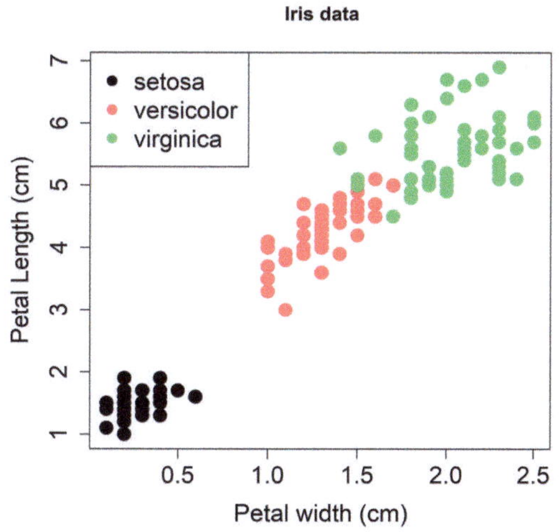

Fig. 4.3 A scatter plot of the petal length and width of the Iris dataset. The different species are represented by different colors: black (Setosa), red (Versicolor), and green (Virginica)

The code below shows some arguments that you can use to change the plot (Fig. 4.3):

```
plot(iris$Petal.Width,iris$Petal.Length,col=iris$Species,
# Type of points (type "help(points)" for more details)
pch=16,
xlab="Petal width (cm)", # Label for the x-axis
ylab="Petal Length (cm)", # Label for the y-axis
# Relative size of point, 2 = two-fold greater than default size
cex=2,
cex.lab=1.5,  # Relative size of x- and y-labels
cex.axis=1.5, # Relative size of the tick labels
main= "Iris data") # Figure title
legend("topleft", legend=levels(iris$Species), pch=16,
col=1:3,cex=1.5)
```

4.1.1 Combining Plots

The function "par" can be used to change graphical parameters. For example, with the parameter "mfrow=c(nrow,ncol)", we can combine several plots in the same window. For example:

```
par(mfrow = c(1,2))
```

will create an empty window with one row and two columns (Fig. 4.4). We can now fill these two columns with two plots:

```
plot(iris$Petal.Width, iris$Petal.Length,col=iris$Species)
plot(iris$Sepal.Width, iris$Sepal.Length,col=iris$Species)
```

Note: restore the window so that for the further plots you only have one window for each plot. To do this, you simply clear your plotting window or type:

```
par(mfrow = c(1,1)) # One row and one column
```

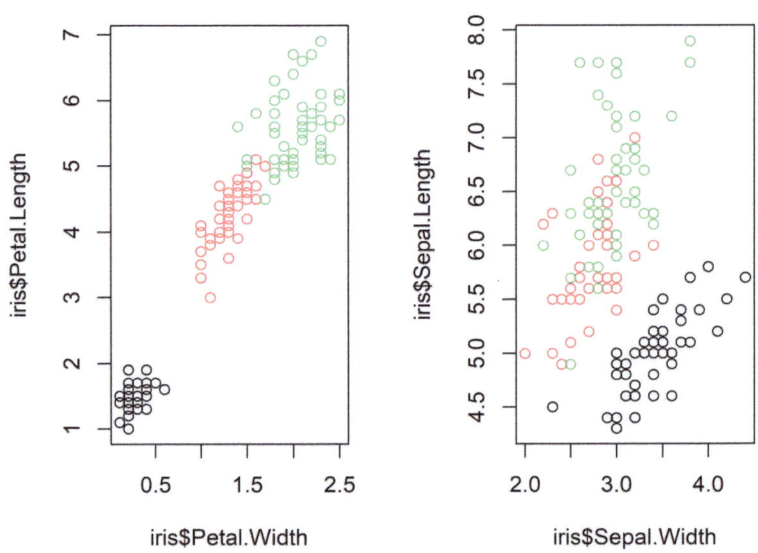

Fig. 4.4 Scatter plot of the petal length and width (left) and sepal length and width (right) of the Iris dataset. The different species are represented by different colors: black (Setosa), red (Versicolor), and green (Virginica)

4.1.2 Scatter Plot with ggplot2

We will now create similar scatter plots by using the **ggplot2** package. **ggplot2** is built on the grammar of graphics concepts, which allows us to create complex plots through a layered approach. We first need to load the package:

```
library(ggplot2)
```

Let's first run the following line of code to see what happens:

```
ggplot(data=iris, aes(x = Petal.Width, y = Petal.Length))
```

We can so far not see any data points in the plot (Fig. 4.5). The code we have just run basically just initializes the plot. We have supplied the Iris data as input (data=iris) and defined that we like to plot the column Petal.Width on the x-axis and the column Petal.Length on the y-axis. We see that the x- and y-axes have automatically been set to appropriate ranges for the values of these two variables. The only thing we need to do is to add the points to this plot and change the labels a bit. The trick is to use the "+" sign, which will add layers or components to an existing plot, such as:

```
ggplot(data=iris, aes(x = Petal.Width, y = Petal.Length)) +
  geom_point() + # Add the points
  # Change the labels
  labs(x = "Petal Width (cm)", y = "Petal Length (cm)")
```

Note that you need to run all lines at the same time to generate the scatter plot in Fig. 4.6. With this code, we first create a plot, then we add the data points with the function "geom_point". Finally, we modify the labels of the x-axis and y-axis.

To put colors for the three different species, we can set "color" in the "aes" function equal to the variable Species:

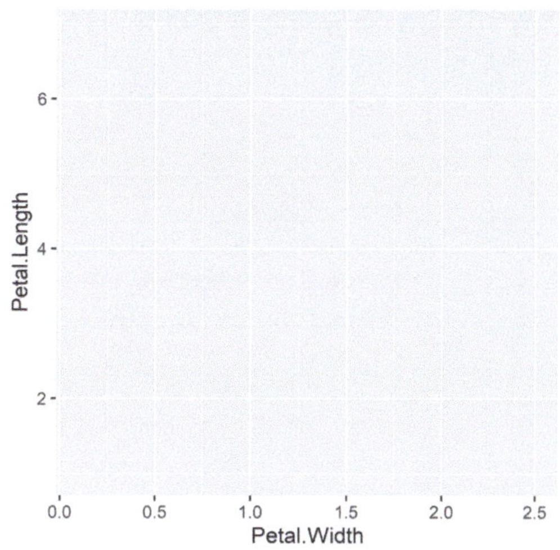

Fig. 4.5 An empty plot initialized by the "ggplot" function

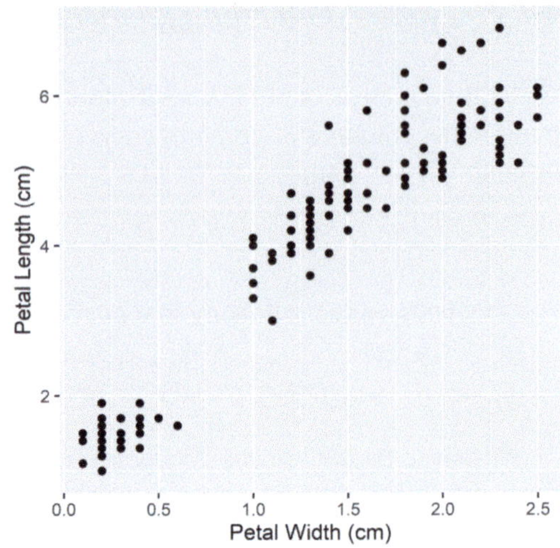

Fig. 4.6 A scatter plot of the petal length and width, using the **ggplot2** package

```
ggplot(data=iris, aes(x = Petal.Width, y = Petal.Length,
color = Species)) +
  geom_point() +
  labs(x = "Petal Width (cm)", y = "Petal Length (cm)")
```

To further change this plot (Fig. 4.7), we can use the functions “theme_minimal” and “theme” to change the style and size of the labels in the plot, as well as adjust the positions of the labels by using “margin” (Fig. 4.8):

```
ggplot(data = iris, aes(x = Petal.Width, y = Petal.Length,
color = Species)) +
  geom_point(size = 3) +
  labs(x = "Petal Width (cm)", y = "Petal Length (cm)",
  title = "Iris data") +
  # Use a minimalistic design (e.g. white background)
  theme_minimal() +
  theme(
    axis.title.x = element_text(size = 12,
    margin = margin(t = 10)),  # Push x-axis label down
    axis.title.y = element_text(size = 12,
    margin = margin(r = 10)),  # Push y-axis label left
    # Size of the tick labels
    axis.text = element_text(size = 12),
    # Remove title in the legend
    legend.title = element_blank(),
    # Adjust legend text size
    legend.text = element_text(size = 12)
  )
```

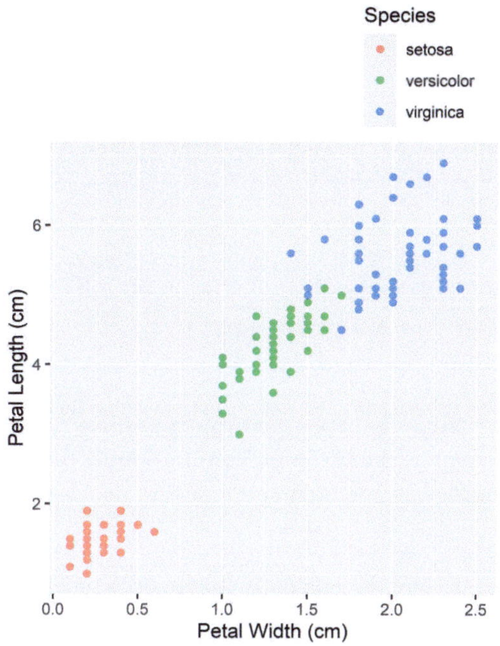

Fig. 4.7 A scatter plot of the petal length and width where the species are represented by different colors, using the **ggplot2** package

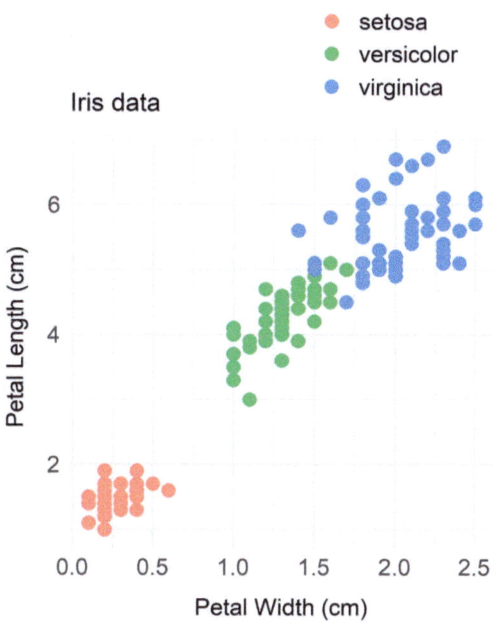

Fig. 4.8 A scatter plot of the petal length and width with a white background, using the **ggplot2** package

To put two plots next to each other, we first create the two plots and save them in objects that we, for example, name plot1 and plot2:

```
# First plot
plot1 = ggplot(iris, aes(x = Petal.Width, y = Petal.Length,
color = Species)) +
  geom_point()

# Second plot
plot2 = ggplot(iris, aes(x = Sepal.Width, y = Sepal.Length,
color = Species)) +
  geom_point()
```

Note that when you run the above code, nothing will be plotted. To plot, for example, the first plot, you can simply run:

```
plot1
```

To plot the two plots next to each other (Fig. 4.9), we can use the function "grid. arrange" in the **gridExtra** package:

```
library(gridExtra)
grid.arrange(plot1, plot2, ncol=2)
```

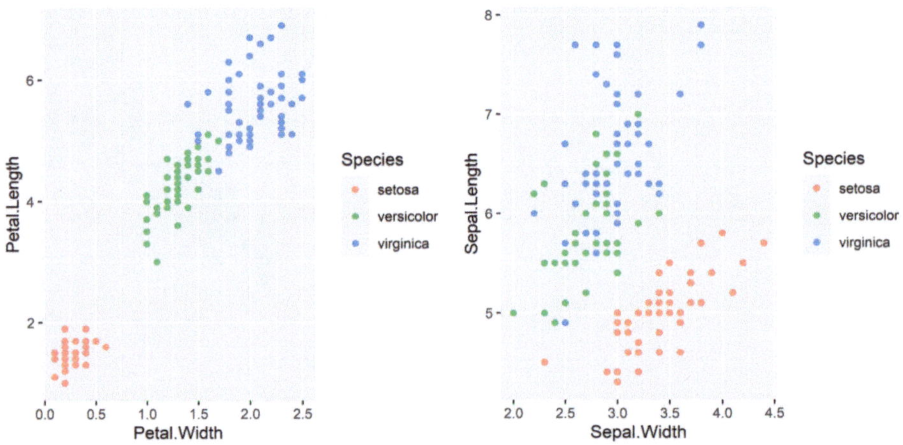

Fig. 4.9 Scatter plots of the petal length and width (left) and the sepal length and width (right) where the species are represented by different colors, using the **ggplot2** package

4.2 Boxplots

Boxplots are very useful for displaying the spread of a variable where we can also separate the categories. Let's plot the petal length for the three different species with different colors by using the argument "border":

```
boxplot(Petal.Length ~ Species,data=iris,ylab="Petal length",
border = 1:3)
```

The horizontal line in the box represents the median of the variable (Fig. 4.10). The box spans from the first quartile to the third quartile, which gives the interquartile range (IQR) that covers about 50% of the data points. The lower whisker represents the smallest data point in the data, whereas the upper whisker represents the largest data point in the dataset given that no outlier is present. Any data point that is very far away from the box is defined as an outlier, which is represented as a dot or a circle in the plot. In Fig. 4.10 we have two outliers, one Setosa and one Versicolor with very short petal lengths.

If we like to see the petal length of the individual flowers, we could add points on top of the boxplot with the function "points" so that we get a mixture of a one-dimensional scatter plot and a boxplot (Fig. 4.11). Note that the argument "outline" in the "boxplot" function is set to FALSE so that we do not display the outlier to avoid that the same data point is plotted twice. We use the argument "jittering" on the x-axis to prevent points from being plotted on the same x-coordinate:

```
boxplot(Petal.Length ~ Species,data=iris,
ylab="Petal length",border = 1:3, outline = FALSE)
points(x = jitter(as.numeric(iris$Species)),
y = iris$Petal.Length,col=iris$Species)
```

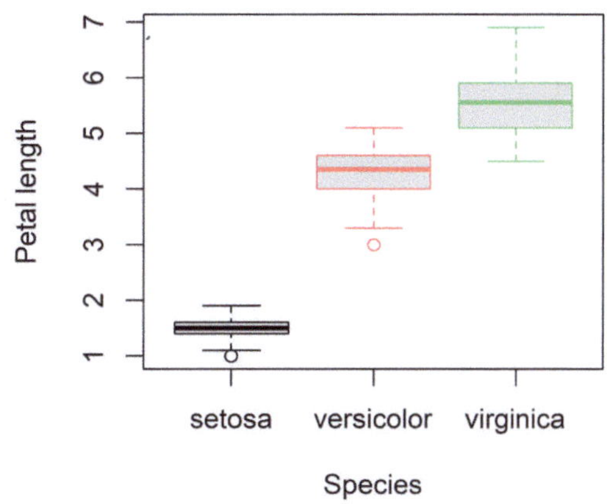

Fig. 4.10 A boxplot of the petal length in the Iris dataset

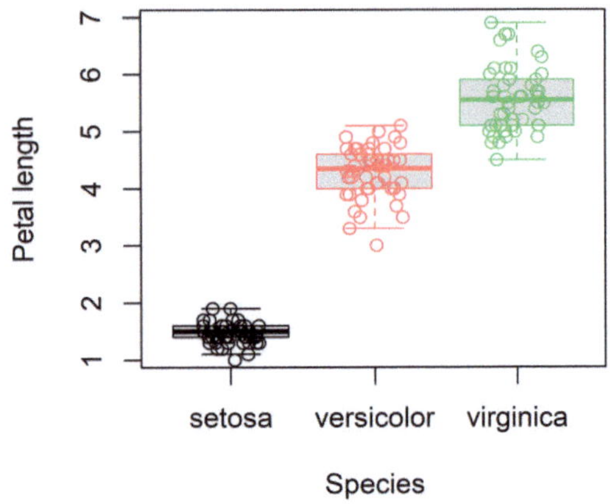

Fig. 4.11 A boxplot combined with a one-dimensional scatter plot of the petal length in the Iris dataset

Let's plot all variables in the same window:

```
par(mfrow = c(2, 2))
boxplot(Petal.Length ~ Species,data=iris,
ylab = "Petal Length", col="white", outline = FALSE)
points(x = jitter(as.numeric(iris$Species)),
y = iris$Petal.Length,col=iris$Species)

boxplot(Sepal.Length ~ Species,data=iris,
ylab = "Sepal Length", col="white", outline = FALSE)
points(x = jitter(as.numeric(iris$Species)),
y = iris$Sepal.Length,col=iris$Species)

boxplot(Petal.Width ~ Species,data=iris,ylab = "Petal Width",
col="white", outline = FALSE)
points(x = jitter(as.numeric(iris$Species)),
y = iris$Petal.Width,col=iris$Species)

boxplot(Sepal.Width ~ Species,data=iris,ylab = "Sepal Width",
col="white", outline = FALSE)
points(x = jitter(as.numeric(iris$Species)),
y = iris$Sepal.Width,col=iris$Species)
```

From these plots (Fig. 4.12), we can identify important patterns in the data. First of all, we see that the Setosa flowers are clearly separated from the other species based on the petal length and petal width. To separate Versicolor from Virginica, the petal length and petal width seem to be the best variables.

```
par(mfrow = c(1, 1)) #Restore normal window size
```

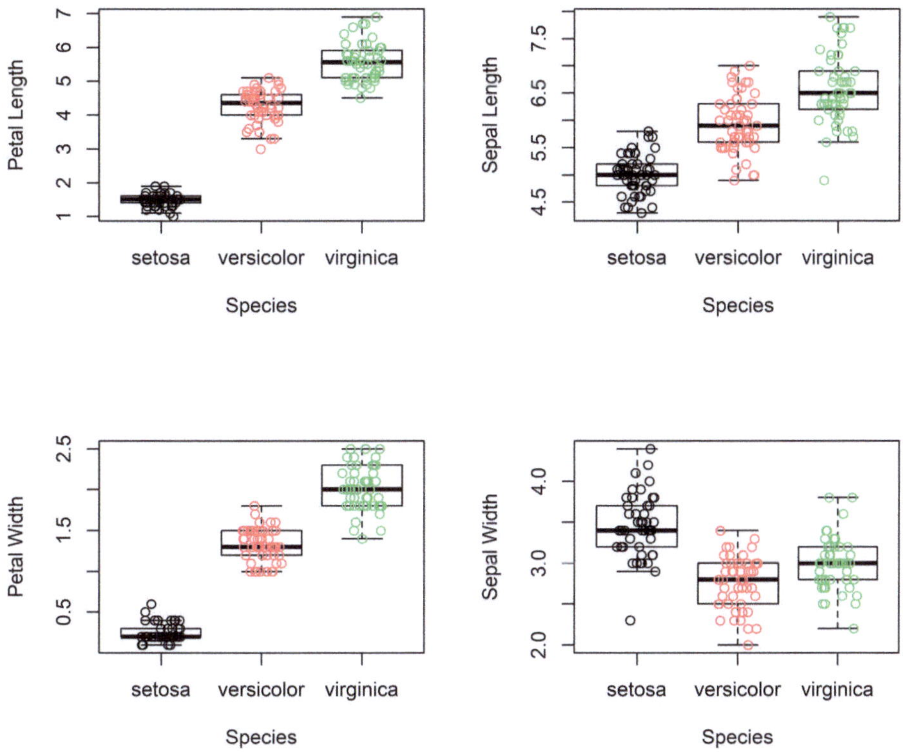

Fig. 4.12 Boxplots combined with one-dimensional scatter plots of all numeric variables in the Iris dataset

So far, we have created boxplots of one variable separated based on the species. If we instead like to make boxplots for all numeric variables, we can use:

```
boxplot(iris[,1:4])
```

From this plot (Fig. 4.13), we can see that the variable petal length has the largest spread in the data. Later, we will use **ggplot2** to create a similar boxplot where we also separate the species. If your variables are highly skewed, it might improve the visibility by using a log scale on the y-axis, such as boxplot(iris[,1:4],log="y").

4.2.1 Boxplots with ggplot2

To create a boxplot in **ggplot2**, we use basically the same code as we used to make a scatter plot. The main difference is that we here use the function "geom_boxplot" to add boxes instead of points in the plot:

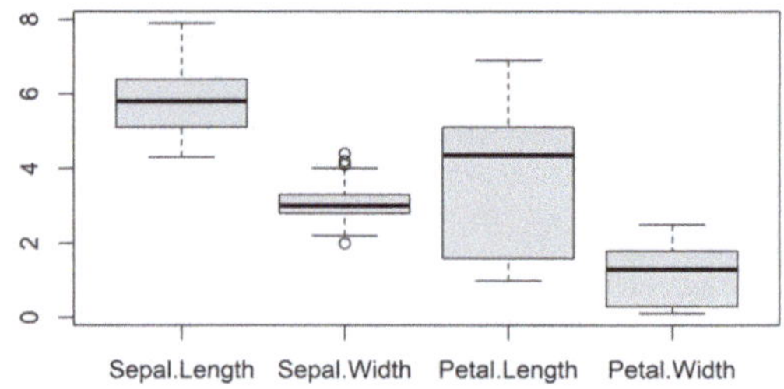

Fig. 4.13 A boxplot of all numeric variables in the Iris dataset

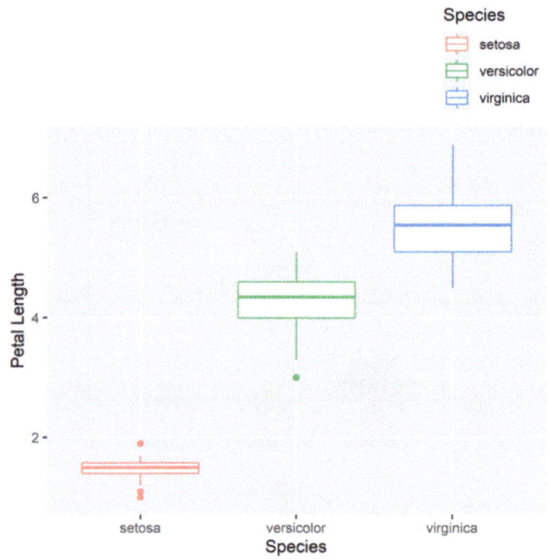

Fig. 4.14 A boxplot of the petal length in the Iris dataset, using the **ggplot2** package

```
library(ggplot2)
ggplot(data=iris, aes(x = Species, y = Petal.Length,
color=Species)) +
  geom_boxplot() + # Add boxes to the plot
  labs(y = "Petal Length")
```

Note that the "geom_boxplot" function defines outliers with a different method compared to the "boxplot" function we used earlier, which explains why there now are two additional outliers among the Setosa flowers (Fig. 4.14).

To instead fill the boxes with colors, we use "fill" instead of "color" in the function "aes". We can also remove the redundant legend if we set "legend.position" to "none":

```
library(ggplot2)
ggplot(data=iris, aes(x = Species, y = Petal.Length,
fill=Species)) +
  geom_boxplot() + # Add boxes to the plot
  labs(y = "Petal Length") +
  theme(legend.position = "none") # Remove legend
```

To add the data points to the previous plot (Fig. 4.15) by using jittering, we can add the function "geom_jitter" to the previous code, where we set width and height to 0.1 and 0, respectively, so that we only use horizontal jittering. Alpha controls the transparency of the points and shape = 21 creates filled circles, whereas aes(color="black") sets the border color of the points to black color:

```
library(ggplot2)
ggplot(data=iris, aes(x = Species, y = Petal.Length,
fill=Species)) +
  geom_boxplot(outlier.shape = NA) + # Suppress outliers
  geom_jitter(aes(color = "black"),size=2,width=0.1,height=0,
  alpha = 0.5, shape = 21) +
  labs(y = "Petal Length") +
  theme(legend.position = "none")
```

By adding the row names on top of the points, we can identify which Iris flowers that are defined as outliers in the boxplot (Fig. 4.16). Since we use jittering to randomly spread out the data points horizontally, we need to set a seed so that the text and the points are placed on the same coordinates:

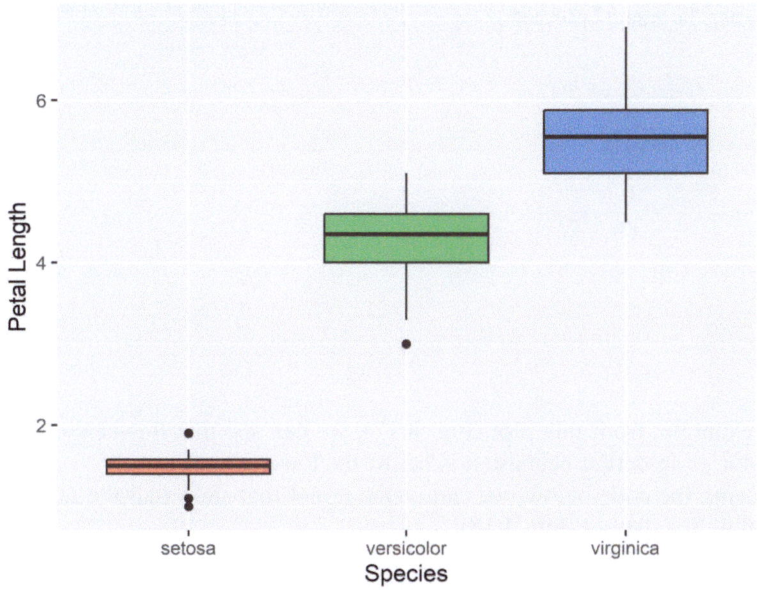

Fig. 4.15 A boxplot of the petal length in the Iris dataset, with filled boxes using the **ggplot2** package

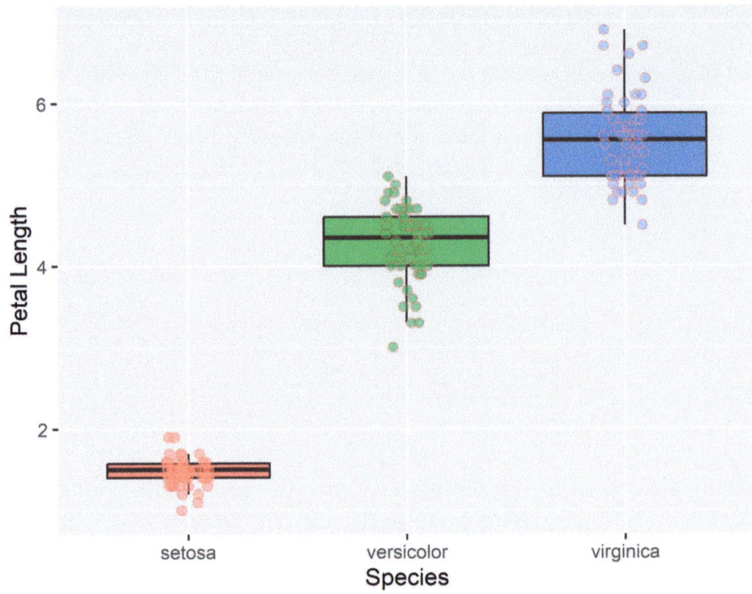

Fig. 4.16 A boxplot combined with a one-dimensional scatter plot of the petal length in the Iris dataset, using the **ggplot2** package

```
ggplot(data=iris, aes(x = Species, y = Petal.Length,
fill=Species)) +
  geom_boxplot(outlier.shape = NA) + # Suppress outliers
  geom_point(position = position_jitter(width = 0.2,
  height = 0, seed = 2),color="green") +
  geom_text(aes(label = rownames(iris)), size = 3,
  color = "black",
           position = position_jitter(width = 0.2, height = 0,
           seed = 2)) +
  theme(legend.position = "none") # Do not show the legend
```

For example, from this plot (Fig. 4.17), we can see that flower 99, which is a Versicolor, is an outlier because it is below the lower whisker.

By using the code below, we can create a plot that shows all the numeric variables in the Iris dataset (Fig. 4.18):

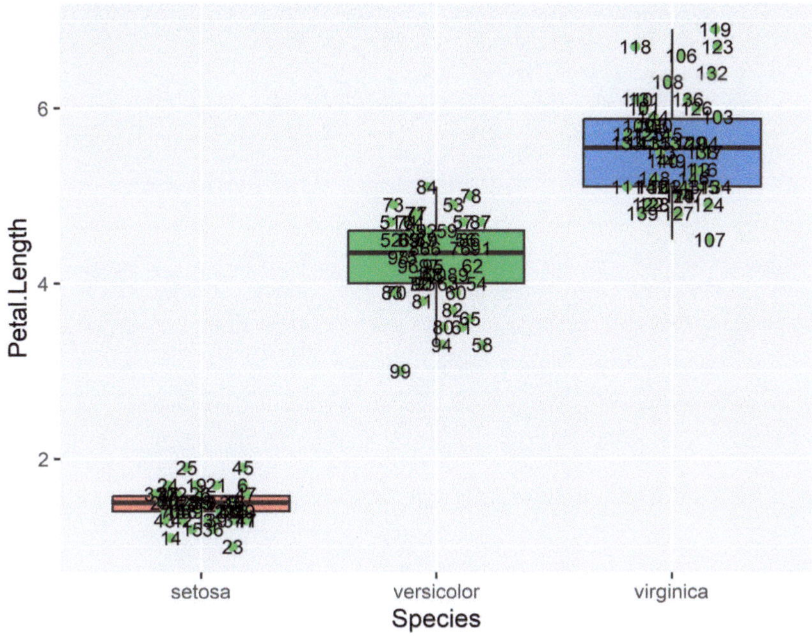

Fig. 4.17 A boxplot combined with a one-dimensional scatter plot of the petal length in the Iris dataset, using the **ggplot2** package with row labels on the points

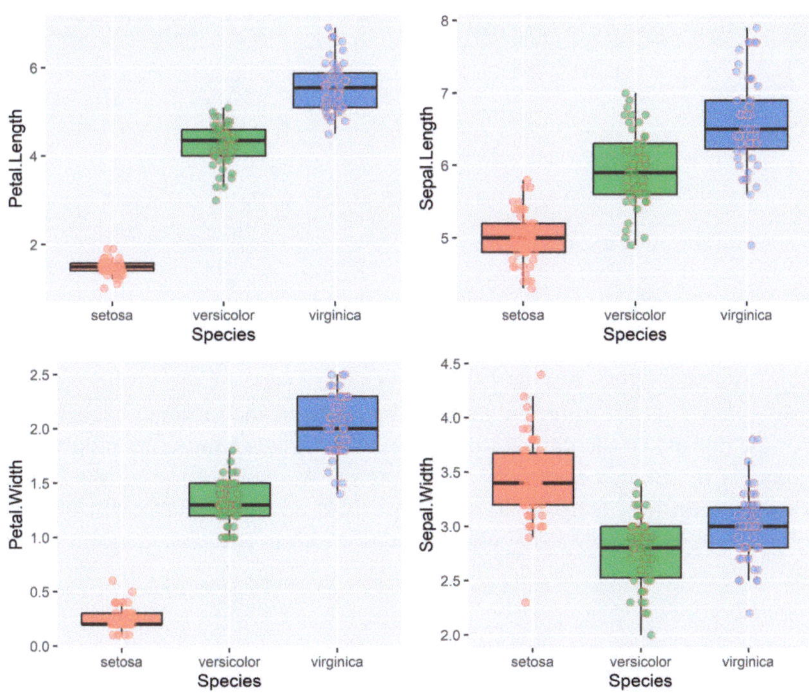

Fig. 4.18 Boxplots combined with one-dimensional scatter plots of all numeric variables in the Iris dataset, using the **ggplot2** package

```
plot1=ggplot(data=iris, aes(x = Species, y = Petal.Length,
fill=Species)) +
  geom_boxplot(outlier.shape = NA) +
  geom_jitter(aes(color = "black"),size=2,width=0.1,height=0,
  alpha = 0.5, shape = 21) +
  theme(legend.position = "none")

plot2=ggplot(data=iris, aes(x = Species, y = Petal.Width,
fill=Species)) +
  geom_boxplot(outlier.shape = NA) +
  geom_jitter(aes(color = "black"),size=2,width=0.1,height=0,
  alpha = 0.5, shape = 21) +
  theme(legend.position = "none")

plot3=ggplot(data=iris, aes(x = Species, y = Sepal.Length,
fill=Species)) +
  geom_boxplot(outlier.shape = NA) +
  geom_jitter(aes(color = "black"),size=2,width=0.1,height=0,
  alpha = 0.5, shape = 21) +
  theme(legend.position = "none")

plot4=ggplot(data=iris, aes(x = Species, y = Sepal.Width,
fill=Species)) +
  geom_boxplot(outlier.shape = NA) +
  geom_jitter(aes(color = "black"),size=2,width=0.1,height=0,
  alpha = 0.5, shape = 21) +
  theme(legend.position = "none")

library(gridExtra)
grid.arrange(plot1, plot3, plot2,plot4, ncol=2)
```

4.3 Violin Plots

Violin plots are quite similar to boxplots. The shape of the violin represents the density of the data at different values. The width of the violin at each y-value indicates the density of the data at that value, which gives a more detailed view of how the data is distributed compared to a boxplot. We can use the **ggplot2** package to create a violin plot (Fig. 4.19) where we also add the data points on top of the violins. In the code below, we use the Sepal width to illustrate a violin plot:

```
ggplot(data=iris, aes(x = Species, y = Sepal.Width,
fill=Species)) +
  geom_violin(trim=FALSE) +
  geom_jitter(size=2,width=0.1,height=0)
```

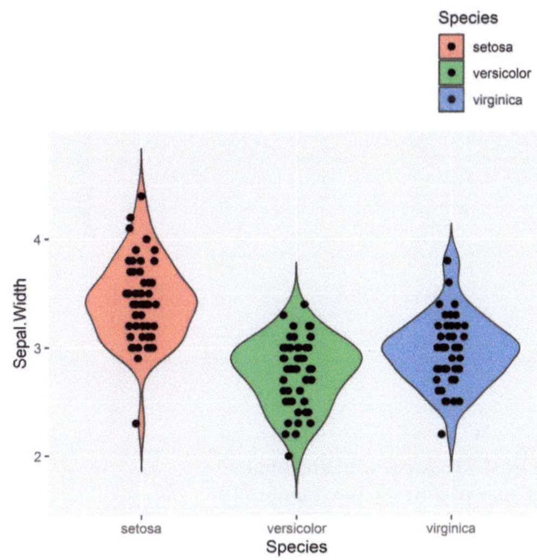

Fig. 4.19 A violin plot combined with a one-dimensional scatter plot of the sepal width in the Iris dataset, using the **ggplot2** package

4.4 One-Dimensional Scatter Plots

To produce a one-dimensional scatter plot where points are plotted for each category, we can use the function "stripchart":

```
stripchart(Petal.Length~Species,data=iris,vertical = TRUE,
method="jitter",pch=1, col=c(1:3), ylab="Petal length")
```

If we like to add a line that represents, for example, the mean, we could do this by using the function "segments". We then need to know the coordinates for placing the line. The x-coordinates of the three categories in Fig. 4.20 are simply 1, 2, and 3, whereas the y-coordinates in our case correspond to the mean values (Fig. 4.21):

```
x=1:3 # x-coordinates
# Mean values = y-coordinates
y=tapply(iris$Petal.Length,iris$Species,mean)
# The width of the segment is here set to ±0.2
segments(x-0.2,y,x+0.2,y,lwd=2)
```

To understand the purpose of using jittering, run the code below to produce a one-dimensional scatter plot without jittering and note that it does not look nice because the data points will overlap a lot:

```
stripchart(Petal.Length~Species,data=iris,vertical = TRUE,
pch=1,col=c(1:3),ylab="Petal length")
```

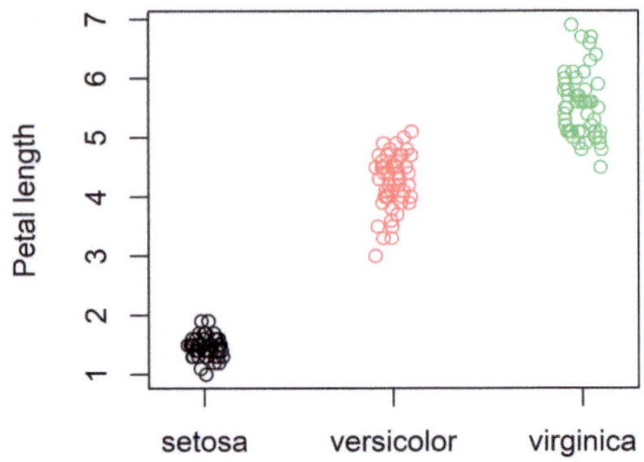

Fig. 4.20 A one-dimensional scatter plot of the petal length in the Iris dataset

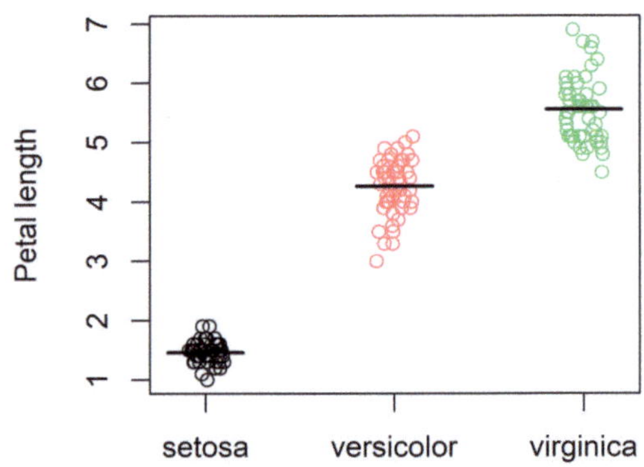

Fig. 4.21 A one-dimensional scatter plot of the petal length in the Iris dataset where the lines represent the mean

We can also use the function "stripchart" to add several plots in the same graph by setting the argument "add" to true. Below we add the different categories one by one by using different colors:

```
stripchart(subset(iris,Species=="setosa")[,-5], vertical = T,
method="jitter",pch=1,col=2, ylim=c(0,8),ylab="size (cm)",
group.names=c("Sepal length","Sepal width","Petal length",
"Petal width"))
stripchart(subset(iris,Species=="versicolor")[,-5],
vertical = T, method="jitter",pch=1,col=3,add = TRUE)
stripchart(subset(iris,Species=="virginica")[,-5],
vertical = T, method="jitter",pch=1,col=4,add = TRUE)
legend("topright", legend=levels(factor(iris[,5])), pch=1,
col=2:4)
```

This plot (Fig. 4.22) clearly shows how the species are separated based on the different measurements, where the petal length and width seem to achieve the best separation between the different species.

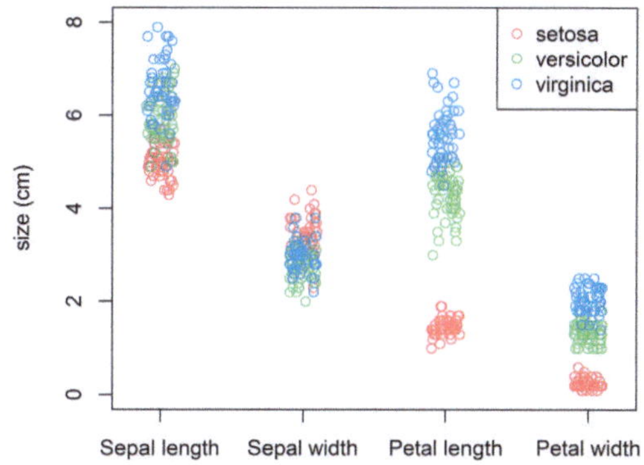

Fig. 4.22 A one-dimensional scatter plot of all the continuous variables in the Iris dataset where the species are identified with colors

4.4.1 A One-Dimensional Scatter Plot in ggplot2

To create a one-dimensional scatter plot in **ggplot2** where we show all species and the different measurements in the same plot as in Fig. 4.22, we first need to reshape the Iris data frame into a long format, which means that we stack the four numeric columns, so that there is only one value on each row, by using the function "pivot_longer" in the **tidyr** package:

```
library(tidyr)
iris_long = iris %>%
  pivot_longer(cols = 1:4, names_to = "variable",
  values_to = "size")
```

Note that the previous Iris data frame has been converted to a tibble by the "pivot_longer" function and that this tibble contains 600 rows since we have stacked the four columns with 150 values on top of each other. Print the tibble and note the difference from our previous data frame. We can now create a one-dimensional scatter plot (Fig. 4.23) based on the long format by the following code:

```
library(ggplot2)
ggplot(data=iris_long, aes(x = variable, y = size,
color = Species)) +
  geom_jitter(size=2,width=0.1,height=0,alpha = 0.5) +
  labs(y = "Size (cm)", x = "") +
  theme(legend.position = "top")
```

Similarly, we can put boxplots next to each other to illustrate the difference in length and width of the three species where "position_dodge(width = 0.8)" determines how far apart the boxes should be for the three species (Fig. 4.24):

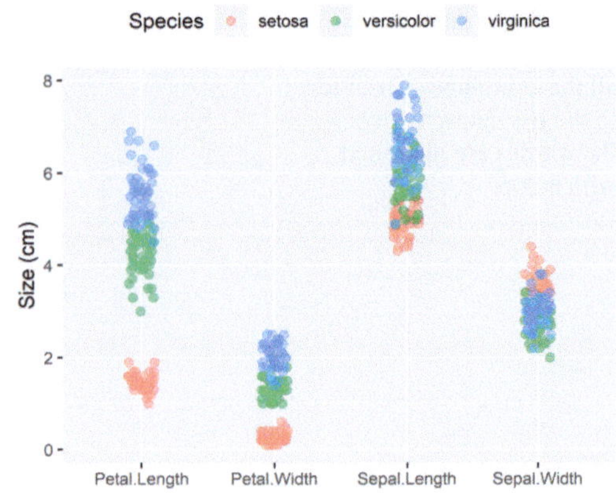

Fig. 4.23 A one-dimensional scatter plot of all the numeric variables in the Iris dataset where the species are identified with colors, using the **ggplot2** package

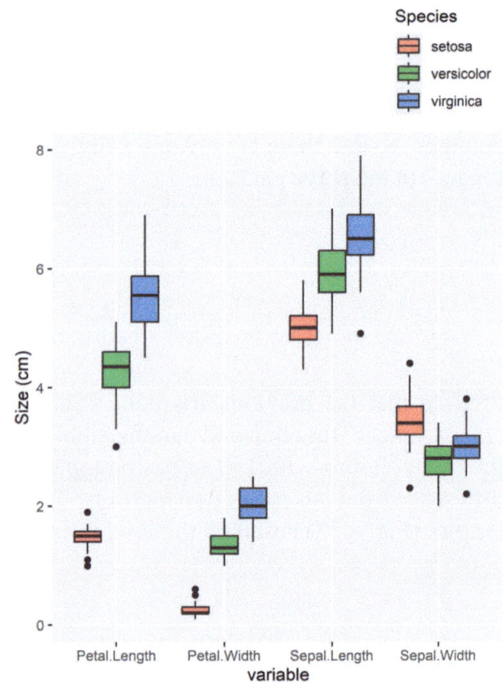

Fig. 4.24 A boxplot of all the numeric variables in the Iris dataset where the species are separated and identified with colors, using the **ggplot2** package

```
ggplot(iris_long, aes(x = variable, y = size,
fill = Species)) +
  # Dodge to separate Species
  geom_boxplot(position = position_dodge(width = 0.8)) +
  labs(y = "Size (cm)", x = "variable", fill = "Species")
```

4.5 Profile Plot

To identify certain patterns in the data, one can use a profile plot or a parallel coordinate plot, which is basically the same as Fig. 4.23 with the exception that lines are drawn between the data points for each flower. One simple way to do this is to use the function "ggparcoord" from the package **GGally**:

```
library(GGally)
ggparcoord(iris, columns=1:4, groupColumn = 5,
scale="globalminmax")
```

We tell the function which columns of the Iris dataset we like to plot (1–4) and which column that includes the grouping variable (the species in column 5). By default, this function standardizes the data so that the variables have a mean of zero and a standard deviation of one. This is useful when the variables have a big difference in their values or if they have different units. However, to be consistent with the previous plots, we do not standardize the variables, which explains why we here set the "scale" argument to globalminmax.

From this plot (Fig. 4.25), we can see that the species Versicolor and Virginica have similar shapes or patterns since the lines of the two groups are roughly parallel. The pattern of Setosa is clearly distinct from the other species, where the main difference in its pattern seems to be in the petal length.

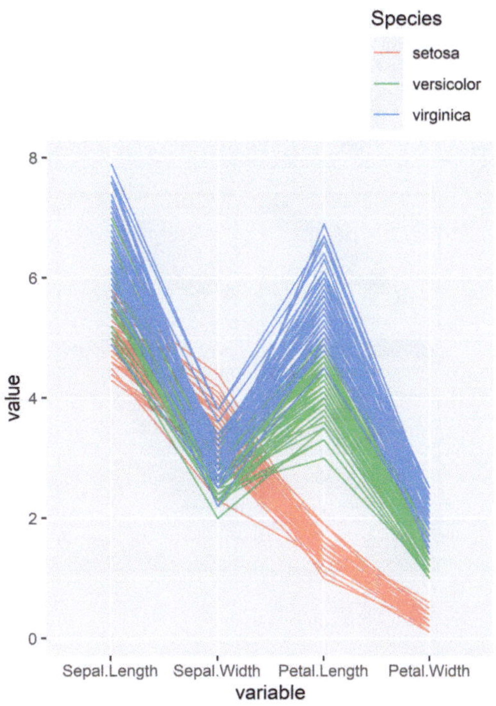

Fig. 4.25 A profile plot of all the numeric variables in the Iris dataset where the species are identified with colors, using the **GGally** package

4.6 Scatter Plot Matrix

A scatter plot matrix is simply several scatter plots that are included in the same figure. If we include four variables in a scatter plot matrix, the plot will show six unique scatter plots. For the numeric variables in the Iris dataset, all possible pairs are shown: (1) sepal length vs sepal width, (2) sepal length vs petal length, (3) sepal length vs petal width, (4) sepal width vs petal length, (5) sepal width vs petal width, and (6) petal length vs petal width. We can plot the numeric variables (columns 1–4 in the data frame) with the function "pairs":

```
pairs(iris[,1:4])
```

Note that the scatter plots below the main diagonal are identical to the ones above the main diagonal (Fig. 4.26). To simplify the interpretation of the plots, we can add

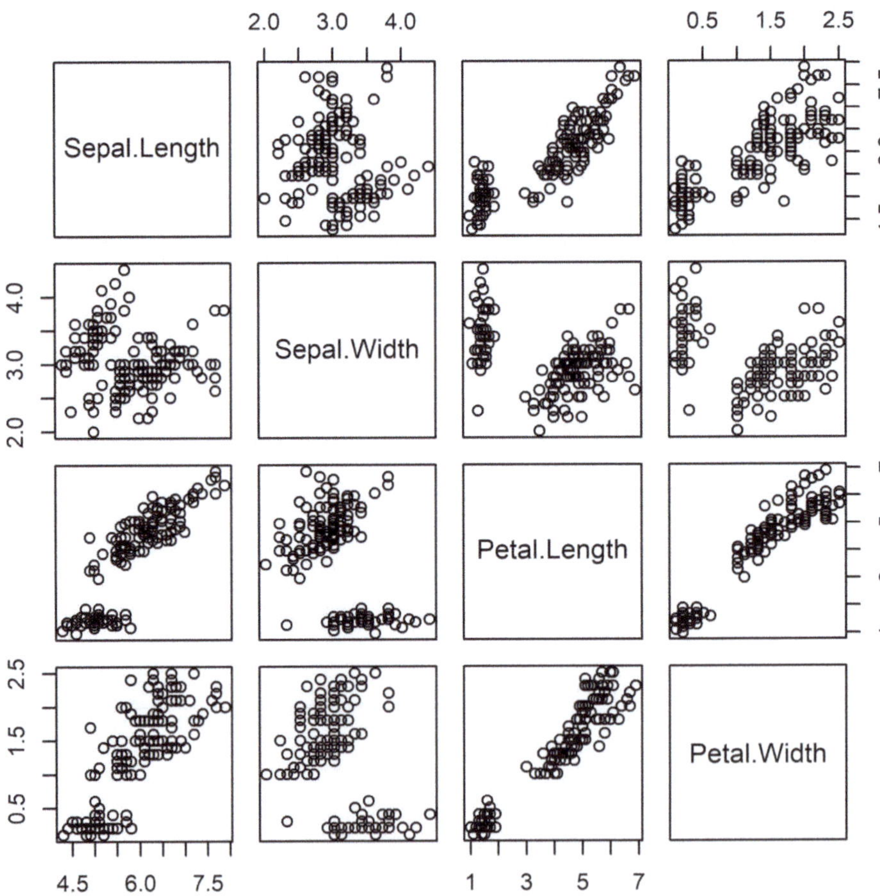

Fig. 4.26 A scatter plot matrix of all the numeric variables in the Iris dataset

colors to the species and only display the scatter plots below the main diagonal to avoid duplicated plots:

```
pairs(iris[,1:4], col = iris$Species, upper.panel=NULL)
```

From this plot (Fig. 4.27), we can see that there is a strong positive linear relationship between the petal length and the petal width. We can also see how the combination of two variables can be used to separate the species in most plots. It seems like Versicolor (red) and Virginica (green) can be separated by combining two variables, except when sepal length and sepal width are combined since the scatter is more or less mixed in this plot. To get a quantitative understanding of how the variables correlate, we can use a correlation matrix that we generate in the next chapter.

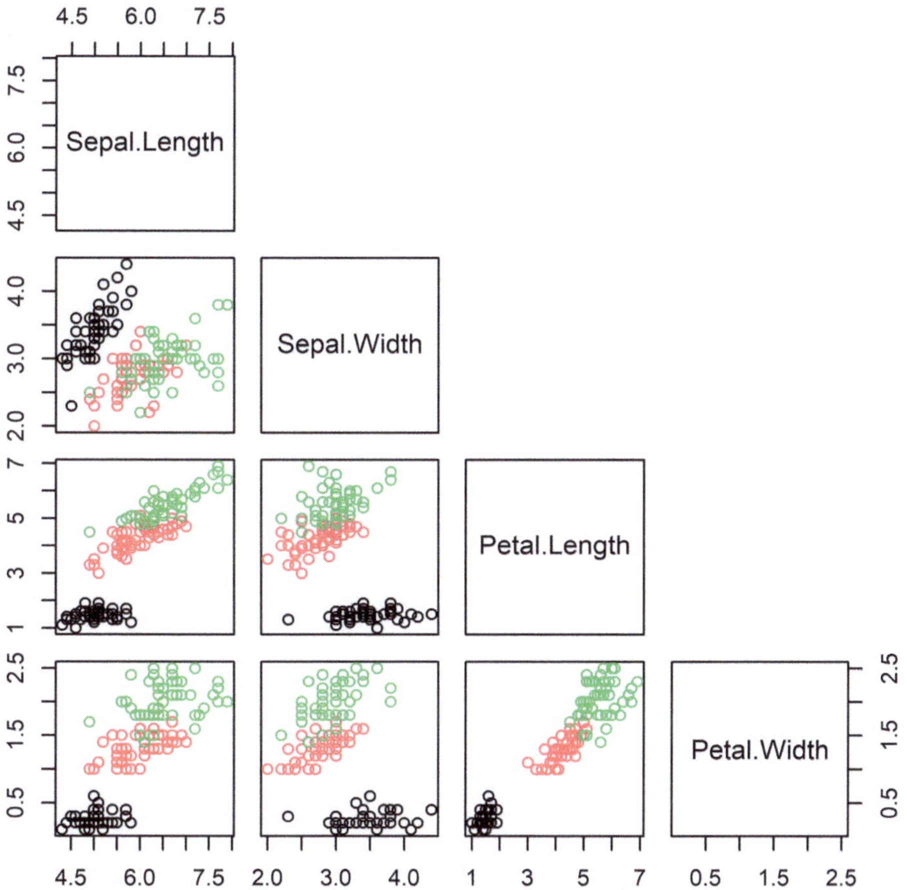

Fig. 4.27 A scatter plot matrix of all the numeric variables in the Iris dataset where the species are identified with different colors: black (Setosa), red (Versicolor), and green (Virginica)

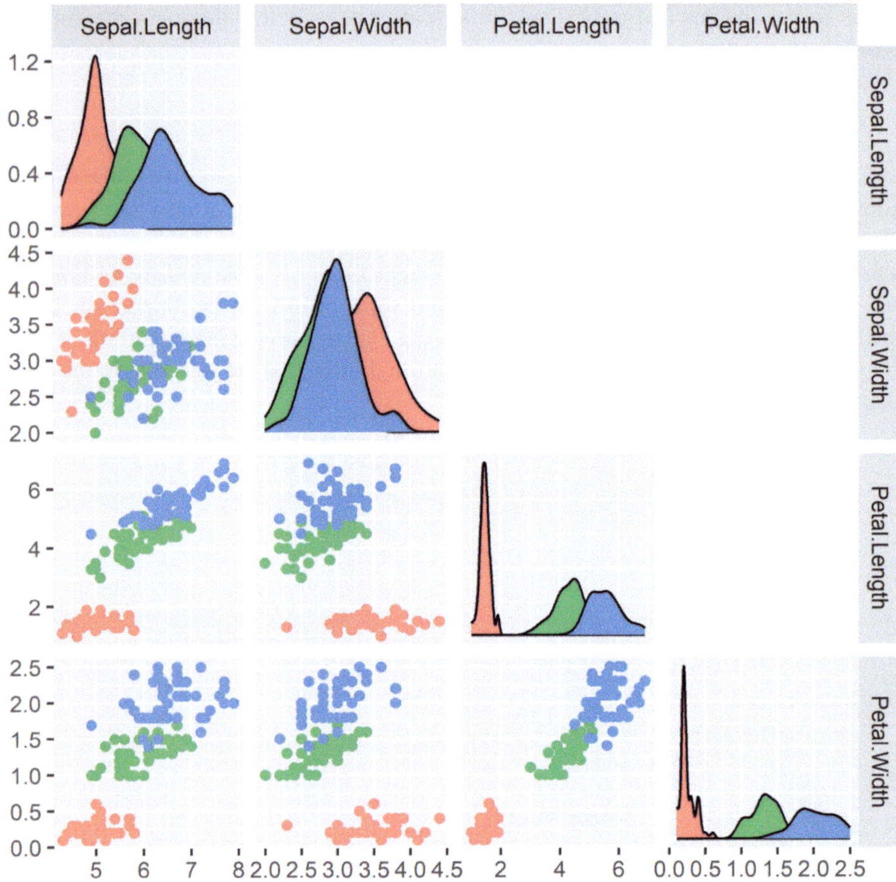

Fig. 4.28 A scatter plot matrix of all the numeric variables in the Iris dataset where the species are identified with different colors: red (Setosa), green (Versicolor), and blue (Virginica), using the **GGally** package

Another way to generate a similar plot as Fig. 4.27 is to use the “ggppairs” function in the **GGally** package. By using this function, we will also get a density plot in the main diagonal for each of the numeric variables in the Iris dataset (Fig. 4.28):

```
library(GGally)
ggpairs(iris, columns = 1:4, aes(color = Species),
upper = list(continuous = "blank"))
```

4.7 Exercises

1. Create a scatter plot of the CW and CL in the Crab dataset and label the variable sex with different colors.
2. Create a boxplot of all the numerical variables in the Crab dataset. Can you identify an outlier in any of the numerical variables?
3. Create a boxplot with **ggplot2** of all the numerical variables in the Crab dataset but where you now plot separate boxes for the blue and orange species.
4. Make a one-dimensional scatter plot including all numerical variables in the Crab dataset and set different colors for the variable species.
5. Make a scatter plot matrix of all the numerical variables in the Crab dataset and set different colors for the variable sex.
6. Create a profile plot of all the numerical variables in the Crab dataset and set different colors for male and female crabs. Which variables in this plot seem to best separate the sex?

Chapter 5
Multivariate Relationships

Covariance and the correlation matrix are important concepts in multivariate statistics, which provide insights into the relationships between the numeric variables in the dataset. Understanding these measures is crucial for detecting associations between multiple variables and for understanding multivariate statistical methods. For example, the calculations involved in PCA are based on the covariance matrix. Watch the video below to learn about the difference between the covariance and the correlation matrix and how to interpret a correlation coefficient.

5.1 Video

https://youtu.be/cAqYNuYXm4c
www.tilestats.com/ml/

5.2 The Dataset

We will here use the Iris dataset that we discussed in Chap. 3. To print the first six lines of the Iris dataset, we can type:

A. Tilevik, *Multivariate Statistics and Machine Learning in R For Beginners*,
https://doi.org/10.1007/978-3-032-01851-9_5

```
head(iris)
  Sepal.Length  Sepal.Width  Petal.Length  Petal.Width  Species
1     5.1          3.5          1.4           0.2       setosa
2     4.9          3.0          1.4           0.2       setosa
3     4.7          3.2          1.3           0.2       setosa
4     4.6          3.1          1.5           0.2       setosa
5     5.0          3.6          1.4           0.2       setosa
6     5.4          3.9          1.7           0.4       setosa
```

We see that the first four columns include numeric variables, whereas the fifth column includes a categorical variable, which tells which species the flower belongs to.

5.3 The Correlation Matrix

A correlation matrix shows the correlation coefficients for all possible pairwise comparisons of the numeric variables that we want to analyze. By using, for example, the function "cor" on the numeric variables of the Iris dataset, with the method "pearson", we will generate the Pearson correlation coefficients between the four variables:

```
cor(iris[,1:4],method="pearson")
             Sepal.Length  Sepal.Width  Petal.Length  Petal.Width
Sepal.Length  1.0000000    -0.1175698   0.8717538     0.8179411
Sepal.Width  -0.1175698    1.0000000    -0.4284401    -0.3661259
Petal.Length  0.8717538    -0.4284401   1.0000000     0.9628654
Petal.Width   0.8179411    -0.3661259   0.9628654     1.0000000
```

From this matrix, we see that the strongest correlation can be found between the petal length and the petal width (r=0.96). The next strongest correlation can be found between the sepal length and the petal length (r= 0.87). If we like to generate a correlation matrix based only on one category, we can simply specify this by defining which rows of the data frame we like to include. For example, a correlation matrix of only the class Versicolor can be generated by:

```
cor(subset(iris,Species=="versicolor")[,1:4],method="pearson")
```

One problem with the Pearson correlation coefficient is that it is highly sensitive to extreme values. If we have extreme values in our dataset, or numeric variables on an ordinal scale, we can instead use Spearman's correlation:

```
cor(subset(iris,Species=="versicolor")[,1:4],
method="spearman")
```

5.3.1 Correlation Plot

The problem with correlation matrices is that they become very hard to read when we have many variables. Thus, it might be difficult to sort out important values in a very big matrix. One way to simplify the analysis is to plot the correlation values. We can do this by using the function "corrplot" in the **corrplot** package:

```
library(corrplot)
# Generate the correlation matrix
cor_mat=cor(iris[,1:4],method="pearson")
corrplot(cor_mat,type = "lower")
```

Figure 5.1 shows strong correlations with bigger circles where positive correlations are indicated by blue color and negative correlations are indicated by red color. We can see that the petal length and petal width have the strongest correlation followed by the petal length and sepal length. Ignore the four blue circles in the main diagonal because these just show the correlation with the variable itself, which is always equal to one (see the above correlation matrix).

5.3.2 Extract Pairs with Strong Correlations

Another alternative to identify strong correlations between pairs of variables is to sort the correlations. To sort the correlations, we first compute the correlation matrix:

```
cor_mat=cor(iris[,1:4],method="pearson")
```

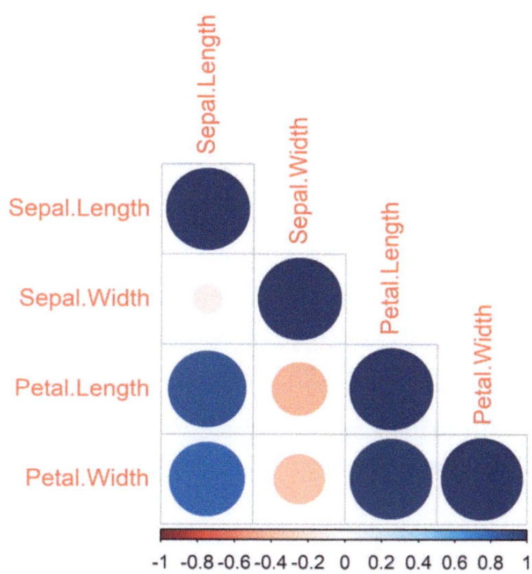

Fig. 5.1 A correlation plot based on all the numeric variables in the Iris dataset. Blue color indicates a positive correlation, whereas red color indicates a negative correlation. The size of the circles represents the strength of the correlation

Since the main diagonal holds correlations of 1 (correlation of the variable with itself), we should remove these values, as well as the duplicated values above or below the main diagonal. We remove these values by first defining them as NAs:

```
diag(cor_mat) = NA
cor_mat[upper.tri (cor_mat)] = NA
cor_mat
             Sepal.Length  Sepal.Width  Petal.Length  Petal.Width
Sepal.Length      NA            NA           NA           NA
Sepal.Width   -0.1175698        NA           NA           NA
Petal.Length   0.8717538   -0.4284401        NA           NA
Petal.Width    0.8179411   -0.3661259    0.9628654        NA
```

Next, we use the “melt” function from the **reshape** package to reshape the matrix and print this matrix without the NAs:

```
library(reshape)
cor_melt=melt(cor_mat)
na.omit(cor_melt) # Print reshaped matrix without NA
          X1              X2          value
2    Sepal.Width    Sepal.Length   -0.1175698
3   Petal.Length    Sepal.Length    0.8717538
4    Petal.Width    Sepal.Length    0.8179411
7   Petal.Length    Sepal.Width    -0.4284401
8    Petal.Width    Sepal.Width    -0.3661259
12   Petal.Width    Petal.Length    0.9628654
```

Next, we extract the correlation coefficients which are, for example, greater or less than 0.8 and -0.8, respectively. Finally, we print the sorted correlation coefficients by the function “order”:

```
index=which(cor_melt$value>0.80 | cor_melt$value<(-0.80))
# Extract correlations that are greater than 0.8 or less than -0.8
most_cor=cor_melt[index,]
# Print sorted correlations
most_cor[order(most_cor$value,decreasing = TRUE),]
          X1              X2          value
12    Petal.Width      Petal.Length   0.9628654
3      Petal.Length    Sepal.Length   0.8717538
4      Petal.Width     Sepal.Length   0.8179411
```

To extract and sort the correlation coefficients, we can also use the functions “filter” and “arrange” in the **dplyr** package:

```
library(dplyr)
most_cor = cor_melt %>%
  filter(!is.na(value), value > 0.80 | value < -0.80) %>%
  arrange(desc(value))
print(most_cor)
           X1            X2         value
1  Petal.Width  Petal.Length    0.9628654
2 Petal.Length  Sepal.Length    0.8717538
3  Petal.Width  Sepal.Length    0.8179411
```

This output is a lot easier to read than a correlation matrix because it clearly shows the pairs of variables with the strongest correlations.

5.3.3 *Significant Correlations*

When we analyze the correlation coefficients, we usually want to know if the correlation coefficients are significantly different from zero. We can use the function "cor.test" for a certain pair of variables. For example, the correlation between the sepal length and sepal width can be computed by:

```
cor.test(iris$Sepal.Length,iris$Sepal.Width)
data:  iris$Sepal.Length and iris$Sepal.Width
t = -1.4403, df = 148, p-value = 0.1519
alternative hypothesis: true correlation is not equal to 0
95 percent confidence interval:
 -0.27269325  0.04351158
sample estimates:
      cor
-0.1175698
```

Since the p-value is greater than 0.05 (and the 95% confidence interval includes the value zero), we can conclude that the correlation coefficient is not significantly different from zero. To generate a matrix with p-values for all pairwise comparisons, we can use the function "rcorr" from the **Hmisc** package:

```
library(Hmisc)
rcorr(as.matrix(iris[,1:4]), type="pearson")
....
....
             Sepal.Length  Sepal.Width  Petal.Length  Petal.Width
Sepal.Length                0.1519        0.0000        0.0000
Sepal.Width     0.1519                    0.0000        0.0000
Petal.Length    0.0000      0.0000                      0.0000
Petal.Width     0.0000      0.0000        0.0000
```

From this output, which shows the p-values below the correlation coefficients, we see that all pairwise correlations have p-values close to zero except for the correlation between the sepal length and the sepal width (p-value = 0.1519). If we like to print only the p-values, we can add "$P" at the end of the line by:

```
rcorr(as.matrix(iris[,1:4]), type="pearson")$P
```

Since we compute six p-values, we should reduce our significant level (or adjust the p-values). A simple method to deal with multiple comparisons is to use Bonferroni correction by multiplying the p-values with the number of correlations we compute. In our example, we would therefore multiply the p-values by six:

```
rcorr(as.matrix(iris[,1:4]), type="pearson")$P*6
             Sepal.Length  Sepal.Width  Petal.Length  Petal.Width
Sepal.Length      NA       9.113888e-01 0.000000e+00 0.000000e+00
Sepal.Width    0.9113888        NA      2.707984e-07 2.443936e-05
Petal.Length   0.0000000   2.707984e-07      NA      0.000000e+00
Petal.Width    0.0000000   2.443936e-05 0.000000e+00      NA
```

None of the adjusted p-values, except for the sepal length VS sepal width, is greater than 0.05. However, it is easier to read this table if we round the values to three decimal places:

```
round(rcorr(as.matrix(iris[,1:4]), type="pearson")$P*6,3)
```

5.4 The Covariance Matrix

The covariance matrix is related to the correlation matrix. A positive covariance means that the variables are positively related, whereas a negative covariance means that the variables are negatively related. We can calculate the covariance matrix by:

```
cov(iris[,1:4])
             Sepal.Length  Sepal.Width  Petal.Length  Petal.Width
Sepal.Length 0.6856935     -0.0424340    1.2743154     0.5162707
Sepal.Width  -0.0424340     0.1899794   -0.3296564    -0.1216394
Petal.Length 1.2743154     -0.3296564    3.1162779     1.2956094
Petal.Width  0.5162707     -0.1216394    1.2956094     0.5810063
```

The main diagonal of this matrix simply shows the sample variance of each variable. For example, the variance of the sepal length can be calculated by:

```
var(iris$Sepal.Length)
0.6856935
```

5.5 Standardize the Variables

For multivariate statistical analyses, we might face the problem of working with variables that have different units. Let's consider the following data (Table 5.1):

```
Gender=factor(c('M','F','F','F','M','M','F'))
Weight=c(80,58,65,70,90,100,50)
Height=c(190,171,175,169,182,183,165)
Temp=c(37.5,38.3,37.0,37.9,38.6,40.1,36.7)
df=data.frame(Gender,Weight,Height,Temp)
```

Our dataset includes three continuous variables: weight in kg, height in cm, and body temperature with the unit of Celsius. However, we could also have expressed the weight in grams, height in meters, and body temperature in Fahrenheit. We would then get different values. The unit that we will use will, for example, affect the size of the variance of each variable. The size of the variance has an important effect in many multivariate methods that we will see later on. By standardizing the variables, we will remove the effect of the units. To standardize a variable (x), we subtract the mean value ($\overline{x}$) from each value (x_i) and divide this difference by the standard deviation (s) of the variable:

$$z_i = \frac{x_i - \overline{x}}{s}$$

After standardizing the variable, the standardized variable (z) will have a mean of zero and a standard deviation of one.

Let's assume that we have the following variable:

```
x=c(10,4,7,9,2)
```

We can standardize this variable by the following calculation:

```
z=(x-mean(x))/sd(x)
z
[1]  1.0709354 -0.7139569  0.1784892  0.7734534 -1.3089211
```

Table 5.1 Example data to be standardized

Person	Gender	Weight (kg)	Height (cm)	Body temperature (Celsius)
1	Male	80	190	37.5
2	Female	58	171	38.3
3	Female	65	175	37.0
4	Female	70	169	37.9
5	Male	90	182	38.6
6	Male	100	183	40.1
7	Female	50	165	36.7

Let's check if the standardized variable (z) has a mean of zero and a standard deviation of one:

```
mean(z)
[1] -9.992007e-17
sd(z)
[1] 1
```

Note that the mean of z is not exactly zero, which is due to rounding effects. To standardize data, we can also use the function "scale":

```
x=c(10,4,7,9,2)
scale(x)
           [,1]
[1,]  1.0709354
[2,] -0.7139569
[3,]  0.1784892
[4,]  0.7734534
[5,] -1.3089211
attr(,"scaled:center")
[1] 6.4
attr(,"scaled:scale")
[1] 3.361547
```

These standardized values are the same as we computed previously. The output from the "scale" function also shows the mean (6.4) and standard deviation (3.36) of the unstandardized data.

To standardize the numeric variables in our previous data frame, we can use the function "scale" to scale/standardize each of the variables in columns 2–4 and then create a data frame of the variable Gender and the standardized data. The function "scale" returns a matrix and if we like to have the standardized data in a data frame, the function "data.frame" is usually used to convert such matrix back to a data frame:

```
dfZ=data.frame(Gender,scale(df[,2:4]))
dfZ
  Gender     Weight         Height         Temp
1    M     0.3779645      1.5241513     -0.4508108
2    F    -0.8604723     -0.6096605      0.2504504
3    F    -0.4664242     -0.1604370     -0.8890990
4    F    -0.1849613     -0.8342723     -0.1001802
5    M     0.9408903      0.6257042      0.5134234
6    M     1.5038161      0.7380101      1.8282882
7    F    -1.3108130     -1.2834959     -1.1520720
```

To check that the scaling has generated a standard deviation of one and a mean of zero, we can use:

```
apply(dfZ[,2:4],2,mean)
       Weight        Height          Temp
-3.687526e-16  1.375884e-15  1.768427e-15
apply(dfZ[,2:4],2,sd)
  Weight Height Temp
     1      1      1
```

The above code requires that we specify the column indexes of the columns we like to standardize. This can be tedious if we have a large dataset with lots of columns. One way to avoid specifying the column number where we have numeric variables that should be standardized is to use the "mutate" function in the **dplyr** package:

```
library(dplyr)
dfZ = df %>%
  mutate(across(where(is.numeric), scale))
```

This code automatically finds the numeric variables and scales them.

5.5.1 Covariance of Standardized Variables

The covariance of standardized variables is identical to the correlation as explained in the video. For example, let's compute the standardized values of the Iris dataset with the function "scale" and compute the covariance of these standardized values:

```
scale_iris=scale(iris[,1:4])
cov(scale_iris)
             Sepal.Length  Sepal.Width  Petal.Length  Petal.Width
Sepal.Length 1.0000000     -0.1175698    0.8717538     0.8179411
Sepal.Width -0.1175698      1.0000000   -0.4284401    -0.3661259
Petal.Length 0.8717538     -0.4284401    1.0000000     0.9628654
Petal.Width  0.8179411     -0.3661259    0.9628654     1.0000000
```

This covariance matrix is identical to the Pearson correlation matrix:

```
cor(iris[,1:4],method="pearson")
             Sepal.Length  Sepal.Width  Petal.Length  Petal.Width
Sepal.Length   1.0000000   -0.1175698    0.8717538     0.8179411
Sepal.Width   -0.1175698   1.0000000    -0.4284401    -0.3661259
Petal.Length   0.8717538   -0.4284401    1.0000000     0.9628654
Petal.Width    0.8179411   -0.3661259    0.9628654     1.0000000
```

5.6 Exercises

1. Calculate the correlation matrix of the numerical variables in the Crab dataset and indicate which correlations that are significantly different from zero. Use Bonferroni correction to adjust the p-values.
2. Print the correlation coefficients as a sorted list where one can easily see which pair that has the strongest positive correlation.
3. Extract only the female crabs and compute a correlation matrix of the variables FL, RW, and CL.

Chapter 6
PCA and PCoA

We will now have a look at principal component analysis (PCA) and principal coordinate analysis (PCoA), which are the most fundamental methods in multivariate statistics. Although PCA and PCoA share similarities in simplifying complex datasets, they are based on different mathematical principles and are suited for specific types of data and distance measures. At the end of this chapter, you will see that these two methods result in the same outcomes if the PCoA is based on Euclidean distances. PCA is a method to combine variables in a way so that the combined variables have maximal variance, which can be seen as the combined variables having maximal information about the original variables. Watch the video below to get an introduction to PCA. If you like, you may also watch the optional second video to understand the mathematical details behind the eigendecomposition method.

6.1 Videos

https://youtu.be/nwwls8Uu7H8
https://youtu.be/0tnBmf8eu3g
www.tilestats.com/ml/

** Note that the weights generated in the second video will not result in the exact same weights as computed below because the calculations by hand in the video are based on rounded values of the covariance matrix.*

A. Tilevik, *Multivariate Statistics and Machine Learning in R For Beginners*,
https://doi.org/10.1007/978-3-032-01851-9_6

6.2 Combine Variables

In this section, we will learn how to combine variables in our dataset with some simple methods before we have a look at PCA. The idea is to reduce the dataset where the smaller dataset is still a good representation of the original dataset.

Let's first have a look at how we can combine two variables into one. In the example data in Table 6.1, one has measured the diastolic (DBP) and systolic blood (SBP) pressures of six individuals.

If we plot these two variables (Fig. 6.1), we see that they have a positive relationship:

```
DBP=c(78,80,81,82,84,86)
SBP=c(126,128,127,130,130,132)
plot(DBP, SBP,xlab="Diastolic BP (mmHg)",
ylab="Systolic BP (mmHg)")
```

To combine these two variables into a single variable that we call blood pressure (BP), we could, for example, calculate the mean or the sum of the two variables:

Table 6.1 Example of blood pressure data

Diastolic BP (mmHg)	Systolic BP (mmHg)
78	126
80	128
81	127
82	130
84	130
86	132

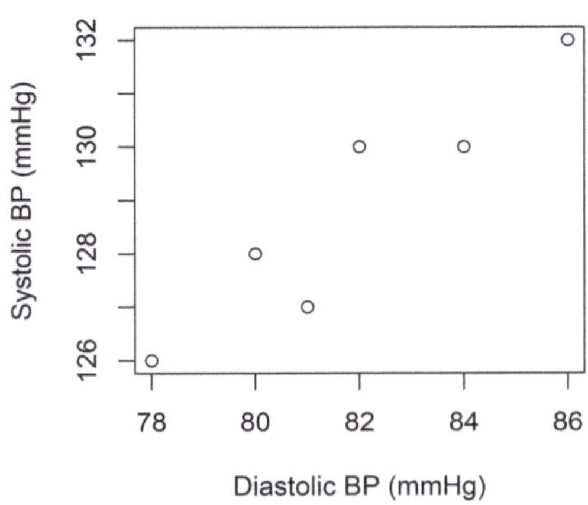

Fig. 6.1 A scatter plot of the diastolic and systolic blood pressure of six individuals

```
BP_mean=(DBP + SBP)/2 # The mean
BP_sum= DBP + SBP      # The sum
data.frame(DBP,SBP,BP_mean,BP_sum)
   DBP   SBP  BP_mean   BP_sum
1   78   126    102      204
2   80   128    104      208
3   81   127    104      208
4   82   130    106      212
5   84   130    107      214
6   86   132    109      218
```

The mean and the sum of the diastolic and systolic BP can be seen as linear combinations of the two variables. A linear combination, Y, of X_1 and X_2, can be formulated as:

$$Y = \alpha_1 X_1 + \alpha_2 X_2$$

where α_1 and α_2 are called weights of the variables X_1 and X_2, respectively. In our example, the linear combination of the mean BP can be written as:

$$\text{MeanBP} = 0.5 \cdot \text{DiastolicBP} + 0.5 \cdot \text{SystolicBP}$$

whereas the sum of the BP can be written as:

$$\text{SumBP} = 1 \cdot \text{DiastolicBP} + 1 \cdot \text{SystolicBP}$$

Note that the difference between the two methods (mean and sum) to form a linear combination is just the values of the weights.

6.3 Principal Component Analysis

Principal component analysis (PCA) is a method to find the linear combination that accounts for as much variation as possible. The more variation that is captured, the more information from the original variables is stored in our linear combination. Hence, PCA aims to reduce the data without losing too much information. If we only have two variables to combine, the aim is to find the optimal values for α_1 and α_2 that generate maximal variance of Y:

$$Y = \alpha_1 X_1 + \alpha_2 X_2$$

with the constraint:

$$\alpha_1^2 + \alpha_2^2 = 1$$

Let's go back to the blood pressure example and test some values for α_1 and α_2. For example, $\alpha_1 = 0.8$, $\alpha_2 = 0.6$ (note that: $0.8^2 + 0.6^2 = 1$) will result in the following linear combination:

```
BP=0.8*DBP + 0.6*SBP
```

Let's calculate the variance of the combined BP:

```
var(BP)
[1] 12.74267
```

Hence, using the weights 0.8 and 0.6 results in a linear combination with a variance of 12.74. Let's try some other values for the weights with the constraint $\alpha_1^2 + \alpha_2^2 = 1$, and compute the variance of the different linear combinations:

```
BP=0.6*DBP + 0.8*SBP
var(BP)
11.84667
BP=0.98*DBP + 0.2*SBP
var(BP)
10.38087
BP=0.2*DBP + 0.98*SBP
var(BP)
7.435587
```

Let's summarize the variances of the four different linear combinations in a table (Table 6.2):

Out of these four different combinations, we can see that the weights that generate the largest variance out of the ones we tested are:

$$\alpha_1 = 0.8, \alpha_2 = 0.6$$

To find the weights that generate the maximum variance of the linear combination, PCA involves the computation of the eigenvectors of the covariance matrix. Below, we will use R's function "eigen" to compute the eigenvectors of the covariance matrix:

Table 6.2 Variance obtained by combining the variables by using arbitrary values of the weights

α_1	α_2	var(Y)
0.8	0.6	12.74
0.6	0.8	11.84
0.98	0.2	10.38
0.2	0.98	7.43

```
data=cbind(DBP,SBP)
COV=cov(data) # Calculate covariance matrix
eig=eigen(COV) # Compute eigenvectors and eigenvalues
eig
eigen() decomposition
$values
[1] 12.7441347   0.3891986

$vectors
          [,1]       [,2]
[1,] -0.7934122  0.6086847
[2,] -0.6086847 -0.7934122
```

The first eigenvector (the first column) gives us the values of the weights that maximize the variance of the linear combination. Hence:

$$Y = -0.79X_1 - 0.61X_2$$

will generate a linear combination with maximal variance. Let's compute the variance of Y with these weights:

```
# Extract value in the first row, first column
alfa1= eig$vectors[1,1]
# Extract value in the second row, first column
alfa2= eig$vectors[2,1]
BP=alfa1*DBP + alfa2*SBP
var(BP)
12.74413
```

The variance of the linear combination is 12.744, which is greater compared to when we tried some arbitrary values. Note that the variance of our linear combination is equal to the so-called eigenvalue, which we previously computed by the "eigen" function:

```
eigen() decomposition
$values
12.7441347   0.3891986
```

6.3.1 Calculating the Principal Components

In PCA, the principal components (PCs) are calculated by first centering the variables so that their means are zero (data is centered around zero). The first principal component (PC1) is similar to our earlier linear combination (Y). The difference is that we here center the variables, which means that we subtract the mean ($\bar{X}$) from the values of each variable (X):

$$PC1 = \alpha_1 \left(X_1 - \bar{X}_1 \right) + \alpha_2 \left(X_2 - \bar{X}_2 \right)$$

Using our weights, the first PC is defined as:

$$PC1 = -0.79\left(\text{DBP} - \overline{\text{DBP}}\right) - 0.61\left(\text{SBP} - \overline{\text{SBP}}\right)$$

We will also have a second principal component (PC2), which will hold the remaining variance that is not included in PC1. We can calculate PC2 based on the second eigenvector: [0.61, -0.79]

$$PC2 = 0.61\left(\text{DBP} - \overline{\text{DBP}}\right) - 0.79\left(\text{SBP} - \overline{\text{SBP}}\right)$$

We can compute the PC scores in R by:

```
PC1=eig$vectors[1,1]*(DBP-mean(DBP)) +
eig$vectors[2,1]*(SBP-mean(SBP))
round(PC1,1) # Print rounded scores
4.8  2.0  1.8 -0.8 -2.4 -5.2
PC2=eig$vectors[1,2]*(DBP-mean(DBP)) +
eig$vectors[2,2]*(SBP-mean(SBP))
round(PC2,1)
-0.1 -0.5  0.9 -0.8  0.4  0.0
```

Another way to compute the scores is to multiply the centered values by the eigenvector matrix (also called the rotation matrix) by:

```
c_data=scale(data,center=TRUE,scale=FALSE) # Center the data
round(c_data%*%eig$vectors,1)
     [,1]  [,2]
[1,]  4.8  -0.1
[2,]  2.0  -0.5
[3,]  1.8   0.9
[4,] -0.8  -0.8
[5,] -2.4   0.4
[6,] -5.2   0.0
```

If we plot these two PCs, we will generate a so-called score plot:

```
plot(PC1,PC2,xlim=c(-6,6),ylim=c(-6,6))
```

We can see that PC1 contains most of the spread (the values range between -5.2 and 4.8), whereas PC2 includes values that only range between -0.8 and 0.9 (Fig. 6.2). Also, note that PC1 and PC2 are completely uncorrelated. The method

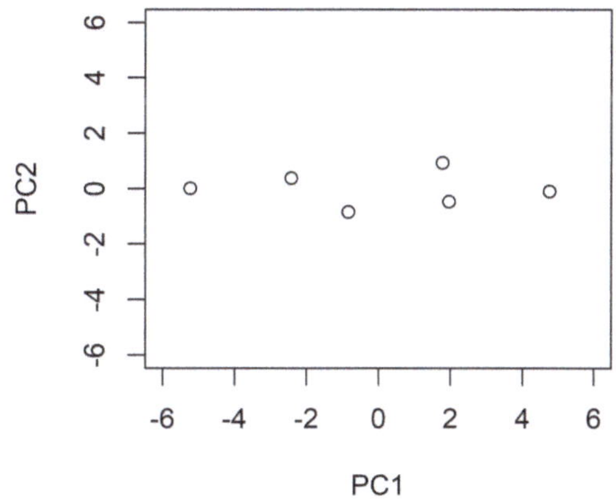

Fig. 6.2 A PCA plot showing the distribution of the six individuals along the two principal components (PC1 and PC2)

has simply rotated the original data in a way so that one of the PCs maximizes its variance (spread). The variance of the two components can be calculated by:

```
var(PC1)
12.74413
var(PC2)
0.3891986
```

6.3.2 *Using the Function prcomp*

To make our coding a bit simpler, we can, for example, use R's function "prcomp", which will do most of the job (note: prcomp uses the singular value decomposition method to compute the PCA, which might give a bit different values compared to if we use the eigenvalue decomposition of the covariance matrix that we used earlier):

```
DBP=c(78,80,81,82,84,86)
SBP=c(126,128,127,130,130,132)
data=cbind(DBP, SBP)
pca=prcomp(data)
pca
Standard deviations (1, .., p=2):
[1] 3.5698928    0.6238579

Rotation (n x k) = (2 x 2):
            PC1          PC2
DBP  0.7934122    0.6086847
SBP  0.6086847   -0.7934122
```

Under "Rotation" and PC1, we find the weights for the first principal component. Note that these weights are positive in comparison to when we computed the eigenvectors of the covariance matrix, which resulted in negative weights. However, as long as the relative differences between the weights are similar, it does not matter if the weights are positive or negative because the PCs will result in the exact same variance.

When we print "pca", only some of the object's information is printed. We can usually extract much more information. To show everything that is stored in the "pca" object, we can use the function "names" in R:

```
names(pca)
"sdev"      "rotation"    "center"    "scale"     "x"
```

To extract, for example, the standard deviation "sdev", we can either use the $ operator or use the [ ] operators:

```
pca[1]
$sdev
3.5698928  0.6238579
pca$sdev
3.5698928  0.6238579
```

To calculate the variances, we simply square the standard deviations:

```
pca$sdev^2 # Variance of the PCs (eigenvalues)
12.7441347  0.3891986
```

Note that the variances of the PCs are exactly the same as the ones we calculated earlier. Our PC scores can be extracted by "pca$x". If we round and print these values:

```
round(pca$x,1) # rounded PCs
       PC1    PC2
[1,]  -4.8   -0.1
[2,]  -2.0   -0.5
[3,]  -1.8    0.9
[4,]   0.8   -0.8
[5,]   2.4    0.4
[6,]   5.2    0.0
```

we see that these values correspond to our previous PC scores. However, the scores of PC1 have opposite signs compared to our previous calculations. If we plot these values:

```
plot(pca$x,xlim=c(-6,6),ylim=c(-6,6))
```

we can see that the data has been rotated in the opposite direction (Fig. 6.3) compared to when we used the weights based on the eigenvector of the covariance

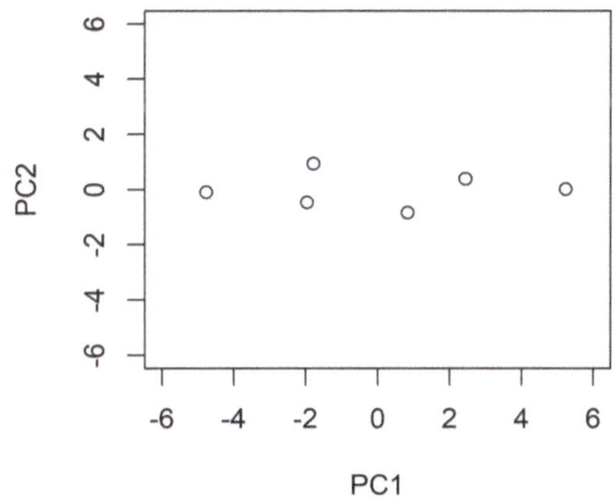

Fig. 6.3 A PCA plot, generated based on the "prcomp" function, showing the distribution of the six individuals along the first two principal components (PC1 and PC2)

matrix (Fig. 6.2). This is due to that the weights of the first PC were positive when we used the "prcomp" function, whereas the corresponding weights from computing the eigenvector of the covariance matrix were negative. This difference does not affect the PCA because the first PC still has the same variance.

6.3.3 How Much "Information" Is Contained in the First PC?

To evaluate the PCs, one usually calculates the ratio of the variance of the principal components and the total variance. The total variance is simply the sum of the variances of all PCs (or the total variance of all original variables).

Let's first calculate the sum of the variances of all PCs:

```
VT=sum(pca$sdev^2)
VT
13.13333
```

Thus, the total variance is 13.1. Hence, we can now calculate the proportion of variance that is captured by, for example, the first PC by:

```
pca$sdev[1]^2/VT
0.9703656
```

Hence, the proportion explained by the first PC is about 97%, whereas the remaining variance explained by the second component is only about 3%. Such a relatively high percentage covered by the first component suggests that this component is a good representation of the two variables because it captures most of the variance.

6.3.4 Plot with ggplot2

To generate a bit nicer score plot, we can use the **ggplot2** package. Try and run the code below:

```
library(ggplot2)
# % Variance of the PCs
prop.pca = (pca$sdev^2/sum(pca$sdev^2))*100
dataset = data.frame(pca$x) # Create a data frame of the PCs
ggplot(dataset) +
  geom_point(aes(PC1,PC2), size = 6,col="orange") +
  geom_text(aes(PC1, PC2,label=1:length(PC1)),size=4) +
  labs(x = paste("PC1 (",round(prop.pca[1]) ,"%)", sep=""),
       y = paste("PC2 (",round(prop.pca[2]) , "%)", sep=""))
```

and note that we now also show the proportion explained by the PCs on the axes (Fig. 6.4). Since the two axes now have different ranges, it is important to account for the proportion explained by each PC. Since PC1 captures almost all variance, we should focus on PC1 when we interpret the plot. For example, although persons

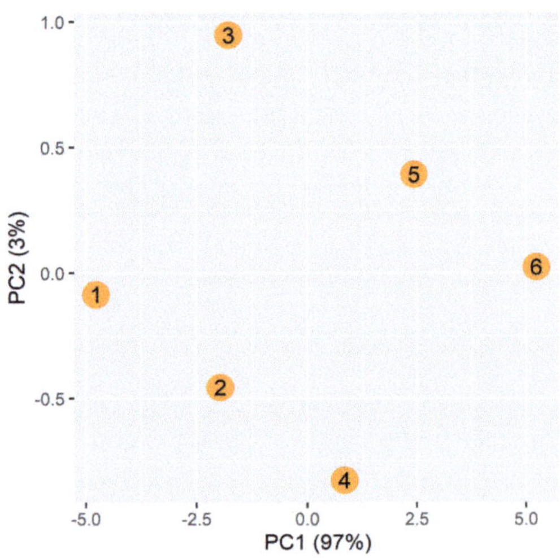

Fig. 6.4 A PCA plot, generated based on the "prcomp" function and the **ggplot2** package, showing the distribution of the six individuals along the two principal components (PC1 and PC2). PC1 explains 97% of the variance, while PC2 explains 3%. The numbers represent the six individuals in the dataset

number 2 and 3 seem to be far away from each other in the plot, they are actually the ones with the most similar blood pressures because they are very close in the horizontal direction, which shows the difference in PC1 that explains most of the variance. This is easier to see if we use the same range of both axes:

```
library(ggplot2)
prop.pca = (pca$sdev^2/sum(pca$sdev^2))*100 # % Variance
dataset = data.frame(pca$x) # Create a data frame of the PCs
ggplot(dataset) +
  geom_point(aes(PC1,PC2), size = 6,col="orange") +
  geom_text(aes(PC1, PC2,label=1:length(PC1)),size=4) +
  labs(x = paste("PC1 (",round(prop.pca[1]) ,"%)", sep=""),
       y = paste("PC2 (",round(prop.pca[2]) , "%)",
       sep="")) +
 ylim(-5, 5) # Manually set y-axis limits
```

In this plot (Fig. 6.5), where the y-axis now also spans between -5 and 5, it is easier to see why persons number 2 and 3 have the most similar blood pressures.

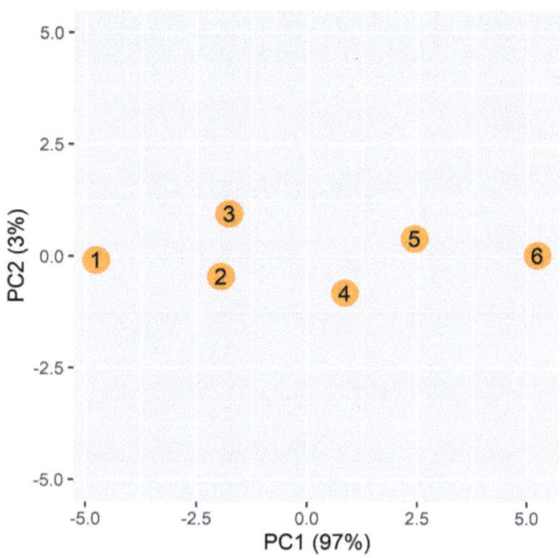

Fig. 6.5 A PCA plot, generated based on the "prcomp" function and the **ggplot2** package, showing the distribution of the six individuals along the two principal components (PC1 and PC2). PC1 explains 97% of the variance, while PC2 explains 3%. The numbers represent the six individuals in the dataset. To more easily visualize the difference in variance between PC1 and PC2, both axes have the same range

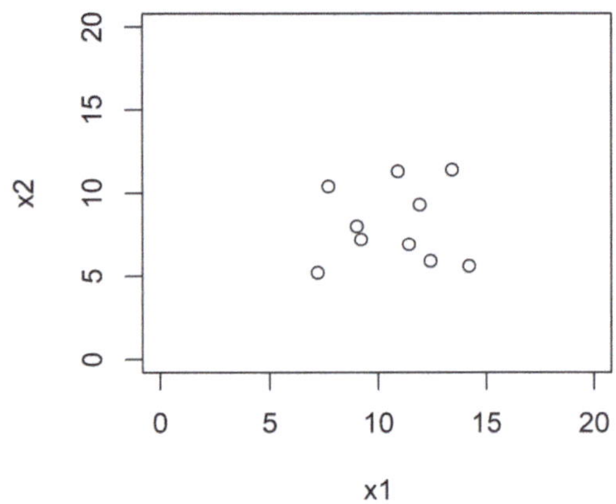

Fig. 6.6 An example of two variables that do not correlate

6.3.5 An Example of When We Cannot Find a Good PC

If two variables are uncorrelated (Fig. 6.6), it is not possible to rotate the data so that most of the variance is kept in one dimension. Running a PCA on such data will generate two PCs that will hold about the same proportion of variance. The first PC will then not be a good representation of the two variables.

For example, if we compute a PCA of the following data:

```
x1=c(14.2, 7.7, 11.9, 9.2, 13.4, 12.4, 10.9,  9.0, 11.4, 7.2)
x2=c(5.6, 10.4, 9.3, 7.2, 11.4, 5.9, 11.3, 8.0, 6.9, 5.2)
plot(x1,x2,ylim=c(0,20),xlim=c(0,20))
data=cbind(x1,x2)
pca=prcomp(data)
# Compute proportion of variance of PC1
pca$sdev[1]^2/sum(pca$sdev^2)
0.5248315
```

the output tells us that the proportion explained by the first PC is only 52.5%, whereas the second PC accounts for 47.5%. Thus, combining two uncorrelated variables into one will result in a major loss of information.

6.4 Exercises

1. Use PCA to combine the two variables Sepal length and Petal length in the Iris dataset, using both the “manual” way where you compute the eigenvector of the covariance matrix and by using the “prcomp” function. You do not need to standardize or center the data. How much variance is explained by the first PC?

2. Show the linear equation for the first PC.
3. Compute a PCA based on all numerical variables in the Iris dataset and plot PC1 vs PC2. Standardize the variables before you compute the PCA. Add colors to this plot so that one can identify the three different species and the row numbers so that one can also identify individual flowers.

6.5 Standardization and How to Extract Components

We will now discuss the importance of first standardizing the variables before we run PCA and then learn how many components that are appropriate to extract. Watch the video below the learn how standardizing the data affects the results and how to use three different methods to know how many components we should extract.

6.5.1 *Video*

https://youtu.be/WyPcFTVX6PU
www.tilestats.com/ml/

6.5.2 *Standardization*

When we have several variables with different units, such as the ones in Table 6.3, we know from the video that PCA works best if we first standardize the variables. Let's first read in the data:

Table 6.3 Example data

Diastolic BP (mmHg)	Systolic BP (mmHg)	Weight (kg)	Height (cm)
82.6	132.1	71	172
79.1	129.9	79	180
81.7	131.2	78	172
80.7	132.1	66	166
74.9	125.0	70	173
79.1	129.1	64	162
83.8	133.1	60	164
78.4	127.0	67	165
82.3	131.6	64	164
79.4	129.2	77	179

```
DBP=c(82.6, 79.1, 81.7, 80.7, 74.9, 79.1, 83.8, 78.4,
82.3, 79.4)
SBP=c(132.1, 129.9, 131.2, 132.1, 125.0, 129.1, 133.1, 127.0,
131.6, 129.2)
Weight=c(71, 79, 78, 66, 70, 64, 60, 67, 64, 77)
Height=c(172, 180, 172, 166, 173, 162, 164, 165, 164, 179)
data=data.frame(DBP,SBP,Weight,Height)
```

To standardize the data, we can use the function "scale":

```
sdata=scale(data)
round(sdata,2) # Print rounded values
         DBP     SBP    Weight     Height
 [1,]   0.93    0.82     0.21       0.36
 [2,]  -0.43   -0.05     1.43       1.60
 [3,]   0.58    0.46     1.28       0.36
 [4,]   0.19    0.82    -0.55      -0.57
 [5,]  -2.05   -1.98     0.06       0.51
 [6,]  -0.43   -0.37    -0.85      -1.19
 [7,]   1.39    1.21    -1.46      -0.88
 [8,]  -0.70   -1.19    -0.39      -0.73
 [9,]   0.81    0.62    -0.85      -0.88
[10,]  -0.31   -0.33     1.12       1.44
…
```

We now run PCA on the standardized data with the function "prcomp" (it is also possible to run on the raw data if we set the argument scale to TRUE in the prcomp function, such as pca=prcomp(data,scale=TRUE)):

```
(pca=prcomp(sdata))
summary(pca)
Importance of components:
                          PC1     PC2     PC3      PC4
Standard deviation      1.5524  1.2030  0.31632  0.20730
Proportion of Variance  0.6025  0.3618  0.02501  0.01074
Cumulative Proportion   0.6025  0.9642  0.98926  1.00000
```

Note that the first PC captures about 60% of the variance, whereas PC2 captures about 36%. In total, these two components capture 96.42% of the total variance. We can compute the variances of each component by:

```
pca$sdev^2
2.40980543  1.44716422  0.10005521  0.04297515
```

Let's print the weights:

```
round(pca$rotation,2)
          PC1    PC2    PC3    PC4
DBP     -0.53  -0.46   0.14  -0.70
SBP     -0.50  -0.52  -0.16   0.68
Weight   0.48  -0.52   0.69   0.12
Height   0.49  -0.50  -0.69  -0.18
```

and the scores:

```
round(pca$x,2)
        PC1    PC2    PC3    PC4
 [1,] -0.62  -1.14  -0.10  -0.14
 [2,]  1.73  -1.32  -0.16   0.14
 [3,]  0.26  -1.35   0.65   0.00
 [4,] -1.05   0.06  -0.09   0.46
 [5,]  2.35   1.68  -0.28   0.00
 [6,] -0.59   1.43   0.23   0.16
 [7,] -2.47  -0.06  -0.40  -0.17
 [8,]  0.41   1.51   0.32  -0.24
 [9,] -1.58   0.19   0.03  -0.09
[10,]  1.58  -1.00  -0.20  -0.13
```

6.5.3 How Many Components Should We Use?

The number of components that are generated will be the same as the number of variables we include in the PCA. If we keep all components from the PCA, we have not reduced the number of dimensions which is the main purpose of the analysis. The analysis aims to have as few components as possible that can still explain most of the variance. There are basically three techniques to determine the final number of components that can be used as an approximation of the original data:

1. Take the smallest number of components that explain 80–90% of the variance in the data.
2. Use Kaiser's criterion, where we retain components whose eigenvalues (variance) are greater than the average of the eigenvalues.
3. Use a scree plot.

Let's apply these three different methods to our previous standardized data.

1. From our previous calculations,

```
(pca=prcomp(sdata))
summary(pca)
Importance of components:
                          PC1     PC2     PC3      PC4
Standard deviation     1.5524  1.2030  0.31632  0.20730
Proportion of Variance 0.6025  0.3618  0.02501  0.01074
Cumulative Proportion  0.6025  0.9642  0.98926  1.00000
```

   we know that the first two PCs explain about 96% (60% + 36%) of the variance. Hence, according to the first method, we would only keep the first two PCs.
2. When we standardize the variables, the mean of the eigenvalues (variances) will be equal to 1. Hence, for standardized variables, we keep only components with an eigenvalue greater than 1 when we use Kaiser's criterion. From our previous example:

```
pca$sdev^2
2.40980543   1.44716422   0.10005521   0.04297515
mean(pca$sdev^2)
1
```

   we see that only PC1 and PC2 have eigenvalues (variances) greater than 1. Hence, using Kaiser's criterion suggests that we should only keep the first two PCs.
3. The third option to extract the number of components is to study a scree plot. This plot simply shows how the variance declines from the first PC to the last PC:

```
plot(pca,type="l")
```

In our example, we only have four PCs. Generally, the ideal scree plot generates a steep curve followed by a slow decrease. One usually retains the components that are involved in the steep section of the curve. From the scree plot (Fig. 6.7), we

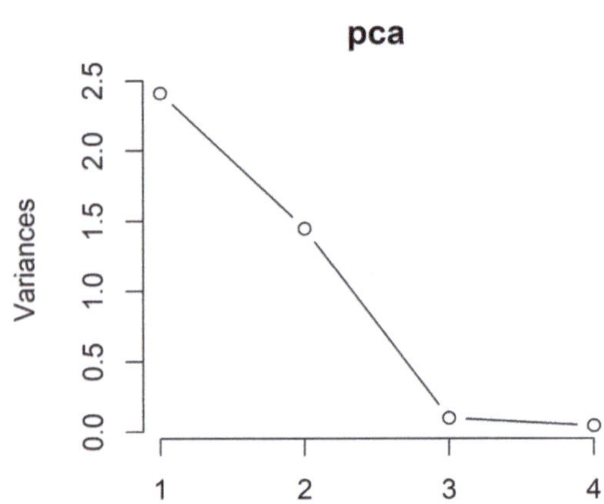

Fig. 6.7 A scree plot displaying the variance explained by each principal component. The x-axis represents the principal components, and the y-axis shows the variance

would consider only components 1 and 2 to be involved in the steep part of the curve. Thus, all three methods, in this case, indicate that we should only keep the first two PCs. However, the three different methods usually result in different numbers of components to keep, which means that you have to select one of the three methods to select the final number of components to extract.

6.6 Exercises

1. Use PCA and the "prcomp" function to combine the four numeric variables in the Iris dataset. Standardize the variables before you compute the PCA. How many PCs should you extract according to the three methods we have discussed in this section?
2. Do the same as in the previous question but use the numeric variables in the Crab dataset.

6.7 Loadings and Varimax Rotation

We will here focus on the difference between the weights and the so-called loadings and how to interpret the values of these loadings. We will also see how Varimax rotation can be used to increase the interpretation of the PCA. Watch the video below to learn about how the weights can be rescaled into loadings, which represent the Pearson correlation coefficients between the variables and the components, and how Varimax rotation is used to increase the interpretation of the PCA.

6.7.1 *Video*

https://youtu.be/MUs4jdEZTfM
www.tilestats.com/ml/

6.7.2 *Varimax Rotation*

As we saw in our previous example:

```
round(pca$rotation,2)
          PC1    PC2    PC3    PC4
DBP     -0.53  -0.46   0.14  -0.70
SBP     -0.50  -0.52  -0.16   0.68
Weight   0.48  -0.52   0.69   0.12
Height   0.49  -0.50  -0.69  -0.18
```

the PCA on the standardized data has about the same absolute weights for the first two components. It is therefore hard to separate the variables based on these values. Usually, one wants to define which variable that loads onto the extracted components. From the previous analysis, we know that we should extract the first two PCs. Let's use Varimax rotation on our two extracted components:

```
varmax=varimax(pca$rotation[,1:2])
varmax
 Loadings:
              PC1          PC2
DBP         -0.699
SBP         -0.715
Weight                    -0.709
Height                    -0.704
...
```

The Varimax rotation shows that the blood pressure variables load on PC1, whereas Weight and Height load on PC2. Hence, the Varimax rotation improves the interpretation of the components. Note that, per default, the "varimax" function does not display weights smaller than 0.1. To view all weights, we can use:

```
print(loadings(varmax),cutoff=0)
Loadings:
              PC1          PC2
DBP         -0.699        0.043
SBP         -0.715       -0.019
Weight      -0.022       -0.709
Height       0.000       -0.704
...
```

which now shows all weights.

6.7.3 Loadings

We have previously seen that the sum of the squared weights is constrained to one. For example, in our previous example, the sum of the squared weights of the first components should be equal to 1.

$$\alpha_1^2 + \alpha_2^2 + \alpha_3^2 + \alpha_4^2 = 1$$

We can see that this is true for the weights of the first PC:

```
sum(pca$rotation[,1]^2)
1
```

However, other software tools such as SPSS and the function "principal" in the **psych** package use the following constraint that was explained in the video:

$$\sum_{i=1}^{n}\alpha_{ki}^{2}=V\left(Y_{k}\right)$$

where $V(Y_k)$ is the variance (or eigenvalue) of component k. Let's extract the variance of the first component:

```
pca$sdev[1]^2
2.409805
```

Hence, the constraint of PC1 from our previous example could be written as:

$$\alpha_1^2+\alpha_2^2+\alpha_3^2+\alpha_4^2=2.41$$

By using this constraint, the weights of the first PC are now allowed to be bigger than we have seen previously. Also, these kinds of weights are called loadings. To compute such loadings, we will use the "principal" function in the **psych** package, which uses this constraint:

```
library(psych)
pr=principal(data, nfactors = 2, rotate = "none")
pr
          PC1    PC2    h2    u2     com
DBP       0.82   0.55   0.98  0.023  1.8
SBP       0.77   0.62   0.98  0.022  1.9
Weight   -0.75   0.63   0.95  0.049  1.9
Height   -0.77   0.60   0.95  0.049  1.9

                     PC1   PC2
SS loadings          2.41  1.45
Proportion Var       0.60  0.36
Cumulative Var       0.60  0.96
...
```

We see that the loading values are greater than the weights obtained by using the "prcomp" function. The eigenvalues (variances) are shown on the row "SS loadings", which correspond to the sum of the squared loadings:

```
sum(pr$loadings[,1]^2)
2.409805
sum(pr$loadings[,2]^2)
1.447164
```

One nice feature of using this constraint is that our loadings now correspond to the Pearson's correlation coefficients between the PCs and the variables. For example, the loading of the DBP for PC1 is 0.82, which is equivalent to the correlation between the scores of PC1 and the DBP:

```
cor(pr$scores[,1],DBP)
0.8190301
```

Hence, the interpretation of the loadings now becomes easier because they can be related to correlation coefficients. The diastolic blood pressure has a strong positive correlation (0.819) to the first PC. We can extract the eigenvalues (variance) for each component by:

```
pr$values
2.40980543 1.44716422 0.10005521 0.04297515
```

which shows that the first two components have an eigenvalue greater than 1. Using the Varimax option where we extract the first two PCs:

```
pr_varmax=principal(data, nfactors = 2, rotate = "varimax")
pr_varmax
            PC1      PC2     h2     u2      com
DBP         0.97    -0.18   0.98   0.023    1.1
SBP         0.98    -0.10   0.98   0.022    1.0
Weight     -0.09     0.97   0.95   0.049    1.0
Height     -0.12     0.97   0.95   0.049    1.0
...
```

now results in a much easier interpretation, where the DBP and SBP clearly load on the first component (because these variables are associated with high absolute loading values), whereas the variables Weight and Height load on the second component. As a rule of thumb, variables with loading values above |0.3| are often considered to load meaningfully. However, one usually tries to find a cutoff value so that the variables load on unique components. The cutoff value is therefore usually set arbitrarily. For example, a cutoff value of 0.9 can be used to determine which variables load on PC1 or PC2. Since the absolute loadings of DBP and SBP on PC1 are greater than 0.9, we can say that these two variables load on PC1. In contrast, since the absolute loadings of Weight and Height on PC2 exceed 0.9, we can say that these two variables load on PC2. In the case studies (Chap. 14), paper 1, we will see how a good cutoff value can be determined based on many variables.

As before, the loadings from the Varimax rotation correspond to the correlation between the components and the variables. For example, the loading of DBP for PC1 is equivalent to the correlation between the PC1 scores from the Varimax rotation and the DBP:

```
cor(pr_varmax$scores[,1],DBP)
0.971276
```

We can print the scores generated by the "principal" function by:

```
round(pr_varmax$scores,2)
         RC1   RC2
 [1,]   0.95  0.39
 [2,]  -0.02  1.56
 [3,]   0.67  0.91
 [4,]   0.45 -0.51
 [5,]  -2.06  0.07
 [6,]  -0.56 -1.11
 [7,]   1.17 -1.08
 [8,]  -1.07 -0.70
 [9,]   0.61 -0.83
[10,]  -0.14  1.30
```

6.8 Exercises

1. Use a PCA on the standardized numerical variables in the Iris dataset. Extract the two first principal components and print the weights/loadings after Varimax rotation. Which variables load on PC1 and PC2?
2. Compute a correlation matrix of the numerical variables in the Iris dataset and try and understand why your answer in the previous question can be explained by the correlation coefficients.

6.9 Principal Coordinates Analysis

Similar to PCA, principal coordinate analysis (PCoA) is a dimensionality reduction technique. The difference is that PCoA is based on a distance matrix. Note that classical multidimensional scaling (MDS) is the same as PCoA. By using PCoA, we can reduce the dimensions based on any distance metric that we think is appropriate for the data. Watch the video below to understand the differences between PCA and PCoA and to understand how PCoA is computed based on a distance matrix.

6.9.1 Video

https://youtu.be/lcaxd88sJO4
www.tilestats.com/ml/

We will here compute a PCoA based on the same dataset as in the video, where we like to combine the four variables diastolic blood pressure (DBP), systolic blood pressure (SBP), body mass index (BMI), and the cholesterol level (Chol). We first read in and standardize the data:

```
rm(list=ls()) # Clear environment
DBP=c(82,    86,  98,    85,    87)
SBP=c(132,  133, 145,   139,   145)
BMI=c(18,    20,  35,    22,    28)
Chol=c(192, 240, 140,   170,   218)
data=data.frame(DBP,SBP,BMI,Chol)
sdata=scale(data) # Standardize the data
```

Let's first compute a PCA and plot the first two principal components (Fig. 6.8):

```
pca=prcomp(sdata) # Compute PCA
library(ggplot2)
dataset = data.frame(pca$x) # Create a data frame of the PCs
ggplot(dataset) +
  geom_point(aes(PC1,PC2), size = 6,color="orange") +
  geom_text(aes(PC1, PC2,label=1:length(PC1)),size=4)
```

From the video, we know that a PCoA based on Euclidean distances will result in the same results as a PCA. To show this, we will here first compute the Euclidean distances between the data points and then use the function "cmdscale" to compute a PCoA based on the distance matrix. We here set k to 2 because we like to extract only the first two dimensions:

```
D = as.matrix(dist(sdata, upper=T, diag=T))
MDS=cmdscale(D,k=2)
```

Next, we make a plot of the scores that are saved in the object "MDS":

```
library(ggplot2)
dataset = data.frame(MDS1=MDS[,1],MDS2=MDS[,2])
ggplot(dataset) +
  geom_point(aes(MDS1,MDS2), size = 6, color="orange") +
  geom_text(aes(MDS1,MDS2,label=1:length(MDS1)),size=4)
```

Note that the PCoA plot (Fig. 6.9) is identical to the PCA plot (Fig. 6.8). Thus, PCoA and PCA will result in the same scores if the PCoA is based on Euclidean distances. However, PCA or PCoA directions are arbitrary in terms of signs, which means that they may result in scores of opposite signs as explained in the video.

Fig. 6.8 A PCA plot, generated based on the "prcomp" function and the **ggplot2** package, showing the distribution of the five individuals along the first two principal components (PC1 and PC2)

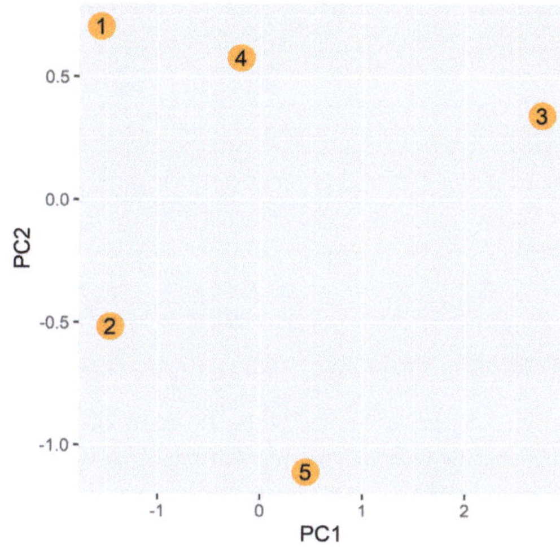

Fig. 6.9 An MDS plot (or a PCoA plot) showing the relative distances between the individuals based on their pairwise dissimilarities. The x-axis and y-axis represent the first two dimensions of the MDS solution

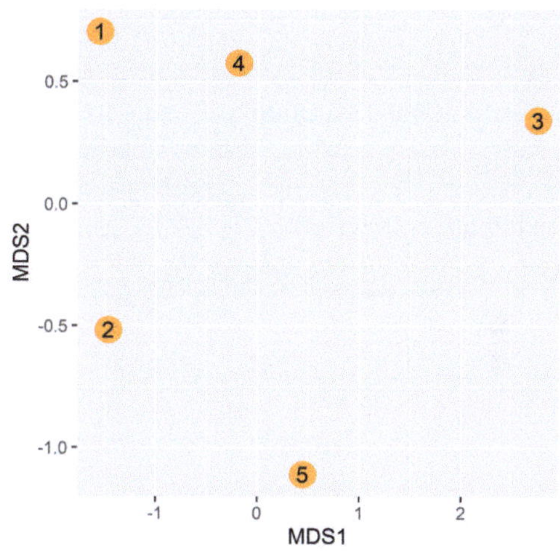

6.9.2 *The Bray–Curtis Dissimilarity Index*

One of the most common applications of PCoA in biology is to compare species composition at different locations. We will here use the same simple example data (Table 6.4) as shown in the video where four fish species have been counted in four different locations.

To compare species composition in two different locations, one common measure to use is the Bray–Curtis dissimilarity index:

Table 6.4 Example data of counts of four fish species in four different locations

Location	Goldfish	Guppy	Rainbow fish	Neon tetra
1	82	132	18	192
2	86	133	20	240
3	98	145	35	140
4	85	139	22	170

$$BC_{jk} = 1 - \frac{2\sum_{i=1}^{p} \min\left(N_{ij}, N_{ik}\right)}{\sum_{i=1}^{p}\left(N_{ij} + N_{ik}\right)}$$

where N_{ij} in this case is the number of fish of species i at site j, whereas N_{ik} is the number of fish of species i at site k. p is the total number of species in the samples. For example, if we would calculate the Bray–Curtis dissimilarity index between locations 1 and 4:

$$BC_{1,4} = 1 - \frac{2\left(82+132+18+170\right)}{\left(82+85\right)+\left(132+139\right)+\left(18+22\right)+\left(192+170\right)} = 0.04285714$$

we see that the dissimilarity is equal to about 0.0428. The index is bounded between 0 and 1, where a value close to 0 indicates that the species composition is similar, whereas a value close to 1 indicates that the species composition is dissimilar. Let's read in the data into R:

```
rm(list=ls()) # Clear environment
Goldfish=c(82,    86,   98,    85)
Guppy=c(132,   133, 145,   139)
Rainbow=c(18,    20,   35,    22)
Neon=c(192, 240, 140,   170)
df=data.frame(Goldfish,Guppy,Rainbow,Neon)
```

To compute the Bray–Curtis dissimilarity between the four different locations, we will here use the "vegdist" function from the **vegan** package:

```
library(vegan)
D = vegdist(df, method="bray")
D
           1             2                3
2   0.06090808
3   0.11638955    0.15496098
4   0.04285714    0.08826816       0.07434053
```

This matrix shows the Bray–Curtis dissimilarity index between all four locations. Note that the distance between locations 1 and 4 corresponds to the distance we calculated by hand above. We will now compute and plot a PCoA based on the above distances:

```
MDS=cmdscale(D, k=2)
library(ggplot2)
dataset = data.frame(MDS1=MDS[,1],MDS2=MDS[,2])
ggplot(dataset) +
  geom_point(aes(MDS1,MDS2), size = 6, color="orange") +
  geom_text(aes(MDS1,MDS2,label=1:length(MDS1)),size=4)
```

To be able to interpret this plot (Fig. 6.10), we should add the variance explained by each MDS dimension to the axes. If we update the previous code with:

```
MDS=cmdscale(D,k=2, eig = TRUE)
# Proportion explained
prop_explained = MDS$eig / sum(MDS$eig) * 100
library(ggplot2)
dataset = data.frame(MDS1= MDS$points[,1],
MDS2= MDS$points[,2])
ggplot(dataset) +
  geom_point(aes(MDS1,MDS2), size = 6, color="orange") +
  geom_text(aes(MDS1,MDS2,label=1:length(MDS1)),size=4) +
  labs( x = paste("MDS1 (", round(prop_explained[1], 1),
  "%)", sep = ""),
    y = paste("MDS2 (", round(prop_explained[2], 1), "%)",
    sep = "")
)
```

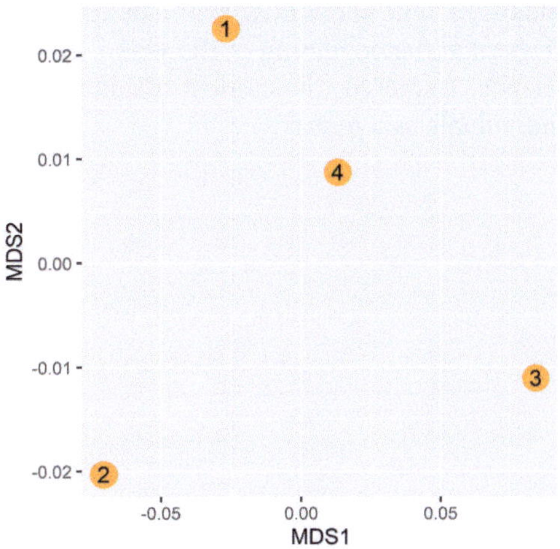

Fig. 6.10 An MDS plot (or PCoA plot) showing the relative distances between the four different locations based on their pairwise dissimilarities, using the Bray–Curtis dissimilarity index, in species composition. The x-axis and y-axis represent the first two dimensions of the MDS solution

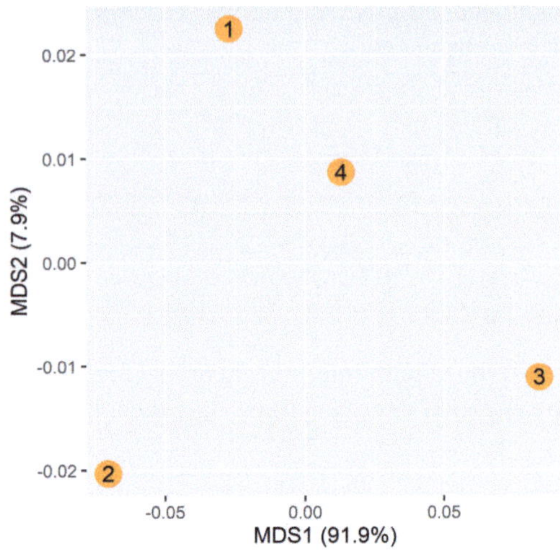

Fig. 6.11 An MDS plot (or PCoA plot) based on the Bray–Curtis dissimilarity index, showing the distribution of locations in the first two MDS dimensions. MDS1 explains 91.9% of the variation in the data, while MDS2 captures 7.9% variation

We will generate the plot shown in Fig. 6.11.

From this plot (Fig. 6.11), we see that we should focus mainly on MDS1 because it captures most of the information about the distances between the locations. For example, although locations 2 and 3 are close in MDS2 (the vertical distance), they are far away in MDS1 (the horizontal distance). These two locations have the most dissimilar species compositions if we study the Bray–Curtis dissimilarity matrix that we created previously. To help interpret the MDS plot (or PCoA plot), it is always good to study also the distance matrix.

6.9.3 *Create a Map*

Finally, I will show how you can create a map (Fig. 6.12) by using PCoA as I showed at the beginning of the video. To create a map between me and some of my friends, I entered the shortest distance (the Euclidean distance) between the five individuals as a matrix:

```
rm(list = ls())
D = matrix(0, 5, 5)
# From me to John, Mike, James, Toby
D[c(2, 3, 4, 5), 1] = c(11.4, 35.8, 20.1, 119.1)
# From John to Mike, James, Toby
D[c(3, 4, 5), 2] = c(23.9, 10.3, 119.7)
D[c(4, 5), 3] = c(17.6, 130.8) # From Mike to James, Toby
D[5, 4] = 118.6 # From James to Toby
D = as.matrix(as.dist(D))
```

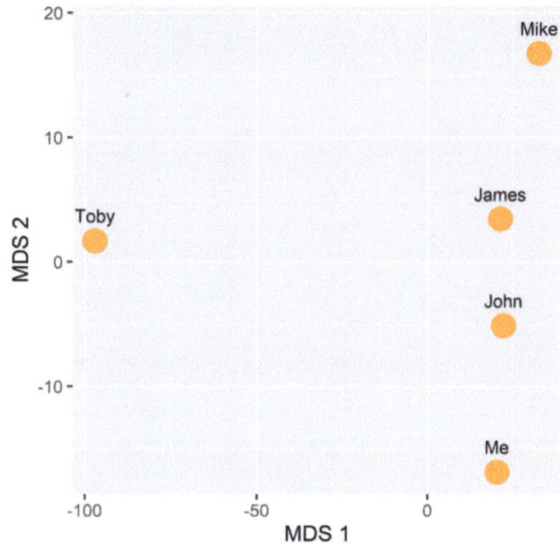

Fig. 6.12 An MDS plot that represents the distances between me and some of my friends

Then I computed a PCoA based on these distances. To rotate the plot so that it aligns with a map orientation where the top points to the north, I here multiplied the MDS scores by -1:

```
MDS=cmdscale(D,k=2)
library(ggplot2)
dataset = data.frame(MDS1 = MDS[, 1]*(-1), MDS2 = MDS[,
2]*(-1),
          friends = c("Me", "John", "Mike", "James", "Toby"))
ggplot(dataset) + geom_point(aes(MDS1,MDS2), size = 5.5,
color="orange") +
  geom_text(aes(MDS1,MDS2+2,label=friends),size=3.2,
  col="black") +
  labs(x = "MDS 1",y ="MDS 2")
```

6.10 Exercises

1. Use a PCoA, based on the Euclidean distances, on the standardized numerical variables of the Iris dataset. Show a PCoA plot where you identify the species with colors and flowers with numbers.
2. Modify the PCoA plot so that it becomes identical to the PCA plot based on the Iris dataset.

Chapter 7
Linear Discriminant Analysis

7.1 Linear Discriminant Analysis

Linear discriminant analysis (LDA) is a statistical technique used for classification and dimensionality reduction. In comparison to PCA, which seeks to find a linear combination of the variables that maximizes the variance, LDA seeks to find a linear combination that best separates the classes in the dataset. Thus, LDA requires that we have a categorical variable in the dataset where the aim is to maximize the separation between the categories. PCA can therefore be seen as an unsupervised learning method that identifies groups in the data, whereas LDA is a supervised learning method that uses predefined groups, or labeled data, to maximize the separation between the groups. Watch the video below to get an idea of how LDA maximizes the between-group variance (the distance between group means) while minimizing the within-group variance (the spread of the data within each group).

7.1.1 Video

https://youtu.be/vR0gOhbQTMk
www.tilestats.com/ml/

To learn how LDA works, we will first see how to calculate the LDA "by hand" and then use the "lda" function to do the same calculations with just one line of code. The dataset in Table 7.1 is the same data as used in the video where one has measured two variables: the CRP level in blood and the body temperature in six patients with a viral infection and six patients with a bacterial infection.

It would be of great clinical value if we could use parameters such as CRP or body temperature to distinguish between viral and bacterial infection since these parameters can be obtained by a quick test. Let's first enter and plot the data:

A. Tilevik, *Multivariate Statistics and Machine Learning in R For Beginners*,
https://doi.org/10.1007/978-3-032-01851-9_7

Table 7.1 Example data for LDA

Infection	CRP (mg/L)	Temp (C)
Viral	40.0	36.0
Viral	11.1	37.2
Viral	30.0	36.5
Viral	21.4	39.4
Viral	10.7	39.6
Viral	3.4	40.7
Bacterial	42.0	37.6
Bacterial	31.1	42.2
Bacterial	50.0	38.5
Bacterial	60.4	39.4
Bacterial	45.7	38.6
Bacterial	17.3	42.7

```
Temp=c(36.0, 37.2, 36.5, 39.4, 39.6, 40.7,37.6, 42.2, 38.5,
39.4, 38.6, 42.7)
CRP=c(40.0, 11.1, 30.0, 21.4, 10.7, 3.4,42.0, 31.1, 50.0,
60.4, 45.7, 17.3)
Group=factor(c(rep("Virus",6),rep("Bacteria",6)),
levels=c("Virus","Bacteria"))
df=data.frame(CRP,Temp,Group)
par(mfrow=c(1,2))
stripchart(CRP~Group,data=df,ylim=c(0,80),ylab="CRP(mg/L)",
vertical = TRUE,xlim=c(0.5,2.5))
stripchart(Temp~Group,data=df,ylim=c(35,43),ylab="Temp(C)",
vertical = TRUE,xlim=c(0.5,2.5))
```

As can be seen in Fig. 7.1, neither the CRP nor the body temperature are good markers to distinguish between bacterial or viral infection because there is no clear horizontal line that can separate the data points in the two groups. However, let's plot the CRP and the body temperature in a scatter plot where we display the two groups by different colors:

```
plot(df$Temp,df$CRP,col=df$Group)
legend("topright", legend=levels(df$Group),pch=1, col=1:2)
```

From Fig. 7.2, we see that it would be possible to separate bacterial from viral infections if both variables were considered. A line that spans from the top-left corner to the bottom right corner would separate the data points quite well.

Similar to the principal component analysis, we can combine the two variables into a linear combination. However, in contrast to PCA, which combines variables by maximizing the variance, we would now like to combine the variables to

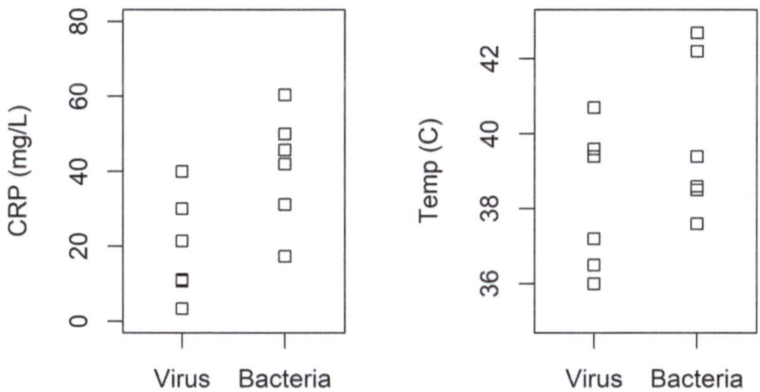

Fig. 7.1 One-dimensional scatter plots of the CRP (left) and body temperature (right) separated by the type of infection

Fig. 7.2 A scatter plot of the CRP and body temperature. The type of infection is indicated with different colors

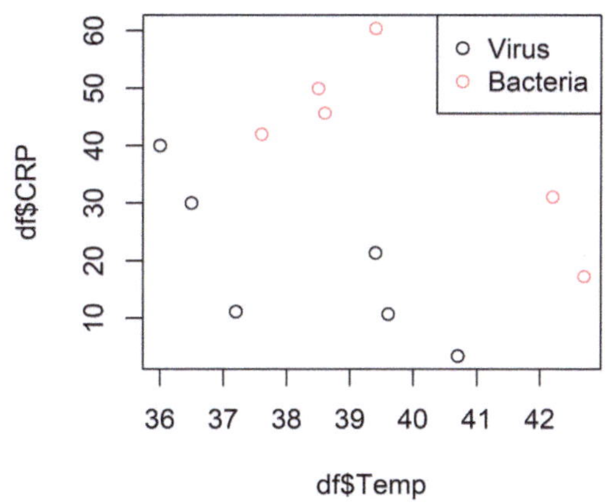

maximize the separation between the two groups. From the video, we know that a measure of separation can be expressed as:

$$\text{Separation} = \frac{\text{Between-group covariance}}{\text{Within-group covariance}}$$

$$S = W^{-1}B$$

Matrix S is our target matrix. We will compute the eigenvectors of this matrix in order to get our weights to use in the LDA. Let's first calculate the pooled within-group covariance matrix (W):

$$W = \frac{(n_1 - 1)\operatorname{cov}(A) + (n_2 - 1)\operatorname{cov}(B)}{n_1 + n_2 - 2}$$

```
# Split data into groups and compute W
# Extract patients with a viral infection
Virus_data=subset(df[,1:2], Group=="Virus")
# Extract patients with a bacterial infection
Bacteria_data=subset(df[,1:2], Group=="Bacteria")
# Sample size of the two groups
n1=nrow(Virus_data);n2=nrow(Bacteria_data)
W=((n1-1)*cov(Virus_data)+(n2-1)*cov(Bacteria_data))/
(n1+n2-2)
W
           CRP        Temp
CRP    208.14017  -22.463333
Temp   -22.46333    4.066667
```

We can also calculate the total covariance, T, by simply calculating the covariance matrix on all data points:

```
T=cov(df[,1:2])
T
           CRP        Temp
CRP    317.05174  -10.973939
Temp   -10.97394    4.395152
```

Since the total covariance T is the sum of the between-group covariance (B) and the within-group covariance (W):

$$T = W + B$$

we can calculate the between-group covariance simply by:

$$B = T - W$$

```
B=T-W
B
           CRP        Temp
CRP    108.91158  11.4893939
Temp    11.48939   0.3284848
```

If we multiply the inverse of the within-group covariance matrix by the between-group covariance matrix:

$$S = W^{-1}B$$

then we will have a matrix S, for which we can find coefficients that maximize the separation. The weights (α_1 and α_2) of the discriminant function:

$$D = \alpha_1 \cdot CRP + \alpha_2 \cdot Temp$$

which maximizes the separation between the groups can be found by calculating the eigenvector of matrix S:

```
S=solve(W)%*%B
eig=eigen(S)
eig
$values
[1]  3.09661985      -0.09090909

$vectors
          [,1]              [,2]
[1,]  0.1496165     -0.07370201
[2,]  0.9887441      0.99728031
```

Our first eigenvector holds the weights of the first discriminant function:

$$D = 0.1496 \cdot CRP + 0.9887 \cdot Temp$$

which maximizes the separation between the two groups. If we like, we can now compute the standardized weight as we did in the video. We first calculate the pooled variance of the discriminant scores by:

```
alfa1=eig$vectors[1,1]
alfa2=eig$vectors[2,1]
D=alfa1*CRP+alfa2*Temp # Discriminant scores
# Variance of the discriminant scores for each group
Vars=tapply(D,Group,var)
pooled_var=((n1-1)*Vars[1]+(n2-1)*Vars[2])/(n1+n2-2)
```

Then we divide the weights by the pooled standard deviation:

```
eig$vectors[,1]/sqrt(pooled_var)
[1] 0.1060934  0.7011204
```

The discriminant scores can now be calculated by the following equation:

$$D = 0.106 \cdot CRP + 0.701 \cdot Temp$$

Computing the discriminant scores with the standardized weights will result in the same separation between the groups as if we use the unstandardized weights because the ratio of the weights is still the same ($0.9887/0.1496 \approx 0.701/0.106 \approx 6.6$).

7.1.2 Using the "lda" Function

To simplify our code for computing LDA, we can use the "lda" function from the **MASS** package:

```
library(MASS)
fit = lda(Group ~ CRP + Temp, data=df)
fit
...
Coefficients of linear discriminants:
              LD1
CRP       0.1060934
Temp      0.7011204
```

Note that this function generates the exact same standardized coefficients as we calculated earlier. Let's extract the weights and compute the discriminant scores:

```
alfa1=fit$scaling[1]  # Discriminant coefficient for CRP
alfa2=fit$scaling[2]  # Discriminant coefficient for Temp
D=alfa1*CRP+alfa2*Temp # Discriminant scores
D
29.48407 27.25932 28.77370 29.89454 28.89957 28.89632
30.81805 32.88678 32.29780 34.03218 31.91171 31.77326
```

We can see that the combined variable generally has greater values for the bacteria group (the last six values) compared to the virus group (the first six values). We can also calculate the centered discriminant scores by:

```
# same as D-mean(D)
D=alfa1*(CRP-mean(CRP))+alfa2*(Temp-mean(Temp))
D
-1.0932056 -3.3179595 -1.8035791 -0.6827330 -1.6777079 -1.6809571
0.2407737 2.3095099  1.7205291  3.4549085  1.3344396
1.1959815
```

However, these centered discriminant scores can also be computed by using the "predict" function on the output object from the "lda" function:

```
D1=predict(fit)$x # Discriminant scores
D1
-1.0932056 -3.3179595 -1.8035791 -0.6827330 -1.6777079 -1.6809571
0.2407737 2.3095099  1.7205291  3.4549085  1.3344396
1.1959815
```

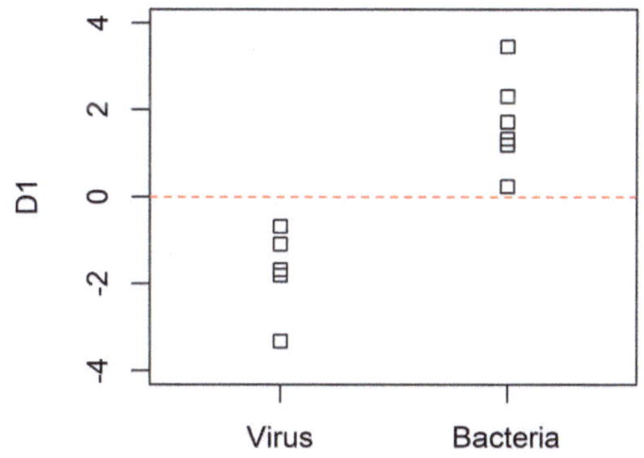

Fig. 7.3 A one-dimensional scatter plot of the centered discriminant scores

An appropriate cutoff value that can be used to separate the groups based on the centered discriminant scores is zero, since that is the mean of the scores. Let's plot the variable D1 (the centered discriminant scores) with the cutoff value zero:

```
stripchart(D1~Group,ylim=c(-4,4),vertical = TRUE,
xlim=c(0.5,2.5))
abline(h=0,col="red",lty=2)
```

We see that a cutoff value of zero separates the two groups perfectly when CRP and temperature are combined into a single variable (Fig. 7.3). All individuals in the viral group have a combined CRP and temperature that is lower than zero, whereas all individuals in the bacteria group have values greater than zero.

We will in Chap. 11 use LDA again and compare it with other supervised machine learning methods.

7.2 Exercises

1. Combine the four numerical variables of the Iris dataset with LDA so that you optimize the separation between the three species in this dataset. Show the equation for calculating the scores of the first discriminant function (you do not need to center the scores).
2. Plot LD1 vs LD2. Compare with a similar PCA plot where you plot PC1 vs PC2. Do you think that LDA provides a better separation between the groups compared to PCA?
3. Combine all the numerical variables of the Crab dataset by using LDA in order to maximize the separation between male and female crabs. Show the equation to calculate the discriminant scores.
4. Plot the discriminant scores with a one-dimensional scatter plot where you separate male and female crabs.

Chapter 8
Distances in Space

Many multivariate statistical methods use different methods to calculate the distance between the data points. For example, the Euclidean distance can be used in hierarchical clustering and K-nearest neighbor classification, whereas the Mahalanobis distance can be used to compute the Hotelling's T-square statistics and to identify outliers in a multivariate space. In addition, centroids are, for example, used in K-means clustering. Watch the video below to learn how the Euclidean distance is calculated and how it differs from the Mahalanobis distance.

8.1 Video

https://youtu.be/AOD-nZF3SWs

www.tilestats.com/ml/

8.2 The Euclidean Distance

The Euclidean distance is used to calculate the shortest distance between two points in space. In two dimensions, the Euclidean distance (d) is given by:

$$d = \sqrt{(x_1 - x_2)^2 + (y_1 - y_2)^2}$$

For example, let's calculate the distance between the two data points with the coordinates (x=2,y=2) and (x=3,y=4) in Fig. 8.1.

$$d = \sqrt{(x_1 - x_2)^2 + (y_1 - y_2)^2} = \sqrt{(2-3)^2 + (2-4)^2} = \sqrt{5} = 2.236$$

A. Tilevik, *Multivariate Statistics and Machine Learning in R For Beginners*,
https://doi.org/10.1007/978-3-032-01851-9_8

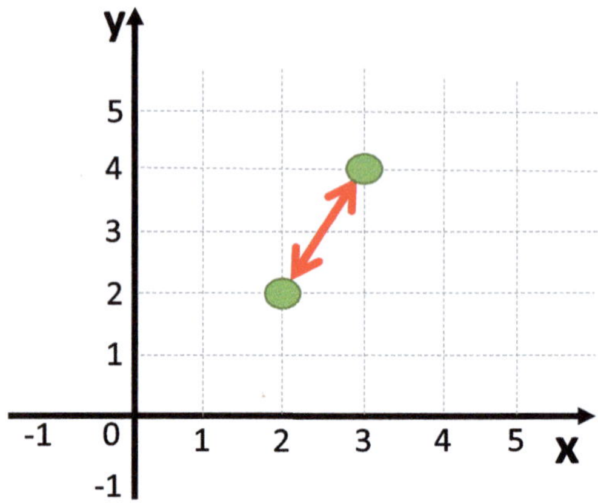

Fig. 8.1 An illustration of the distance in a two-dimensional space between two data points

Hence, the Euclidean distance between the two points is about 2.2. To calculate the Euclidean distance in R, we can use the function "dist":

```
x=c(2,3) # x-coordinates of the two points
y=c(2,4) # y-coordinates of the two points
data1=data.frame(x,y)
dist(data1, method = "euclidean")
            1
2       2.236068
```

For example, let's calculate the Euclidean distances between seven individuals based on their heights and weights. We first plot the data by labeling each individual with a number (row number):

```
Weight=c(80,58,65,70,90,100,50)
Height=c(190,171,175,169,182,183,165)
df=data.frame(Weight,Height)
plot(Weight,Height,ylim=c(160,max(Height)+5))
# Put the number above (+2 in the y-direction) the point
text(Weight,Height+2,1:7,col="red")
```

From this plot (Fig. 8.2), we see that persons 2, 3, and 4 seem to be close. Person 1 seems to have the longest distance to its closest neighbor. Let's calculate the Euclidean distances:

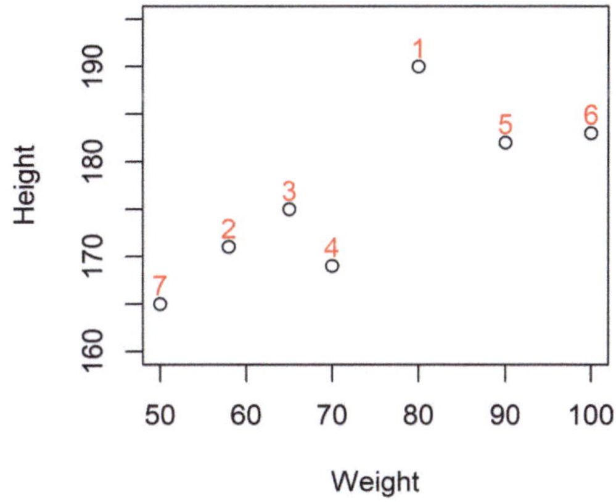

Fig. 8.2 A scatter plot of the variables Height and Weight that shows the distance in space between the seven individuals

```
dist_mat=dist(df, method = "euclidean")
round(dist_mat,1)
     1       2       3       4       5       6
2  29.1
3  21.2    8.1
4  23.3   12.2    7.8
5  12.8   33.8   26.0    23.9
6  21.2   43.7   35.9    33.1    10.0
7  39.1   10.0   18.0    20.4    43.5    53.1
```

From this matrix with Euclidean distances, we can, for example, see that individual 1 has the shortest Euclidean distance (12.8) to person number 5. The shortest distance between all individuals is 7.8, which is between individuals 3 and 4. However, when we calculate the Euclidean distance between points in a space based on variables on different scales, this may cause problems. Variables with larger values will dominate the Euclidean distance calculation. One therefore usually standardizes the variables before the distances are calculated to ensure that all variables contribute equally to the distance metric, regardless of their original scale. Let's compute the distance matrix based on standardized variables by using the function "scale":

```
dist_mat=dist(scale(df), method = "euclidean")
round(dist_mat,1)
     1    2    3    4    5    6
2  2.5
3  1.9  0.6
4  2.4  0.7  0.7
5  1.1  2.2  1.6  1.8
6  1.4  2.7  2.2  2.3  0.6
7  3.3  0.8  1.4  1.2  3.0  3.5
```

From this matrix with Euclidean distances based on standardized data, we can see that the shortest distance between all individuals is now 0.6, which is between individuals 2 and 3 and between individuals 5 and 6.

8.3 The Centroid

A centroid (or a mean vector) is the mean position of all data points in all directions. If we have a scatter plot of two variables (Fig. 8.3), x and y,

then the centroid is simply the mean of x and the mean of y:

$$\text{Centroid} = \begin{pmatrix} \overline{x} \\ \overline{y} \end{pmatrix}$$

Let's calculate the centroid of the data points in Fig. 8.3 by calculating the mean of x and y:

```
x=c(2,2,3,5)
y=c(2,4,2,4)
df=data.frame(x,y)
colMeans(df)
x    y
3    3
```

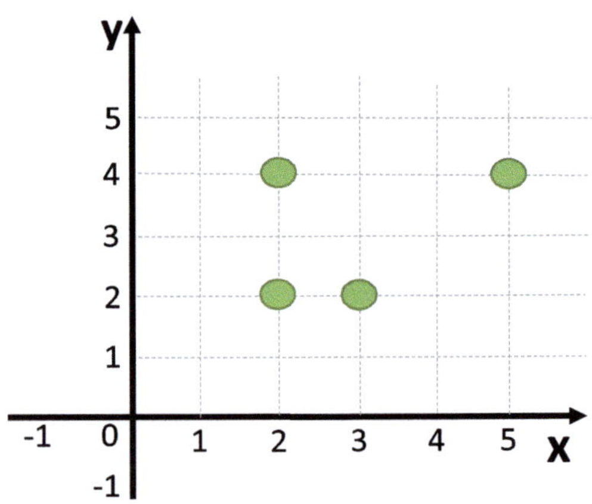

Fig. 8.3 An illustration of four arbitrary data points in a two-dimensional space

8.4 The Mahalanobis Distance

The Mahalanobis distance is a distance measure that considers the correlation between the variables. The Mahalanobis distance can be used to detect outliers in a multivariate space. Let's consider the following data in Fig. 8.4 in a two-dimensional space.

To this dataset (green points in Fig. 8.4), we have added two arbitrary data points (data points 1 and 2).

Let's calculate the Euclidean distance between the two data points and the centroid (the orange point in Fig. 8.4) of the green points:

```
rm(list=ls()) # Clear environment
x=c(4.6, 4.4, 3.9, 3.9, 3.8, 3.5, 3.8, 3.4, 3.0, 2.7, 3.7,
3.0, 2.5, 2.2, 2.9, 2.5, 2.3, 2.1, 2.1, 1.5)
y=c(4.6, 4.1, 4.5, 3.9, 3.5, 4.0, 3.3, 3.2, 3.7, 3.5, 2.1,
2.7, 3.1, 3.2, 2.3, 2.0, 2.3, 1.8, 1.4, 1)
df=data.frame(x,y)
centroid=colMeans(df)
p1=c(5,5) # Data point 1
p2=c(5,1) # Data point 2
dist(rbind(p1,centroid), method = "euclidean")
centroid 2.758297
dist(rbind(p2,centroid), method = "euclidean")
centroid 2.77276
```

We can see that the two data points have about the same Euclidean distance to the centroid. In comparison, the Mahalanobis distance takes into account the correlation structure of the data when it computes the distance to the centroid:

$$MD = \sqrt{\begin{pmatrix} x-\overline{x} \\ y-\overline{y} \end{pmatrix}^{T} W^{-1} \begin{pmatrix} x-\overline{x} \\ y-\overline{y} \end{pmatrix}}$$

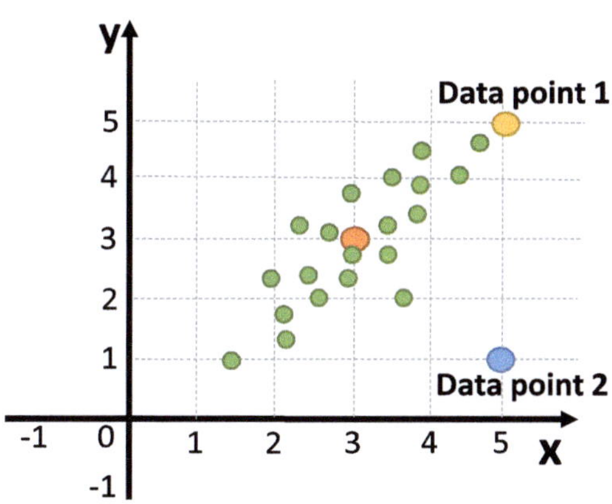

Fig. 8.4 An illustration of some data points in a two-dimensional space. The orange point represents the centroid of the green data points. The distance between data points 1 and 2 to the centroid will be evaluated

where x and y are our coordinates of the data point of interest, $\overline{x}$ and $\overline{y}$ are the means (coordinates of the centroid), and W^{-1} is the inverse of the covariance matrix. Let's calculate the inverse of the covariance matrix:

```
W=cov(df) # Covariance matrix
W1=solve(W) # Inverse of the covariance matrix
```

Next, we check the Mahalanobis distance between data point 1 and the centroid and between data point 2 and the centroid:

```
sqrt(t(p1-centroid)%*%W1%*%(p1-centroid))
2.262389
sqrt(t(p2-centroid)%*%W1%*%(p2-centroid))
6.485741
```

We can also use R's function "mahalanobis" to compute the same thing. The function generates the squared Mahalanobis distance, which means that we need to take the square root of the output to calculate the Mahalanobis distance:

```
# Squared Mahalanobis distance
MD2=mahalanobis(p1,centroid, W)
sqrt(MD2) # Mahalanobis distance
2.262389
# Squared Mahalanobis distance
MD2=mahalanobis(p2,centroid, W)
sqrt(MD2) # Mahalanobis distance
6.485741
```

We see that we get the exact same distances as we previously calculated. By using the Mahalanobis distance, data point 1 is now considered to be much closer to the centroid compared to data point 2.

8.5 The Error Ellipse and Multivariate Outliers

Let's draw a 95% error ellipse around our previous data (the green data points in Fig. 8.4) by using the function "ellipse" from the **ellipse** package.

```
plot(x,y,xlim=c(0,6),ylim=c(0,6))
library(ellipse)
alfa=0.05 # To get a 95% error ellipse
lines(ellipse(cor(df),scale=c(sd(x),sd(y)),centre=centroid,
level=1-alfa),col="red",lwd=4)
```

We will now calculate the squared Mahalanobis distance between all the data points and the centroid to compute p-values based on a Chi-square distribution with the degrees of freedom equal to the number of variables, which is two in our example. Then we order the Mahalanobis distances to easily identify possible outliers.

```
MH2=mahalanobis(df, centroid, cov(df))
p_val=1-pchisq(MH2,df=2)
data3=data.frame(df,MH2,p_val)
# Print the first 6 rows of the sorted data
head(data3[order(data3$MH2,decreasing = TRUE),])
     x    y    MH2       p_val
11   3.7  2.1  6.131468  0.04661962
20   1.5  1.0  4.129075  0.12687695
14   2.2  3.2  3.805684  0.14914417
1    4.6  4.6  3.211719  0.20071699
19   2.1  1.4  2.494115  0.28734914
2    4.4  4.1  2.429122  0.29684024
```

We see that data point 11 has a p-value of about 0.0466. This p-value is less than 0.05, which explains why it is outside the ellipse in Fig. 8.5. Given that the data is normally distributed, we expect that 5% of the data points to be outside the 95% error ellipse due to chance. If we use a threshold of 0.001 to detect outliers in the multivariate space, none of the data points would be considered as an outlier because they are all associated with p-values greater than 0.001. The threshold we select should depend on the sample size in our experiment. A larger sample size should

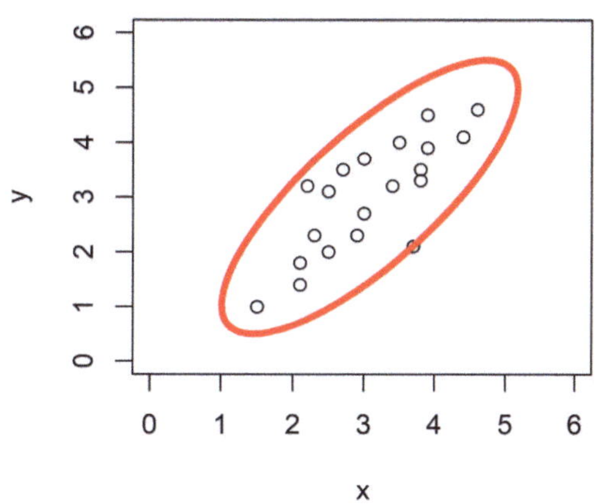

Fig. 8.5 An illustration of some data points and a 95% error ellipse

have a lower threshold because more data points will then be outside the 95% error ellipse due to chance. One way to determine an appropriate threshold is to use the Bonferroni method, where the cutoff is based on the general significance level of 0.05, divided by the number of data points we have. In our case, we would use a threshold of 0.0025.

$$Threshold = \frac{\alpha}{n} = \frac{0.05}{20} = 0.0025$$

Thus, any data point with an associated p-value less than 0.0025 can be considered as an outlier.

8.6 Exercises

1. Use the Mahalanobis distance in order to identify possible outliers in the numerical variables of the Crab dataset. Use a cutoff value based on the Bonferroni method.

Chapter 9
Multivariate Statistical Tests

Multivariate statistical tests are powerful tools used to analyze and interpret data with multiple outcome variables. Unlike univariate tests, which examine only one dependent variable at a time, multivariate tests consider the relationships and interactions between multiple dependent variables simultaneously. Multivariate statistical tests are essential when analyzing complex datasets, where variables may not act independently but instead exhibit correlations or shared structures. In this chapter, we will cover the Hotelling's T-square test and MANOVA, which can be seen as the multivariate counterparts of the t-test and ANOVA, respectively. We will also discuss PERMANOVA, which can be seen as the non-parametric alternative to MANOVA. Finally, we will have a look at canonical correlation analysis, which is a multivariate method for analyzing the correlation between two sets of variables.

9.1 Hotelling's T-Square and MANOVA

We will first have a look at the Hotelling's T-square test and MANOVA. Watch the videos below to learn how the two methods are computed and what kind of assumptions they rely on.

9.1.1 Videos

https://youtu.be/btonaMqu9eA

https://youtu.be/NIFHW8AZrK0

www.tilestats.com/ml/

A. Tilevik, *Multivariate Statistics and Machine Learning in R For Beginners*,
https://doi.org/10.1007/978-3-032-01851-9_9

As explained in the videos, Hotelling's T-square is a multivariate statistical test that can be used when we like to compare two groups, whereas MANOVA can be used if we have two or more groups. We will here use the same example data as in the videos. Our null hypothesis for this example can be stated as:

$$H_0 : \begin{array}{l} \overline{CRP}_{virus} = \overline{CRP}_{bacteria} \\ \overline{Temp}_{virus} = \overline{Temp}_{bacteria} \end{array}$$

This hypothesis means that the centroids of the two populations have the same location. To test this hypothesis, we can use Hotelling's T-square or MANOVA because we here have only two groups (Virus vs Bacteria). Let's read in the data:

```
Temp=c(36.0, 37.2, 36.5, 39.4, 39.6, 40.7,37.6, 42.2, 38.5,
39.4, 38.6, 42.7)
CRP=c(40.0, 11.1, 30.0, 21.4, 10.7, 3.4,42.0, 31.1, 50.0,
60.4, 45.7, 17.3)
Group=factor(c(rep("Virus",6),rep("Bacteria",6)),
levels=c("Virus","Bacteria"))
df=data.frame(CRP,Temp,Group)
```

We will now use R's function "manova" to test if there is a significant difference between viral and bacterial infections based on the two variables CRP and body temperature:

```
fit = manova(cbind(CRP,Temp) ~ Group,data=df)
summary(fit)
          Df  Pillai  approx F  num Df  den Df    Pr(>F)
Group      1 0.77809    15.778       2       9  0.001142 **
Residuals 10
```

Since the p-value is less than 0.05, we can reject the null hypothesis and conclude that there is a significant difference in CRP and body temperature between patients with a viral or bacterial infection. Thus, the centroids of these two groups have a significantly different location.

9.1.2 Assumptions for MANOVA

MANOVA relies on the following assumptions:

1. Multivariate normality
2. No outliers
3. Homogeneity of variance–covariance matrices
4. No multicollinearity
5. Linear relationship of the dependent variables

9.1.3 Multivariate normality

Multivariate normality means, in this example, that the two dependent variables CRP and Body temperature show a normal distribution in a two-dimensional plane. We can check this assumption by using the "mshapiro.test" function in the package **mvnormtest**. Note that the null hypothesis of this test states that the variables show multivariate normality. Below, we check if we fulfill this assumption for both groups. Note that "mshapiro.test" expects the input to be a matrix where rows represent variables and columns represent the individuals. We therefore first need to transpose our data when we use this function:

```
# We first split the groups
V=subset(df,Group=="Virus")
B=subset(df,Group=="Bacteria")

library(mvnormtest)
# Check multivariate normality of the viral data
mshapiro.test(as.matrix(t(V[,1:2])))
    Shapiro-Wilk normality test

data:  Z
W = 0.90473, p-value = 0.4027
# Check multivariate normality of the bacterial data
mshapiro.test(as.matrix(t(B[,1:2])))
    Shapiro-Wilk normality test

data:  Z
W = 0.89379, p-value = 0.3385
```

We see that the multivariate normality tests result in p-values greater than 0.05 for both groups. Thus, we do not reject the null hypothesis about multivariate normality and therefore conclude that we fulfill the assumption of multivariate normality.

9.1.4 Outliers

To check for outliers in a multivariate space, we can compute the squared Mahalanobis distances and their corresponding p-value from a Chi-square distribution as we discussed in Chap. 8:

```
MD_V=mahalanobis(V[,1:2], colMeans(V[,1:2]), cov(V[,1:2]))
MD_B=mahalanobis(B[,1:2], colMeans(B[,1:2]), cov(B[,1:2]))
1-pchisq(MD_V,df=2)
        1         2         3         4         5         6
0.3247704 0.1978959 0.6622269 0.4834522 0.7706478 0.4249111
1-pchisq(MD_B,df=2)
        7         8         9        10        11        12
0.3077667 0.5138578 0.8066937 0.2288042 0.8261654 0.2793981
```

If we use a cutoff of 0.05/6 = 0.0083, based on the Bonferroni method, we see that none of the p-values in each group is less than this value. We can therefore conclude that we have no outliers in our dataset.

9.1.5 Homogeneity of variance–covariance matrices

Similar to ANOVA, the variance within the different groups should be equal (homogeneity of variance). Homogeneity of variance–covariance matrices means that the covariance matrices of the dependent variables are equal across groups. This assumption can be tested with Box's M-test. The function "boxM" in the **biotool** package can be used to test for homogeneity of the covariance matrices:

```
library(biotools)
boxM(df[,1:2], df[,3])
Chi-Sq (approx.) = 0.17925, df = 3, p-value = 0.9809
```

The null hypothesis of this test states that the population covariance matrices of the dependent variables are equal across the groups. Since the p-value is greater than 0.05, the null hypothesis of equal population covariance matrices is not rejected. Thus, we can therefore assume that we fulfill the assumption of homogeneity of variance–covariance matrices.

9.1.6 No multicollinearity

The correlation of our dependent variables should not be too strong (absolute value greater than 0.9) since multicollinearity is problematic for MANOVA. We can check the correlation simply by running a Pearson's correlation on the dependent variables:

```
cor(Temp,CRP)
-0.2939751
```

The correlation coefficient is not greater than 0.9, or less than -0.9, which means that there is no strong correlation between the two variables.

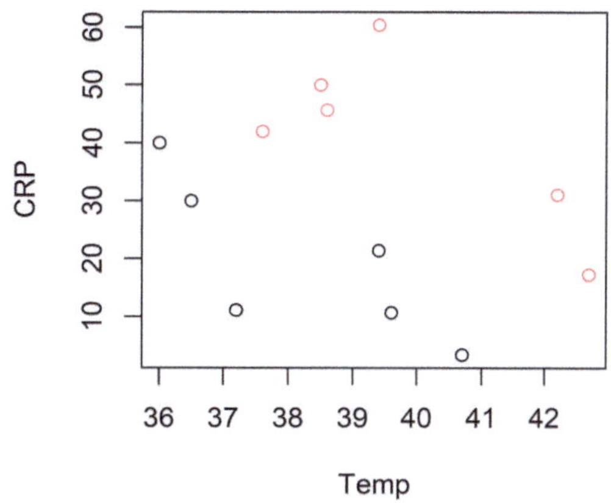

Fig. 9.1 A scatter plot of CRP and body temperature of six individuals with viral infections (black circles) and six individuals with bacterial infections (red circles)

9.1.7 Linear relationship of the dependent variables

The final assumption is that each pair of our dependent variables should be linearly related within each group. We can check this simply by a scatter plot:

```
plot(Temp,CRP,col=Group)
```

According to this plot (Fig. 9.1), there is no indication that the dependent variables are not linearly related within the two groups (it is not possible to identify any clear non-linear trend in the data). Since we have quite a few data points in this example, it is, however, hard to identify any pattern in the data.

Thus, it seems like we fulfill all assumptions for the MANOVA.

9.1.8 Calculate the Hotelling's T-square by hand (optional)

We will here see how to calculate the p-value from the Hotelling's T-square by hand. From the video, we know that we should first calculate the centroid of each group by:

```
# Extract data for the virus group
Group1=subset(df[,1:2], Group=="Virus")
# Extract data for the bacteria group
Group2=subset(df[,1:2], Group=="Bacteria")
# Calculate the mean of each column (variable)
Centroid_G1=colMeans(Group1)
# Calculate the mean of each column (variable)
Centroid_G2= colMeans(Group2)
```

Then we calculate the pooled within-group covariance matrix by:

```
# Sample size of group 1 and 2
n1=nrow(Group1);n2=nrow(Group2)
# Pooled covariance matrix
W = ((n1-1)*cov(Group1)+(n2-1)*cov(Group2))/(n1+n2-2)
```

Next, we calculate the squared Mahalanobis distance and the T^2 score by:

```
MD2=mahalanobis(Centroid_G1, Centroid_G2, W)
T2=((n1*n2)/(n1+n2))*MD2
```

Finally, we compute the F-ratio and the p-value by:

```
p=2 # Number of dependent variables
F=((n1+n2-p-1)/(p*(n1+n2-2)))*T2
# Compute p-value from an f-distribution
1-pf(F,p , (n1+n2-p-1))
0.001142398
```

We see that this p-value is exactly the same as shown in the output from the "manova" function. The Hotelling's T-square can also be calculated by the "HotellingsT2" function in the **ICSNP** package.

```
library(ICSNP)
HotellingsT2(cbind(Temp, CRP) ~ Group)
   Hotelling's two sample T2-test
data:  cbind(Temp, CRP) by Group
T.2 = 15.778, df1 = 2, df2 = 9, p-value = 0.001142
```

9.1.9 *Calculate the MANOVA by hand (optional)*

To calculate the MANOVA by hand, we first center the variables by:

```
cCRP=CRP-mean(CRP)
cTemp=Temp-mean(Temp)
```

Then we can calculate the sums of squares and cross-product matrix by:

```
mat=cbind(cCRP,cTemp)
sscpT=t(mat)%*%mat
sscpT
            cCRP        cTemp
cCRP    3487.5692   -120.71333
cTemp   -120.7133     48.34667
```

Next, we calculate the within-groups sums of squares and cross-product matrix by:

```
# Extract numeric variables in the virus group
V=subset(df,Group=="Virus")[,-3]
# Extract numeric variables in the bacteria group
B=subset(df,Group=="Bacteria")[,-3]

mV=scale(V,center = TRUE, scale = FALSE) # Center data
mB=scale(B,center = TRUE, scale = FALSE) # Center data
sscpW1=t(mV)%*%mV
sscpW2=t(mB)%*%mB
sscpW=sscpW1+sscpW2
sscpW
           cCRP           cTemp
cCRP    2081.4017    -224.63333
cTemp   -224.6333      40.66667
```

Next, we calculate the between-groups sums of squares and cross-product matrix:

```
sscpB=sscpT-sscpW
sscpB
          cCRP        cTemp
cCRP    1406.168    103.92
cTemp    103.920      7.68
```

Finally, we compute the eigenvalues of the target matrix S:

$$S = SSCP_W^{-1} \cdot SSCP_B$$

by:

```
S=solve(sscpW)%*%sscpB
eigen(S)
eigen() decomposition
$values
[1]  3.506282e+00   -2.220446e-16
...
```

Our eigenvalues are therefore:

$$\lambda_1 = 3.51 \ \lambda_2 = 0.0$$

We can now calculate different test statistics of the MANOVA. For example, we will here calculate Wilk's lambda by:

$$\text{Wilk's Lambda} = \prod_{K=1}^{K} \frac{1}{1+\lambda_K} = \frac{1}{1+3.51} \cdot \frac{1}{1+0} = 0.22$$

```
prod(1/(1+eigen(S)$values))
[1] 0.2219124
```

This is the exact same test statistic as generated by the "manova" function if we run Wilk's lambda:

```
fit = manova(cbind(CRP,Temp) ~ Group,data=df)
summary(fit,test="Wilks")
          Df   Wilks   approx F  num Df  den Df    Pr(>F)
Group      1  0.22191   15.778      2       9    0.001142 **
Residuals 10
```

We can reproduce the p-value from Wilks lambda (Λ) with the following formula (Navarro, 2016):

$$F = \frac{(f \cdot t - g) \cdot \left(1 - \Lambda^{1/t}\right)}{p \cdot h \cdot \Lambda^{1/t}}$$

where

$$t = \sqrt{\frac{p^2 \cdot h^2 - 4}{p^2 + h^2 - 5}} \left(\text{if } p^2 + h^2 - 5 > 0, \text{otherwise } t = 1\right)$$

$$f = e - 0.5 \cdot (p - h - 1), \text{with } e = n - h - p$$

$$g = \frac{p \cdot h - 2}{2}$$

and n is the sample size, h is the number of groups minus one, and p is the number of dependent variables. The degrees of freedom are calculated by:

$$df_1 = p \cdot h$$

$$df_2 = f \cdot t - g$$

We can compute this in R by:

```
Wilks=prod(1/(1+eigen(S)$values))
h=length(levels(Group))-1 # Number of groups -1
p=2 #Number of dependent variables
n=nrow(df) # Sample size
e=n-h-p
f=e-0.5*(p-h-1)
g=(p*h-2)/2
if(p^2+h^2-5>0){
  t=sqrt(  (p^2*h^2-4)/ (p^2+h^2-5)   )
} else {
  t=1
}
F=(  (f*t-g)*(1-Wilks^(1/t)) ) / (p*h*Wilks^(1/t) )
1-pf(F,p*h ,f*t-g) # Compute p-value from f-distribution
[1] 0.001142398
```

9.2 PERMANOVA

One problem with MANOVA and the Hotelling's T-square is that they rely on several assumptions that might be hard to fulfill, especially if we work with count data that are often highly skewed and might consist of lots of zeros. Permutational multivariate analysis of variance (PERMANOVA) can be seen as the non-parametric alternative to MANOVA. PERMANOVA can therefore be used if we do not fulfill the underlying assumptions in MANOVA. However, PERMANOVA still assumes that the two groups have about the same spread (dispersion) in the data, but the test is quite robust to differences in spread, especially if the groups have equal sample sizes (Anderson and Walsh, 2013). We will first try to reproduce the example as shown in the video below and then test the method on some count datasets.

9.2.1 Video

https://youtu.be/Y5SMcG_bpgk
www.tilestats.com/ml/

Let's first set up the same dataset as in the video where one wants to test if there is a significant difference in the location of the centroids of groups A and B based on the systolic (SBP) and diastolic blood pressure (DBP):

```
SBP=c(124,125,127,127, 132, 130, 132, 133)
DBP=c( 78, 82,83, 79,  84,   87,  89,  88)
n=4 # Sample size in each group
Group=factor(c(rep("A",n),rep("B",n)))
df=data.frame(SBP,DBP,Group)
df
    SBP  DBP   Group
1   124  78        A
2   125  82        A
3   127  83        A
4   127  79        A
5   132  84        B
6   130  87        B
7   132  89        B
8   133  88        B
```

Let's also make a plot of the data, where we add the two centroids:

```
plot(DBP,SBP,pch=16,cex=2,col=c(rep("green",4),rep("orange",
4)),las=1,xlim=c(76,90),ylim=c(124,134))
text(DBP,SBP,1:8,cex=0.7)

# Calculate and add the centroids to the plot
centroids = aggregate(cbind(SBP, DBP) ~ Group, data = df,
mean)
points(centroids$DBP[1],centroids$SBP[1],pch=17,col="green",
cex=2)
points(centroids$DBP[2],centroids$SBP[2],pch=17,col="orange",
cex=2)
legend("topleft", legend = c("Group A", "Group B", "Centroid A",
"Centroid B"),
  col = c("green", "orange", "green", "orange"), pch = c(16,
  16, 17, 17))
```

We see that the two centroids are quite far from each other (Fig. 9.2). We will now use PERMANOVA to test if they have a significant difference in location of the centroids. To compute this test, we will use the package **PERMANOVA** where we first compute the distance matrix. To be consistent with the video, we will use the Euclidean (Pythagorean) distance:

```
library(PERMANOVA)
D = DistContinuous(df[,-3],coef = "Pythagorean")
```

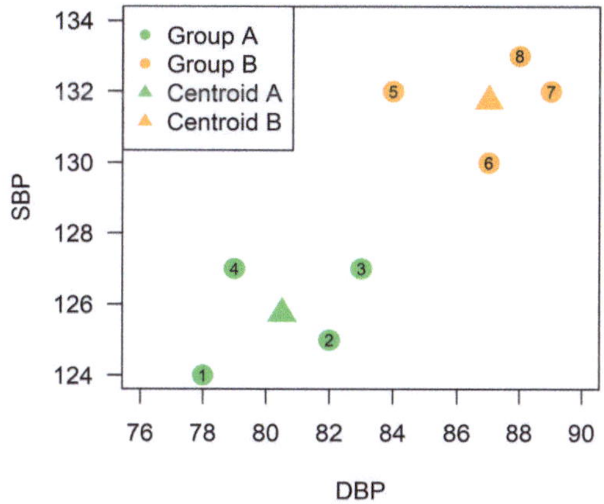

Fig. 9.2 A scatter plot of the systolic blood pressure (SBP) and diastolic blood pressure (DBP) of the eight individuals in two groups: group A (green points) and group B (orange points). The triangles represent the centroids of the two groups

If you print this distance matrix, you will see the Euclidean distance between all data points. Note that we can use other distance measures such as the Bray–Curtis dissimilarity metric as we discussed in Chap. 6. We will now compute the PERMANOVA by using, for example, 2000 permutations:

```
PERMANOVA(D, Group, nperm = 2000, seed=29)
...

MANOVA
            Explained Residual df Num df Denom F-exp     p-value    p-value adj
 Total        156.5     42.5        1       6     2.09412  0.03148426  0.03148426
```

We see that the approximate F-statistic and the p-value are exactly the same as in the video, but note that PERMANOVA involves a random process, which means that we might get different results every time we run the code with a different seed. For example, if we set the seed to 1, we will get a bit smaller p-value:

```
PERMANOVA(D, Group, nperm = 2000, seed=1)
...
MANOVA
          Explained Residual df Num df Denom  F-exp      p-value   p-value adj.
 Total     156.5      42.5      1       6      22.09412  0.02248876  0.02248876
```

In general, we should try to run at least 999 permutations (set nperm to at least 999), but the more permutations we do, the better the precision of p-values we will get. If you run the same test but with different seeds and get different p-values, you can either average the p-values or report the range of the p-values.

We can also compute a PERMANOVA by using the "adonis2" function in the **vegan** package:

```
library(vegan)
set.seed(29) #For reproducibility
adonis2(df[,-3]~Group,method = "euclidian",
permutations = 2000)
         Df   SumOfSqs      R2        F      Pr(>F)
Group     1     156.5     0.78643   22.094   0.03198 *
Residual  6      42.5     0.21357
Total     7     199.0     1.00000
```

We see that we get basically the same result as we got previously when we used a seed of 29. The **vegan** package is simple to use when we like to test for interactions that we will see later on. Also, it comes with a test that can check if we fulfill the assumption of equal dispersion between the groups, which can be thought of as the groups having similar degrees of multivariate scatter. To test this, we can use the function "betadisper":

```
(betadisp_res = betadisper(dist(df[,-3], method = "euclidean"),
type= "centroid", Group))
…
Average distance to centroid:
  A       B
2.369   2.094
...
plot(betadisp_res, hull=FALSE, ellipse=TRUE)
```

This method computes a PCoA and calculates the centroids (or the medians if the argument "type" is set to median). The method then averages the distances between the data points and the centroids in the PCoA space. We see that the average distances of the data points to their given centroids in the two groups are quite similar (Fig. 9.3), which suggests that the two groups have equal dispersion. To test if there is a significant difference in dispersion between the two groups, an ANOVA of the distances to the group centroids can be performed by:

```
anova(betadisp_res)
           Df   Sum Sq    Mean Sq    F value   Pr(>F)
Groups      1   0.15114   0.15114    0.3617    0.5696
Residuals   6   2.50730   0.41788
```

We see that the p-value is larger than 0.05, which suggests that the two groups have equal dispersion. An alternative is to use the function "permutest" to compute a permutation test instead of the ANOVA.

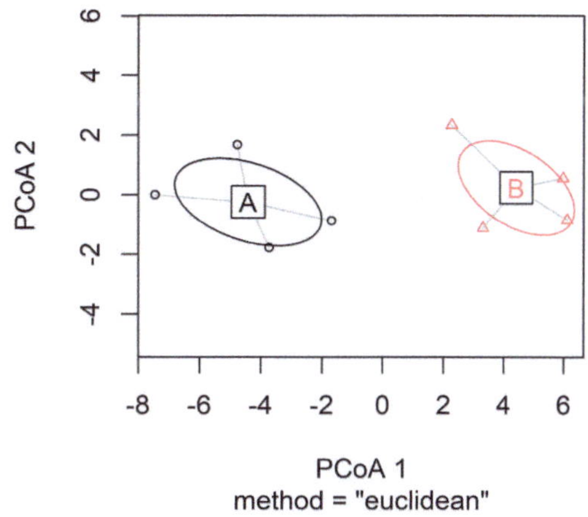

Fig. 9.3 A PCoA plot illustrating the distribution of the eight individuals across the two groups (Group A and Group B). Each point represents an individual and the squares represent the centroids of the two groups. This plot shows the similarities and differences between individuals within and across the two groups based on the Euclidean distance

9.2.2 Standardize the data

Since we have based the PERMANOVA on Euclidean distances, the scales of our variables may bias the test toward variables with larger scales. Thus, differences in the location of the centroids might be based mainly on variables with large values or larger spread. It is therefore important, especially if we have variables on different scales, to standardize the data before computing the PERMANOVA so that all variables have an equal contribution to determining the location of the centroids. Let's try to run the PERMANOVA based on standardized variables:

```
data=data.frame(scale(df[,-3]))
set.seed(29) #For reproducibility
adonis2(data~Group,method = "euclidian", permutations = 2000)
             Df   SumOfSqs       R2        F       Pr(>F)
Group        1    11.1571     0.79694   23.548   0.03198 *
Residual     6     2.8429     0.20306
Total        7    14.0000     1.00000
```

In this case, we happened to get the same p-value although we standardized the continuous variables.

9.2.3 The Dune dataset

The **vegan** package comes with a dataset that is especially suitable for PERMANOVA. We will here analyze the dune meadow vegetation data that can be loaded by:

```
library(vegan)
data(dune)
dune
```

If you print this data frame, you will see that the data has 30 columns that correspond to 30 different species. The rows represent 20 different locations that were analyzed. The values in this dataset are scores from zero to nine, where high scores are related to a high abundance of the species, whereas a score of zero represents that the species is not present in the given location. We can also load the dune.env data by:

```
data(dune.env)
dune.env
```

which gives information about the 20 different locations. For example, the column Management shows the type of farming in the 20 different locations: Biological farming (BF), hobby farming (HF), nature conservation management (NM), and standard farming (SF). Let's test if there is a difference in the species composition between the different farming by using a PERMANOVA based on the Bray–Curtis metric, which is commonly used to quantify the dissimilarity in species composition between different locations:

```
adonis2(dune ~ Management, method = "bray", data = dune.env)
              Df      SumOfSqs      R2          F        Pr(>F)
Management     3      1.4686      0.34161     2.7672    0.003 **
Residual      16      2.8304      0.65839
Total         19      4.2990      1.00000
```

We can see that the species composition significantly differs between the types of farming because the p-value is less than 0.05. To graphically illustrate the difference in the species composition between the types of farming, we can compute a PCoA plot based on the Bray–Curtis metric:

```
dune.dist = vegdist(dune, method="bray")
dispersion = betadisper(dune.dist, group=dune.env$Management)
anova(dispersion) # Check dispersion assumption
plot(dispersion, hull=FALSE, ellipse=TRUE)
```

We see that the combined species composition is different between the different farming and that the nature conservation management (NM) seems to differ quite much from the other farming (Fig. 9.4).

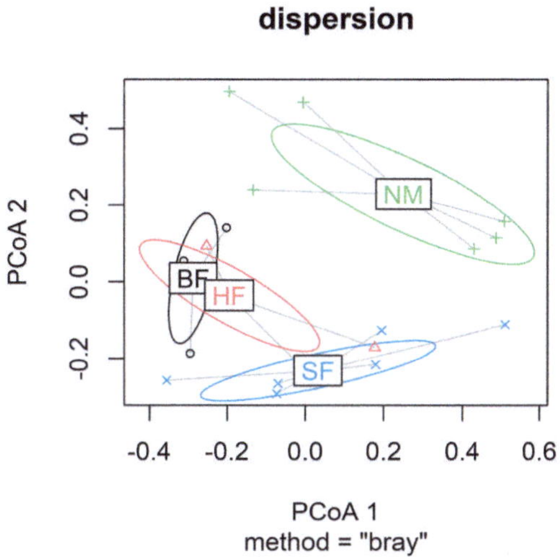

Fig. 9.4 A PCoA plot based on the Dunn data from the **vegan** package, illustrating the distance between the 20 different locations based on the species composition, using the Bray–Curtis metric. The colors represent the different types of farming: Biological farming (BF), hobby farming (HF), nature conservation management (NM), and standard farming (SF)

9.2.4 *Test for interactions*

In MANOVA and PERMANOVA, we can add more than one independent variable on the right-hand side of the equation to test if more variables affect the species composition or to control for confounders. For example, we could add the continuous variable A1, which represents soil thickness in the different locations:

```
set.seed(1) #For reproducibility
adonis2(dune ~ Management + A1, data = dune.env,by = "terms")
             Df   SumOfSqs      R2        F       Pr(>F)
Management    3     1.4686   0.34161   3.0730    0.002 **
A1            1     0.4409   0.10256   2.7676    0.021 *
Residual     15     2.3895   0.55583
Total        19     4.2990   1.00000
```

We see that the variable A1 is also significant, which means that the species composition also depends on the soil thickness. The advantage of including the variable A1 in the model is that we remove the effect of soil thickness when we study management (farming). Thus, management is still significant when we control for the variable A1. We can also test if there is an interaction between A1 and management by:

```
set.seed(1) #For reproducibility
adonis2(dune ~ Management + A1 + Management:A1 , data = dune.env,
by = "terms")
# adonis2(dune ~ Management*A1 , data = dune.env) # Same as above
```

```
               Df   SumOfSqs   R2        F        Pr(>F)
Management     3    1.4686     0.34161   3.2629   0.002 **
A1             1    0.4409     0.10256   2.9387   0.013 *
Management:A1  3    0.5892     0.13705   1.3090   0.192
Residual       12   1.8004     0.41878
Total          19   4.2990     1.00000
```

We see that there is no significant interaction (p-value = 0.192), which means that the effect of management on the species composition does not depend on the variable A1 or vice versa.

9.3 Canonical Correlation Analysis

Canonical correlation analysis (CCA) is a statistical method used to explore the correlation between two sets of variables. It identifies and measures the associations between these variable sets by finding linear combinations that maximize the correlation between them. Watch the video below to learn how CCA works and how to interpret the output from such analysis.

9.3.1 Video

https://youtu.be/0F2yHftqodA
www.tilestats.com/ml/

Let's compute a CCA based on the same example as in the video where the correlation between the two blood pressure variables (systolic blood pressure and diastolic blood pressure) and the two variables that may represent body size (Weight and Height) were calculated:

```
library(CCA)
rm(list=ls()) # Clear environment
SBP=c(120,109,130,121,135,140)
DBP=c(76,80,82,78,85,87)
Weight=c(60,80,70,85,90,87)
Height=c(165,180,170,185,180,187)
data=data.frame(SBP,DBP,Height,Weight)
X=data[,c(1,2)] # Variables for blood pressure
Y=data[,c(3,4)] # Variables for body size
cc(X, Y)
$cor
[1] 0.7206701 0.1953755
...
```

We see that the correlation between the two sets of variables is computed to 0.72. The correlation between the blood pressure variables and the variables that define the body size (Weight and Height) is therefore 0.72. Note that canonical correlation coefficients cannot be negative due to the scaling created by the standardized weights in the linear equation (Sherry & Henson, 2005). The canonical correlation coefficients can therefore only take values between zero and one. Further down in the output, we can find the coefficients, or weights, that are used to combine the two blood pressure variables:

```
$xcoef
            [,1]        [,2]
SBP   0.04210423  -0.1364278
DBP  -0.31846622   0.2205200
```

and the coefficients that are used to combine Weight and Height:

```
$ycoef
               [,1]        [,2]
Height   0.05924242    0.291672
Weight  -0.12586754   -0.183518
```

By using these coefficients, the scores of the combined variables can be calculated. The scores that represent the blood pressure are the ones that are shown below:

```
$scores
$scores$xscores
            [,1]        [,2]
[1,]  1.4528785 -0.38027806
[2,] -0.2841330  2.00250715
[3,] -0.0368765 -0.42143564
[4,]  0.8580503 -0.07566583
[5,] -0.7817540 -0.44201442
[6,] -1.2081652 -0.68311320
```

whereas the scores that represent the body size are shown below:

```
$scores$yscores
            [,1]        [,2]
[1,]  1.58924976 -0.3174559
[2,] -0.03946482  0.3872655
[3,]  0.62678643 -0.6942753
[4,] -0.37259044  0.9280359
[5,] -1.29814024 -1.4479141
[6,] -0.50584069  1.1443440
```

For example, if we would extract these scores and compute the correlation between these:

```
Blood_pressure_scores=cc(X, Y)$scores$xscores[,1]
Body_size_scores=cc(X, Y)$scores$yscores[,1]
cor(Blood_pressure_scores,Body_size_scores)
0.7206701
```

we would obtain the exact same canonical correlation coefficient that is shown at the beginning of the output.

The correlation coefficients in Fig. 9.5 are the ones that are shown below from the output:

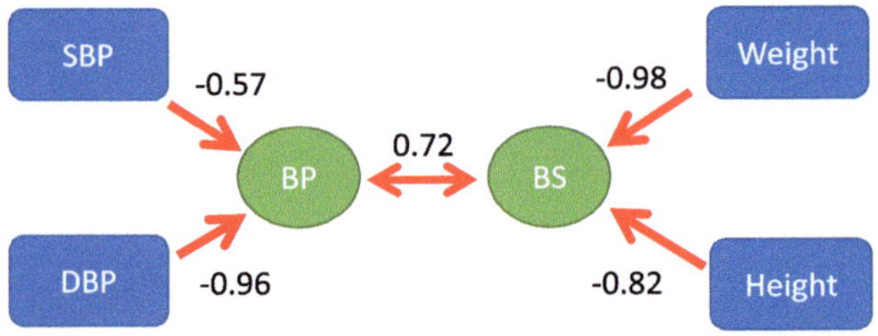

Fig. 9.5 An illustration of the results from a CCA, which shows the correlation between the individual variables and the variates blood pressure (BP; the combination of SBP and DBP) and body size (BS; the combination of Weight and Height). The correlation between the two sets of variables is 0.72

```
$scores$corr.X.xscores
          [,1]        [,2]
SBP   -0.5692857  -0.8221398
DBP   -0.9555297  -0.2948949

$scores$corr.Y.xscores
            [,1]        [,2]
Height  -0.5943171   0.11050631
Weight  -0.7062492   0.03888925

$scores$corr.X.yscores
        [,1]        [,2]
SBP  -0.4102672  -0.16062598
DBP  -0.6886217  -0.05761524

$scores$corr.Y.yscores
          [,1]        [,2]
Height  -0.8246730  0.5656098
Weight  -0.9799896  0.1990487
```

The main interest in this output is usually the correlation coefficient between the two sets of variables at the beginning of the output, which was about 0.72. One way to test if this coefficient is significant is to compute a permutation test. This can be done with the "p.perm" function in the **CCP** package. The advantage of permutation tests is that they do not rely on any assumptions about the underlying distribution. To compute the p-value of the canonical correlation coefficient, we can run the following code:

```
library(CCP)
p.perm.out=p.perm(X, Y, nboot = 1000, type = "Pillai")
plt.perm(p.perm.out)
```

Which will give the plot in Fig. 9.6.

The Pillai's test statistic on the original data was computed to 0.558 (the red dotted line in Fig. 9.6). By using permutations, we use resampling of the original data and compute Pillai's test statistic based on the permuted data. Out of the 1000 permutations, 764 (or 76.4%) resulted in a larger Pillai's test statistic than 0.558 from our original data. Our p-value is therefore 0.764 (Fig. 9.6). Thus, our canonical correlation coefficient of 0.72 is not significant, which is due to the small sample size in this example.

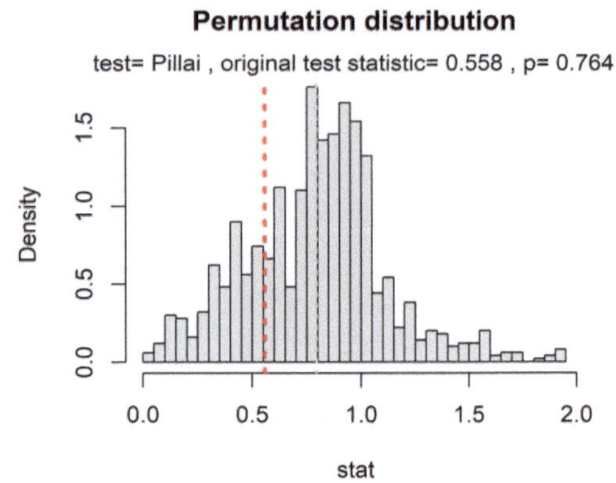

Fig. 9.6 A histogram of the Pillai's test statistics generated from 1000 permutations

9.4 Exercises

1. Use MANOVA on the Crab dataset to test if there is a difference in the means of the numerical variables between male and female crabs. Run t-tests on the individual variables if you reject the null hypothesis.
2. Do you fulfill the assumptions for MANOVA?
3. Compute a PERMANOVA on the Crab dataset, using the Euclidean distance, to test if there is a difference in the numerical variables between male and female crabs. Standardize the continuous variables before you run the PERMANOVA and run 9999 permutations.
4. Run the same PERMANOVA as in the previous question but use both sex and species as independent variables to test if there is a significant interaction between sex and species.
5. In the Iris dataset, we can think of the petal length and petal width as representing the petal size, whereas sepal length and sepal width can be considered as the sepal size of the flowers. Compute the canonical correlation coefficient between petal size and sepal size, using the Iris dataset. Also, compute a p-value by a permutation test.

References

Anderson, M. J., & Walsh, D. C. (2013). PERMANOVA, ANOSIM, and the Mantel test in the face of heterogeneous dispersions: what null hypothesis are you testing? *Ecological Monographs, 83*(4), 557–574.

Navarro, J. A. (2016). *Multivariate statistical methods: A primer*. Chapman and Hall/CRC.

Sherry, A., & Henson, R. K. (2005). Conducting and interpreting canonical correlation analysis in personality research: A user-friendly primer. *Journal of Personality Assessment, 84*(1), 37–48.

Chapter 10
Classification and Performance Metrics

This chapter introduces different performance metrics for clinical tests. We will in Chap. 11 use the same metrics to quantify the success of predictive ML models. We will begin with metrics like sensitivity and specificity, which are especially important in domains like healthcare, where false negatives or false positives may have important consequences. Next, we will explore the receiver operating characteristic (ROC) curve, which provides a graphical representation to determine an appropriate cutoff value and can be used to assess the performance of the test. Finally, we will discuss the concept of validation, which is an essential step to ensure that a clinical test generalizes well to unseen data.

10.1 Diagnostic Metrics

To determine the performance of a clinical test, or how good an ML model predicts, there is a range of different metrics. The most basic metrics involve sensitivity, specificity, and accuracy. Sensitivity measures the test's ability to correctly identify individuals with a disease, whereas specificity measures the test's ability to correctly identify individuals who do not have the disease. Watch the videos below to learn how to calculate the sensitivity and specificity, and how to calculate and interpret other metrics such as the likelihood ratio, the positive predictive value (PPV), and the negative predictive value (NPV).

10.1.1 Videos

https://youtu.be/T8PwFgz1-uo
https://youtu.be/QaP3U09SfCM

A. Tilevik, *Multivariate Statistics and Machine Learning in R For Beginners*, https://doi.org/10.1007/978-3-032-01851-9_10

https://youtu.be/A23Hn2gTPQM
www.tilestats.com/ml/

We will first calculate the sensitivity and specificity based on a small dataset. One biomarker to distinguish between healthy subjects and subjects with prostate cancer is the prostate-specific antigen (PSA). Let's say that we have measured the PSA level of 14 subjects, where we know that seven of these subjects are healthy and that the other seven subjects have prostate cancer. A prostate biopsy has been performed to determine whether the subjects have prostate cancer or not. The PSA levels in prostate cancer subjects and healthy subjects are shown in Table 10.1.

Let's enter the data in R:

```
rm(list=ls()) # Clear environment
C=c(3.8, 3.4, 2.9, 2.8, 2.7, 2.1, 1.6) # Cancer
H=c(2.5, 2.0, 1.7, 1.4, 1.2, 0.9, 0.8) # Healthy
PSA=c(C,H)
Group=factor(rep(c("Cancer","Healthy"),c(7,7)),
levels=c("Healthy","Cancer"))
df=data.frame(Group,PSA)
```

Note that, when we create the grouping factor that defines if a person is healthy or has the disease, we should always set the healthy group as our baseline, which means that the category "Healthy" should always come first. This explains why we use the argument "levels" where we tell R that "Healthy" should be our first category. Per default, R puts the categories in alphabetic order, which means that we need to change the order in this case. If we print the variable "Group":

```
Group
Cancer  Cancer  Cancer  Cancer  Cancer  Cancer  Cancer
Healthy Healthy .....
Levels: Healthy Cancer
```

we see that the row "Levels" now tells us that the category "Healthy" is first, which is exactly what we want. Try and change the order of the categories in the code above and make sure you understand the meaning of the argument "levels". Before you move on, make sure that "Healthy" is your first category. Let's plot the data:

Table 10.1 Example data of PSA levels from 14 individuals

Prostate cancer	NO	NO	NO	NO	NO	NO	NO	YES	YES	YES	YES	YES	YES	YES
PSA level (μg/L)	2.5	2.0	1.7	1.4	1.2	0.9	0.8	3.8	3.4	2.9	2.8	2.7	2.1	1.6

```
stripchart(PSA~Group,data=df,ylim=c(0,4),ylab=c("PSA (µg/L)"),
vertical = T,xlim=c(0.7,2.3) , las=1)
# Add a vertical (v) line in the plot so it looks nicer
abline(v=1.5)
```

We would now like to find a threshold, or cutoff value, that can be used to determine if a patient has prostate cancer or not based on a simple PSA measurement. By studying Fig. 10.1, it seems like an appropriate threshold value is 2.3 µg/L. Let's place a horizontal line in the figure for this cutoff value:

```
# Place a line that represents the cutoff value (2.3 µg/L)
abline(h=2.3,lty=2,col="red")
```

We could now use this cutoff value to predict if a new patient has prostate cancer or not. However, how accurate is such a threshold value? From Fig. 10.2, we see that using such a threshold level on subjects that are known to be healthy or are diagnosed with prostate cancer (e.g., determined by biopsy of the prostate), we misclassify three subjects. One healthy patient is incorrectly classified as having prostate

Fig. 10.1 A one-dimensional scatter plot of the PSA levels of the 14 individuals

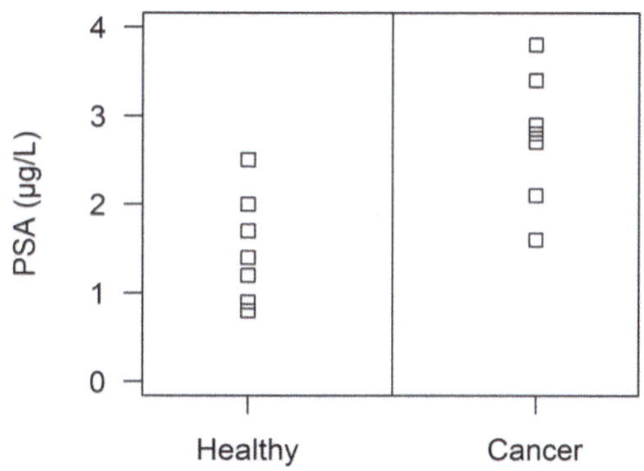

Fig. 10.2 A one-dimensional scatter plot of the PSA levels of the 14 individuals, showing a cutoff line at 2.3

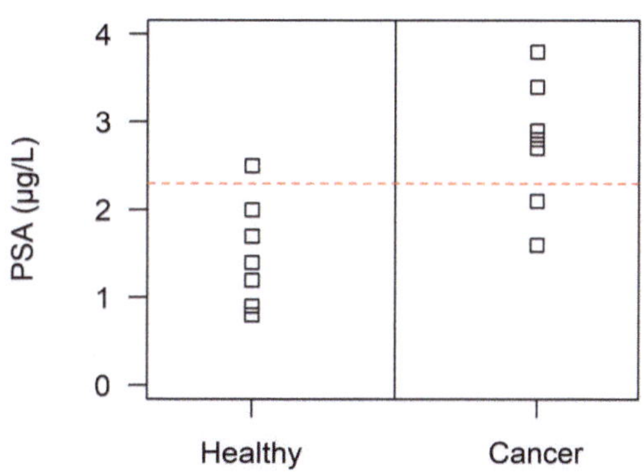

cancer, whereas two subjects with prostate cancer are incorrectly classified as being healthy. Thus, we have four possible outcomes:

TP (true positives): Number of prostate cancer patients predicted as having prostate cancer
TN (true negatives): Number of healthy subjects predicted as being healthy
FP (false positives): Number of healthy subjects **incorrectly** predicted as having prostate cancer
FN (false negatives): Number of prostate cancer patients **incorrectly** predicted as being healthy

10.1.2 The Confusion Matrix

We will now compute a confusion matrix in R. To create such a table, we need a vector that defines how each individual is classified according to the cutoff value. We can use the function "ifelse" to assign the predicted class of the individuals based on whether their PSA levels are greater or less than 2.3 (above or below the cutoff line) and add these predictions to the data frame:

```
pred=factor(ifelse(df$PSA<2.3,"Healthy","Cancer"),
levels=c("Healthy","Cancer"))
df$pred=pred # Add predicted class to the data frame
df
     Group      PSA      pred
1    Cancer     3.8      Cancer
2    Cancer     3.4      Cancer
3    Cancer     2.9      Cancer
4    Cancer     2.8      Cancer
5    Cancer     2.7      Cancer
6    Cancer     2.1      Healthy
7    Cancer     1.6      Healthy
8    Healthy    2.5      Cancer
9    Healthy    2.0      Healthy
10   Healthy    1.7      Healthy
11   Healthy    1.4      Healthy
12   Healthy    1.2      Healthy
13   Healthy    0.9      Healthy
14   Healthy    0.8      Healthy
```

We can generate a table, a confusion matrix, of the two vectors by using the function "table":

```
tab = table(pred,Group)
tab
               Group
pred      Healthy    Cancer
  Healthy       6         2
  Cancer        1         5
```

where the rows represent the predicted class and the columns the actual class. Let's calculate the TP, TN, FN, and FP:

```
TP=tab[2,2] # True positive
FP=tab[2,1] # False positive
TN=tab[1,1] # True negative
FN=tab[1,2] # False negative
# Print the values with the corresponding labels
print(c(TP=TP,FP=FP,TN=TN,FN=FN))
TP FP TN FN
5  1  6  2
```

We can now calculate the metrics for the predicted performance of our cut-off value:

```
Sensitivity=TP/(TP+FN)
Sensitivity
0.7142857

Specificity=TN/(TN+FP)
Specificity
0.8571429

Accuracy=(TP+TN)/(TP+TN+FP+FN) # or sum(diag(tab))/sum(tab)
Accuracy
0.7857143

pLR=Sensitivity/(1-Specificity) # Positive likelihood ratio
pLR
5

nLR=(1-Sensitivity)/Specificity # Negative likelihood ratio
nLR
0.3333333

# Prevalence in sample = % of cancer patients
Prevalence=(TP+FN)/(TP+FN+FP+TN)
Prevalence
```

```
0.5
# Positive predictive value
PPV=(Sensitivity*Prevalence)/
((Sensitivity*Prevalence)+(1-Specificity)*(1-Prevalence))
PPV
0.8333333
# Negative predictive value
NPV=(Specificity*(1-Prevalence))/(((1-Sensitivity)*Prevalence)
+Specificity*(1-Prevalence))
NPV
0.75
```

We can compute the same metrics and much more with the function "confusionMatrix" from the **caret** package. Note that we need to state which of the categories that are defined as a "positive" result. In most cases, this is the disease category, which is why we set the argument "positive" to "Cancer":

```
library(caret)
confusionMatrix(data=pred,reference=Group, positive="Cancer")
Reference
Prediction   Healthy   Cancer
   Healthy      6         2
   Cancer       1         5

               Accuracy : 0.7857
                 95% CI : (0.492, 0.9534)
    No Information Rate : 0.5
    P-Value [Acc > NIR] : 0.02869

                  Kappa : 0.5714
 Mcnemar's Test P-Value : 1.00000

            Sensitivity : 0.7143
            Specificity : 0.8571
         Pos Pred Value : 0.8333
         Neg Pred Value : 0.7500
             Prevalence : 0.5000
         Detection Rate : 0.3571
   Detection Prevalence : 0.4286
      Balanced Accuracy : 0.7857

       'Positive' Class : Cancer
```

We see that the accuracy is 78.57% and that its 95% confidence interval spans between 0.492 and 0.9534. We can also see that a p-value has been computed (P-Value [Acc > NIR]: 0.02869). This p-value has been computed to test whether the accuracy (Acc) is significantly greater than the no information rate (NIR). The NIR corresponds to the accuracy you would achieve by always predicting the majority class. Since we have a balanced dataset with seven individuals in each group, one would correctly predict prostate cancer in 50% of the cases. Since the p-value is less than the general significance level of 0.05, we may conclude, given the cutoff value, that the accuracy is significantly larger than 50% (it is significantly better than what we would achieve by always predicting the majority class).

In addition to the accuracy, Kappa (or Cohen's Kappa) is another measure that is used in classification. Kappa measures the agreement between the predicted groups and the true groups, adjusted for the agreement that could occur by chance. It is given by:

$$\kappa = \frac{P_o - P_e}{1 - P_e} = \frac{0.7857 - 0.5}{1 - 0.5} = 0.5714$$

where P_o is the observed agreement (accuracy) and P_e is the expected agreement by chance, which is 0.5 in this example because there is a 50% chance to correctly predict prostate cancer since we have 7 individuals in each group. Kappa is especially appropriate to use in cases where we have an imbalanced dataset where the classes are not evenly distributed, which provides a better measure of the true performance compared to the accuracy. The value of Kappa spans between zero and one, where a value of zero indicates that a clinical test (or a model) is not better than chance where one always guesses the majority class. A value close to one would imply that the clinical test performs well beyond random chance.

10.1.3 Prior Probability and PPV

Using a cutoff level of 2.3 results in a sensitivity of 71% and a specificity of 86%. For our study, we selected the same sample size for the two groups. However, let's say that out of the ones testing for prostate cancer in a certain population, we know from previous studies that 90% are healthy and 10% have prostate cancer. Thus, our prior probabilities are then 0.9 and 0.1. We can calculate the PPV and NPV with the same code as before but where we now set the prevalence to 0.1:

```
Prevalence=0.1
PPV=(Sensitivity*Prevalence)/
((Sensitivity*Prevalence)+(1-Specificity)*(1-Prevalence))
PPV
0.3571429
```

```
NPV=(Specificity*(1-Prevalence))/(((1-Sensitivity)*Prevalence)
+Specificity*(1-Prevalence))
NPV
0.9642857
```

We can compute the same values by setting the argument "prevalence" to 0.1 in the function "confusionMatrix":

```
library(caret)
confusionMatrix(data=pred,reference=Group, positive="Cancer",
prevalence=0.1)
...
            Sensitivity : 0.7143
            Specificity : 0.8571
         Pos Pred Value : 0.3571
         Neg Pred Value : 0.9643
...
```

From the video about the positive and negative predictive value, we know that the PPV is reduced when the prevalence is reduced. In contrast, a reduced prevalence increases the NPV. When a disease is rare in the population, a negative test result is more likely to be a true negative rather than a false negative.

10.1.4 Using Another Cutoff Value

All our previous calculations were done based on the cutoff value of 2.3 µg/L. However, all the metrics will change if we change the cutoff value. Let's say that we want to increase the sensitivity because we might think that it is really important to identify all individuals with prostate cancer with our PSA test. We can then simply reduce the cutoff value to, for example, 1.5 µg/L:

```
stripchart(PSA~Group,data=df,ylim=c(0,4),
ylab=c("PSA (µg/L)"),vertical = T, xlim=c(0.7,2.3) ,las=1)
# Add a vertical (v) line in the plot so it looks nicer.
abline(v=1.5)
# horizontal (h) line = cutoff value
abline(h=1.5,lty=2,col="red")
```

With this low cutoff value (Fig. 10.3), we will get 100% sensitivity since all prostate cancer patients are classified as having prostate cancer because all data points of the cancer patients are now above the cutoff line. However, a reduced cutoff value will reduce the specificity to about 57%. Note that 100% sensitivity only

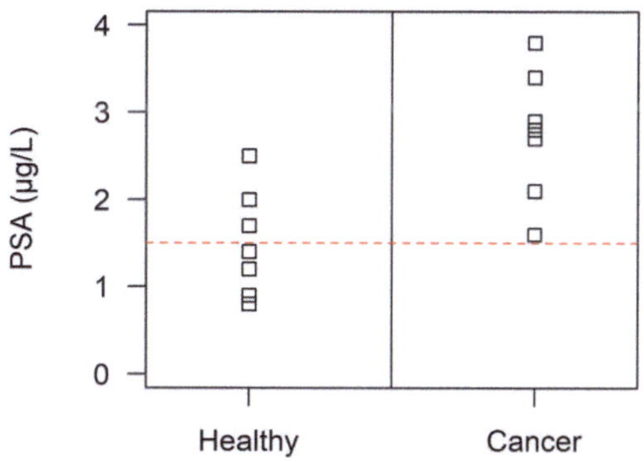

Fig. 10.3 A one-dimensional scatter plot of the PSA levels of the 14 individuals, showing a cutoff line at 1.5

accounts for our sample. If we would use this cutoff value for a new set of data including hundreds of individuals, then a few prostate cancer patients will for sure have a lower PSA level than 1.5 µg/L. We will later see how to validate our classifier that gives a better prediction of the true accuracy. Let's compute the confusion matrix based on a cutoff value of 1.5:

```
cutoff=1.5
pred=factor(ifelse(PSA<cutoff,"Healthy","Cancer"),
levels=c("Healthy","Cancer"))
confusionMatrix(data=pred,reference=Group,positive="Cancer")
                 Reference
Prediction       Healthy     Cancer
   Healthy          4           0
   Cancer           3           7
....
               Accuracy : 0.7857
...
            Sensitivity : 1.0000
            Specificity : 0.5714
...
```

We see that the accuracy is still the same since we still misclassify three individuals. Sensitivity is now 100%, whereas the specificity has been reduced to 57%.

10.2 Exercises

1. Make a one-dimensional scatter plot of the variable body depth (BD) from the Crab data where you separate the two colors (Blue (B) and Orange (O)). Place a cutoff line at 11 and use jittering so that you can see all the data points.

2. Based on the plot you have generated, with the cutoff value of 11, how many false negatives do you have, given that you set the color **blue** as the baseline category (orange is therefore considered as a positive case)?
3. Based on the same data and the cutoff value as in the previous question, compute sensitivity, specificity, PPV, and NPV.

10.3 ROC Curve

We will here have a look at the so-called receiver operating characteristic (ROC) curve, which can be used to find an appropriate cutoff value, given a certain sensitivity and specificity. ROC curves are also commonly used to compare how well different biomarkers (or ML models) perform. Watch the video below to learn how to interpret the ROC curve and how the area under the ROC curve is calculated.

10.3.1 Video

https://youtu.be/GNxpv0Ha_G8
www.tilestats.com/ml/

The ROC curve represents the calculated specificity and sensitivity for different cutoff values. Let's first enter the same data that we have used previously, which was also used in the video:

```
rm(list=ls()) # Clear environment
C=c(3.8, 3.4, 2.9, 2.8, 2.7, 2.1, 1.6) # Cancer
H=c(2.5, 2.0, 1.7, 1.4, 1.2, 0.9, 0.8) # Healthy
PSA=c(C,H)
Group=factor(rep(c("Cancer","Healthy"),c(7,7)) ,
levels=c("Healthy","Cancer"))
df=data.frame(Group,PSA)
```

We will here use the **pROC** package to generate an ROC curve with the function "roc":

```
library(pROC)
roc1=roc(Group, PSA)
Setting levels: control = Healthy, case = Cancer
Setting direction: controls < cases
```

Note that the output tells us that the “Healthy” category has been set as the “control” and the category “cancer” has been set as the “case”. This is exactly what we want because the category healthy should be our baseline. To generate a nice printout of the different sensitivities and specificities for given cutoff values, we can print the output as a data frame:

```
data.frame(roc1$thresholds,roc1$sensitivities,
roc1$specificities)
      roc1.thresholds     roc1.sensitivities     roc1.specificities
1          -Inf                1.0000000               0.0000000
2          0.85                1.0000000               0.1428571
3          1.05                1.0000000               0.2857143
4          1.30                1.0000000               0.4285714
5          1.50                1.0000000               0.5714286
6          1.65                0.8571429               0.5714286
7          1.85                0.8571429               0.7142857
8          2.05                0.8571429               0.8571429
9          2.30                0.7142857               0.8571429
10         2.60                0.7142857               1.0000000
11         2.75                0.5714286               1.0000000
12         2.85                0.4285714               1.0000000
13         3.15                0.2857143               1.0000000
14         3.60                0.1428571               1.0000000
15         Inf                 0.0000000               1.0000000
```

From this output, we can see how different cutoff values affect sensitivity and specificity. If we think that sensitivity and specificity are equally important, an appropriate threshold value seems to be at a PSA level of 2.05 µg/L. If we like to have 100% sensitivity for the test, a threshold value of 1.5 µg/L could be used, although this cutoff reduces the specificity to 57%. However, note that these results only account for our sample and that we need to validate the sensitivity and specificity for a given threshold with test data or by using cross-validation which we will do later on. Let’s generate an ROC curve, which is simply a curve representing the values in the two columns above for sensitivity and specificity:

```
plot(roc1)
```

The thin diagonal line is our reference line (Fig. 10.4). The thick curve represents the ROC curve. What we want is an ROC curve that is approaching the top-left corner so that our clinical test has as high sensitivity and specificity as possible. If the two groups show weak separation (the values from the two groups are completely mixed), then the ROC curve will be close to the reference line.

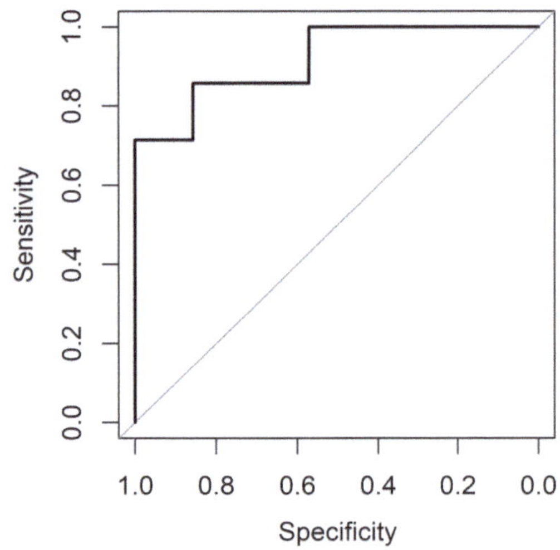

Fig. 10.4 An ROC curve illustrating the performance of PSA to discriminate the healthy controls from patients with prostate cancer. The x-axis represents the specificity, and the y-axis represents the sensitivity for different cutoff values

10.3.2 Optimal Cutoff Value

The package **pROC** includes a function that can help us to select the optimal cutoff value. One such measure is the Youden Index, which selects the cutoff value that maximizes the sum of sensitivity and specificity:

$$J = Sensitivity + Specificity - 1$$

The cutoff values that maximize the above sum are 2.6 and 2.05. By using the function "coords", we can extract the best cutoff according to the Youden Index:

```
coords(roc1,"best", best.method="youden",transpose = FALSE)
  threshold      specificity     sensitivity
  2.6000000      1.0000000       0.7142857
```

Note that the function only reports one threshold, 2.6. Read the documentation of the "coord" function for more information. Another measure is the cutoff value that is closest to the top-left corner of the ROC curve, which can be obtained by finding the cutoff value that results in the minimum value of the following calculation:

$$(1 - Sensitivity)^2 + (1 - Specificity)^2$$

The cutoff value that is closest to the top-left corner is 2.05:

```
coords(roc1, "best", best.method="closest.topleft",
transpose = FALSE)
  threshold         specificity     sensitivity
  2.0500000         0.8571429       0.8571429
```

10.3.3 PPV and NPV

If we know the prevalence of the disease in the population where the PSA test will be used, we can also calculate the PPV and NPV for different cutoff values. Let's say that we know, from earlier studies, that the prevalence of prostate cancer for the ones who will do the test is estimated to be 1%, then the PPV and NPV for the different cutoffs can be calculated by:

```
Prevalence=0.01
Sensitivity=roc1$sensitivities
Specificity=roc1$specificities
PPV=(Sensitivity*Prevalence)/
((Sensitivity*Prevalence)+(1-Specificity)*(1-Prevalence))
NPV=(Specificity*(1-Prevalence))/(((1-Sensitivity)*Prevalence)
+Specificity*(1-Prevalence))
data.frame(roc1$thresholds,PPV,NPV,Sensitivity,
Specificity) # Print
   roc1.thresholds        PPV       NPV  Sensitivity  Specificity
1             -Inf 0.01000000       NaN    1.0000000    0.0000000
2             0.85 0.01164725 1.0000000    1.0000000    0.1428571
3             1.05 0.01394422 1.0000000    1.0000000    0.2857143
4             1.30 0.01736973 1.0000000    1.0000000    0.4285714
5             1.50 0.02302632 1.0000000    1.0000000    0.5714286
6             1.65 0.01980198 0.9974811    0.8571429    0.5714286
7             1.85 0.02941176 0.9979839    0.8571429    0.7142857
8             2.05 0.05714286 0.9983193    0.8571429    0.8571429
9             2.30 0.04807692 0.9966443    0.7142857    0.8571429
10            2.60 1.00000000 0.9971223    0.7142857    1.0000000
11            2.75 1.00000000 0.9956897    0.5714286    1.0000000
12            2.85 1.00000000 0.9942611    0.4285714    1.0000000
13            3.15 1.00000000 0.9928367    0.2857143    1.0000000
14            3.60 1.00000000 0.9914163    0.1428571    1.0000000
15             Inf        NaN 0.9900000    0.0000000    1.0000000
```

In addition to the sensitivity and specificity, this table now shows the PPV and the NPV, given a prevalence of 1%. For example, a cutoff value of 2.05 results in a PPV of only 5.7%, whereas the NPV is 99.8%. Since we have a small sample size in this example, the values vary quite much for each cutoff value. A cutoff value of 2.6 suddenly increases the PPV from about 5% to 100% because such a cutoff value results in a 100% specificity, which causes a dramatic change in the calculation of the PPV due to the small sample size.

10.3.4 The Area Under the ROC Curve

The area under the ROC curve (AUC) is an important measure of how well a test performs. The AUC can vary between one and zero. The area below the reference line is exactly 0.5. What we want is an area that is close to one and at least significantly different from 0.5 (the area below the reference line). We can extract the area under the ROC curve from the output by:

```
roc1$auc
Area under the curve: 0.9184
```

We can generate a 95% CI for the AUC by:

```
ci.auc(roc1)
95% CI: 0.7723-1 (DeLong)
```

We see that the 95% confidence interval does not include the value of 0.5. Hence, we can conclude that the AUC value is significantly greater than 0.5. It is also possible to compute a p-value based on a Mann-Whitney U test. Let's compute a two-sided Mann-Whitney U test to check if our AUC is significantly different from 0.5:

```
wilcox.test(PSA~Group, exact=FALSE, correct=FALSE)
     data:  PSA by Group
W = 4, p-value = 0.008809
```

We see that the p-value is less than 0.05. Since we know that the AUC is larger than 0.5, we can conclude that the area is significantly greater than 0.5.

10.3.5 Comparing ROC Curves

If your dataset includes several variables, you might want to plot an ROC curve for each of the variables and possibly compare such ROC curves. As an example, we will here use the Iris dataset where we only focus on the classes Versicolor and Virginica. We will plot an ROC curve for the petal width and the sepal width. From Fig. 10.5, we can see that Versicolor is more separated from Virginica based on the petal width compared to the sepal width.

Let's first prepare the data where we extract only Versicolors and Virginicas:

```
rm(list=ls()) # Clear environment
# Extract Versicolor and Virginica
Iris=subset(iris,Species=="versicolor"|Species=="virginica")
# Set Species as a factor with two levels
Iris$Species=factor(Iris$Species)
```

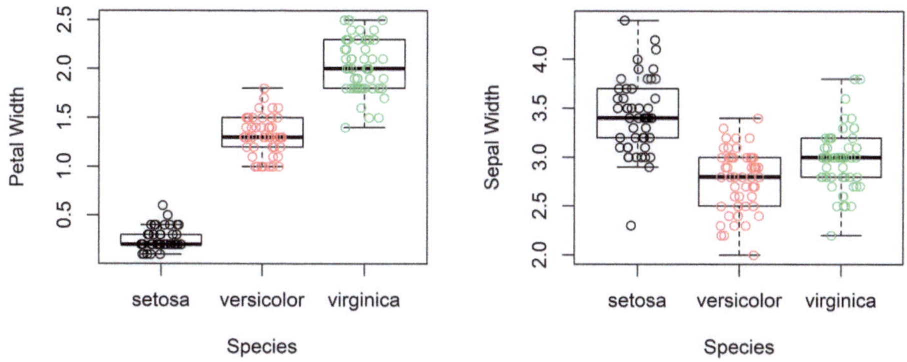

Fig. 10.5 Boxplots combined with one-dimensional scatter plots of the petal width and sepal width of the Iris dataset

Fig. 10.6 ROC curves illustrating the performance of petal width and sepal width to discriminate between the species Versicolor and Virginica in the Iris dataset

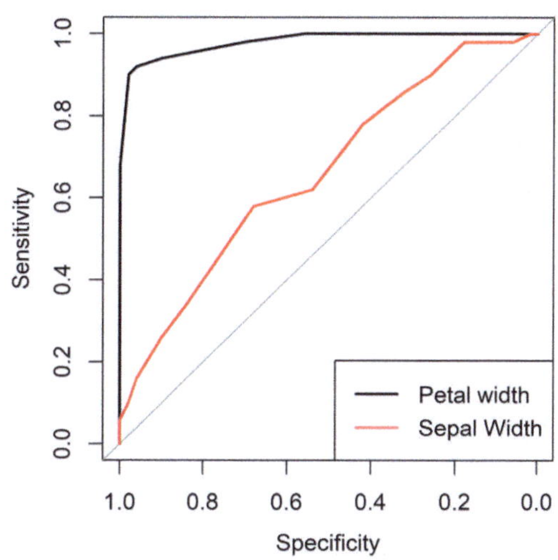

We then plot one ROC curve for the petal width and one curve for the sepal width (Fig. 10.6):

```
(roc1=roc(Iris$Species,Iris$Petal.Width))
…
0.9804

plot(roc1)
(roc2=roc(Iris$Species,Iris$Sepal.Width))
…
0.6636
lines(roc2,col="red")
legend("bottomright",c("Petal width","Sepal Width"),
col=1:2,lty=1,lwd=2)
```

The AUC value for the petal width is 0.98, whereas the AUC value for the sepal width is only 0.66. By using the function "roc.test", we can test if there is a significant difference in AUC between the two curves. Since the two ROC curves are built on variables from the same sample (repeated measures on the same flower), we set the argument "paired" to true:

```
roc.test(roc1,roc2, paired=TRUE)
DeLong's test for two correlated ROC curves
data:  roc1 and roc2
Z = 6.2869, p-value = 3.238e-10
alternative hypothesis: true difference in AUC is not
equal to 0
sample estimates:
AUC of roc1    AUC of roc2
  0.9804         0.6636
```

Since the p-value is less than the general significance level of 0.05, we can conclude that the AUC is significantly larger for the petal width compared to the sepal width.

10.4 Exercises

1. Use the variable body depth (BD) from the Crab dataset to classify the two-color forms (Blue (B) and Orange (O)). Generate an ROC curve of the data and compute the AUC.
2. Calculate the 95% confidence interval of your AUC value. Is your AUC value significantly greater than 0.5?
3. Use the "youden" method to find an appropriate cutoff value. Report the cutoff value and the corresponding sensitivity and specificity based on this cutoff.
4. Create two ROC curves that represent the two variables body depth (BD) and rear width (RW) in the same plot. Use the function "roc.test" to test if there is a significant difference in AUC between the two curves.

10.5 Validation

In this section, we will discuss only the basics of how to validate the performance of a test, or a biomarker, by using either the hold-out method or cross-validation. In the next chapter, we will use ML models to predict, which requires more advanced types of validation methods to deal with, for example, hyperparameter tuning. We will therefore discuss the hold-out method and the cross-validation in more detail in Chap. 11. Watch the video below to get an understanding of the basic validation techniques.

10.5.1 Video

https://youtu.be/JWK6riEiEfc
www.tilestats.com/ml/

We will here learn how to perform validation based on the Iris dataset. To simplify, we will here reduce this dataset so that we only have the petal length and the two species Versicolor and Virginica:

```
rm(list=ls()) # Clear environment
# Extract petal length and exclude Setosa
df=iris[iris$Species!="setosa",c(3,5)]
df$Species=factor(df$Species) # Set to two levels
stripchart(Petal.Length~Species,data=df,ylim=c(2.8,7),
method="jitter",
vertical = T,xlim=c(0.7,2.3) ,las=1)
```

To see how well a single cutoff line can separate the groups (Fig. 10.7), we can use, for example, a cutoff line based on the mean of the two group means:

```
# Calc the mean of the two means
cutoff=mean(tapply(df$Petal.Length,df$Species,mean))
abline(h=cutoff,lty=2,col="red")
```

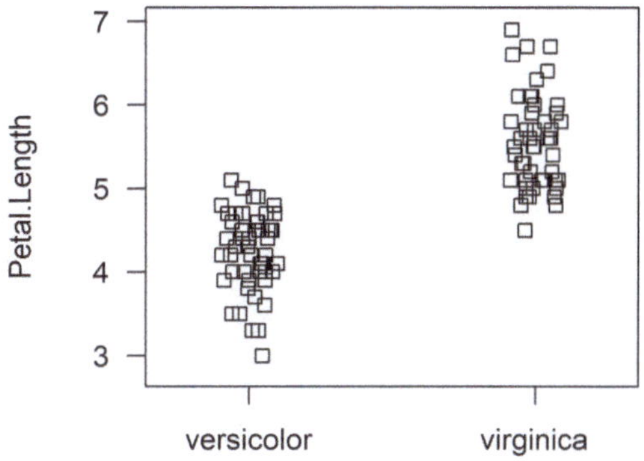

Fig. 10.7 A one-dimensional scatter plot of the petal length in the Iris dataset

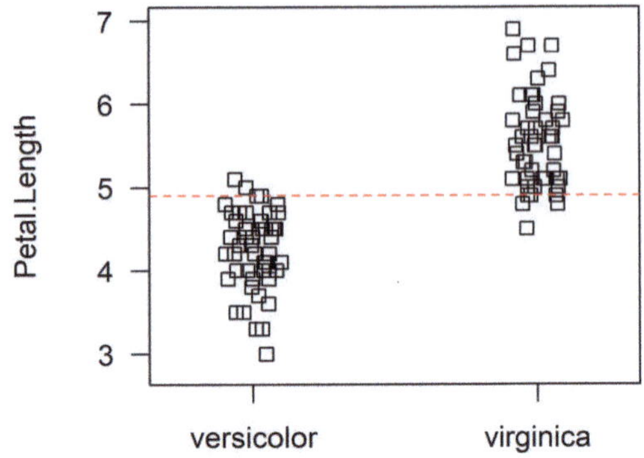

Fig. 10.8 A one-dimensional scatter plot of the petal length in the Iris dataset with a cutoff line calculated based on the mean of the two group means

If we use this cutoff (Fig. 10.8) to calculate the confusion matrix:

```
pred=factor(ifelse(df$Petal.Length<cutoff,"versicolor",
"virginica"))
CT=table(pred,df$Species)
CT
                 Species
pred             versicolor   virginica
  versicolor         48            6
  virginica          2            44
```

we see that six Virginicas are incorrectly predicted as Versicolors, whereas two Versicolors are incorrectly predicted as Virginicas.

10.5.2 Calculating the Accuracy

There are several ways we can calculate the accuracy based on the above confusion matrix (CT). One way is to sum the values in the main diagonal and divide by the sum of all flowers in the table by:

```
sum(diag(CT))/sum(CT)
0.92
```

Another way is to sum how many times the true labels (df$Species) are equal to the predicted labels (pred) in the corresponding indexes and then divide by the total number of flowers, which is the length of the vector with the predicted classes:

```
sum(df$Species==pred)/length(pred)
0.92
```

If the expression “df$Species == pred” is true, the operator returns TRUE, else it returns FALSE. Run the code below to see which flowers that are correctly predicted (TRUE):

```
df$Species==pred
```

Since TRUE is treated as 1 and FALSE as 0 in R, we can also calculate the mean of the ones (true) and zeros (false)

```
mean(df$Species==pred)
0.92
```

which can also be used to calculate the accuracy.

However, by determining the cutoff value on all data and using the same data to predict, we usually overestimate the accuracy because if we use a new dataset, our given cutoff value might not be optimal for that dataset. To get a better estimation of how well a single cutoff value can separate the groups, we need to use some sort of validation method.

10.5.3 The Hold-Out Method

The so-called hold-out method can be used to separate the data into two groups: a training group and a test group. Let’s randomly split the 100 flowers into a training group and a test group. In this example, we use 60% of the data in the training group and 40% in the test group. We can use the function “sample” to generate a random sequence in a certain range. To illustrate how this function works, we will here first generate a random sequence between 1 and 10:

```
set.seed(10) #For reproducibility
sample(1:10)
9  7  8  6  3  2 10  5  4  1
```

Before we run the function “sample”, we use the function “set.seed” with some arbitrary number. If you run these two lines of code several times, you will get the exact same random sequence every time. This is nice because you will then get the same random sequence of numbers as shown in this book. However, if you get different numbers compared to the ones above, you might be using a different R-version compared to the R-version used to generate the above numbers (I used version 4.4.2). This means that you will then not get the same results as shown in this book. Also, different versions of packages might also result in differences in outputs from this book.

To randomly select 60% of the Versicolors for the training data, we can create a sequence of random numbers between 1 and 50 because the Versicolors are located on rows 1–50 in the data frame. We also generate a sequence between 51 and 100 because all the Virginicas are located on these rows.

```
set.seed(150) #For reproducibility
ind_Versicolor=sample(1:50)
ind_Virginica=sample(51:100)
```

Then we take the first 30 numbers of these two random sequences so that we select 30 out of the 50 flowers of each species (60%):

```
ind_train=c(ind_Versicolor[1:30],ind_Virginica[1:30])
ind_train
35 46 19 17  3 20 15  7 21  8 11 29 14 42 18 27 13 34 23 10
43 30 25 33 32  6 41 24  5 50 96 56 68 66 74 61 62 97 72 59
64 87 78 88 89 71 82 99 83 90 91 63 53 51 80 75 69 84 58 93
```

The random numbers you see above will be used to select the rows of the data frame to be used in our training data:

```
train=df[ind_train,]
# Check how many flowers we have in the training data
nrow(train)
60
```

We see that we have selected 60 out of the 100 flowers for our training data. For the test data, we will select all the flowers that were not included in the training data. This can be done by simply using a minus sign in front of "ind_train":

```
test=df[-ind_train,]
nrow(test)
40
```

A simpler way to do the same thing as above is to use the function "createData-Partition" in the **caret** package. The first argument takes a vector of the outcomes, which are the species in our example. This makes sure that we select equal proportions of data points from the groups. The argument *p* sets the proportion of data that should be used as training data. If we run the code below, we will get the following numbers:

```
library(caret)
set.seed(3) #For reproducibility
ind = createDataPartition(df$Species, p = 0.6, list=FALSE)
ind
          Resample1
 [1,]         2
 [2,]         5
 [3,]         6
 [4,]         8
 [5,]         9
...
```

that we can use to extract the training data from the original data:

```
training = df[ind,]
```

For example, in the printout above, we can see that flower numbers 2, 5, 6, 8, etc. will be included in the training data. Since the numbers 1, 3, 4, 7, etc. are not included in the above sequence, these flowers will be included in the test data. We can create the test data by extracting all rows that were not included in the training data:

```
testing = df[-ind,]
```

Note that when we supply a categorical variable (df$Species) to the "createDataPartition" function, it creates a random sequence of numbers so that we get the same proportions from each group. To check if we have equal proportions of species in the two datasets, we can run:

```
table(training$Species)
versicolor  virginica
   30          30
table(testing$Species)
versicolor  virginica
   20          20
```

We will now compute an appropriate cutoff value based on the training data by, for example, calculating the mean of the two group means:

```
cutoff=mean(tapply(training$Petal.Length,
training$Species,mean))
cutoff
4.93
```

Next, we will use this cutoff value to see how well it can separate the two species based on the test dataset. According to Fig. 10.8, we know that we should predict a new flower as Virginica if the petal length is larger than the cutoff because these flowers generally have longer petals.

```
pred=factor(ifelse(testing$Petal.Length<cutoff,"versicolor",
"virginica"))
table(pred,testing$Species)
pred              versicolor    virginica
  versicolor          19            5
  virginica           1             15
sum(diag(table(pred, testing$Species)))/nrow(testing)
0.85
```

We see that the accuracy is 85% if we use the hold-out method in comparison to when we used all the data (92%). An accuracy that is based on the test data is a better estimation of the true accuracy because such data was not used to identify the most optimal cutoff value.

10.5.4 k-fold Cross-Validation

Another type of validation approach is the *k*-fold cross-validation where the data is divided into multiple subsets (folds). In each subset, the data is split into training data and test data. Data points that are included in the test data in one subset are used as training data in all other subsets. The test data in one subset is used to evaluate how well a cutoff value, determined by the training data, can separate the groups. The cross-validation is then repeated *k*-folds, where the accuracy of each subset is calculated. The accuracy will then be averaged over the *k*-fold cross-validations. *k* should be adjusted based on the sample size. A small sample size requires larger *k*s. When *k* equals the sample size, the cross-validation is called leave-one-out cross-validation (LOOCV). We will here implement the cross-validation algorithm with a simple for-loop. In every loop, we split the data into training data and test data. Then we calculate a new cutoff value based on the mean of the training data and test if the data points that were left out as a test dataset are correctly predicted given the cutoff. To illustrate how the code works, we will here set "n_fold" to 100 so that we first run the LOOCV:

```
library(caret)
set.seed(150) #For reproducibility
n_folds = 100 # Number of cross-validation folds
folds = createFolds(df$Species, k = n_folds,
returnTrain = TRUE)
```

Note that "n_folds" is here set to 100, which is equal to our sample size. Thus, we will here use the LOOCV where a single data point is set aside as the test data in each iteration. The function "createFolds" returns indices (row numbers) that should be used to extract the training dataset. For example, if we print "folds"

```
folds
$Fold001
 [1]   2   3   4   5   6   7   8   9  10  11  12  13  14  15
 16  17  18  19  20  21  22  23  24  25
[25]  26  27  28  29  30  31  32  33  34  35  36  37  38  39
40  41  42  43  44  45  46  47  48  49
[49]  50  51  52  53  54  55  56  57  58  59  60  61  62  63
64  65  66  67  68  69  70  71  72  73
[73]  74  75  76  77  78  79  80  81  82  83  84  85  86  87
88  89  90  91  92  93  94  95  96  97
[97]  98  99 100
...
```

we see that we have 100 folds, or 100 subsets, of indices. In the first subset, "$Fold001", we see that the numbers 2–100 are included. Thus, 1 is excluded in the first subset, which means that the first flower will be used in the test data, whereas all other flowers will be used in the training data. If you study "$Fold002" in the output, note that flower number 2 has been excluded and that flower number 3 has been excluded in "$Fold003" and so forth. We will now loop through each of these 100 subsets where we use the training data to calculate the cutoff based on the mean of the two group means and then use the single flower that was left out to test if it is correctly predicted or not:

```
Accuracy=NULL  # Create a vector to save accuracy
for (i in seq_along(folds)) {
  ind_train = folds[[i]] # Get the training indices

  # Split the data into training and test sets
  train = df[ind_train, ]
  test = df[-ind_train, ]

  # Calculate the cutoff and predict the test data
  cutoff=mean(tapply(train$Petal.Length,train$Species,mean))
  pred=factor(ifelse(test$Petal.Length<cutoff,"versicolor",
  "virginica"),levels = levels(df$Species))
  Accuracy[i]=sum(diag(table(pred, test$Species)))/nrow(test)
}
# Print the results
mean(Accuracy)
0.9
```

By using the LOOCV, we get an accuracy of 90%. Try and change the parameter "n_folds" to, for example, 5 and note that the function has generated 5 subsets of data. You will then run a 5-fold cross-validation where 20 data points will be used in the test dataset in each of the 5-folds.

10.6 Exercises

1. Use the hold-out method as a validation method to compute the accuracy of how well the variable body depth (BD) can classify the two-color forms (Blue (B) and Orange (O)). Use the training data (60% of the total data) to compute an appropriate cutoff value based on the ROC curve, using the Youden method. Then use the test data to see how well this cutoff value can discriminate the two groups. Calculate the accuracy.
2. Use the LOOCV to compute the accuracy of the variable body depth (BD), using all crabs, to classify the two-color forms (Blue (B) and Orange (O)), using the Youden method to determine the cutoff value in every iteration.

Chapter 11
Supervised Machine Learning

In the previous chapter, we only used one variable with a certain cutoff value to classify if a person had prostate cancer or not. When we deal with just one variable, we do not need a classification model. However, if we want to use more than one variable/feature to predict the group membership, we need some kind of method that can combine the variables in a way so that the model predicts as well as possible. In this chapter, we will have a look at different supervised machine learning (ML) models that can be used for classification. The first video of this book explains why some ML models perform better than other models due to the distribution of the data. Supervised ML is a type of ML where the model is trained on labeled data (known group membership) so that it learns how to classify new data with unknown labels. For example, if we have data on patients with a certain disease and data on similar healthy persons, we can train the model so that it can be used to predict if a new person has the disease or not. To know how well the trained model can predict new data, we usually evaluate the model with a test dataset. Before we have a look at the different ML models, we will first discuss how to validate and evaluate a model.

11.1 Validation and Evaluation

Validation and evaluation are critical steps in the development of an ML model. Validation and evaluation are distinct processes used in the development and assessment of models. Validation occurs during the model development phase and focuses on assessing the ability of the model to generalize to new data. This is typically achieved by splitting the data into training and validation data or by using techniques like cross-validation. The goal is usually to ensure that the model predicts as good as possible and at the same time make sure that it does not overfit. In contrast, evaluation takes place after the model is finalized and involves testing its

A. Tilevik, *Multivariate Statistics and Machine Learning in R For Beginners*, https://doi.org/10.1007/978-3-032-01851-9_11

performance on a completely unseen test dataset. Unlike validation, evaluation is used to predict how well the model performs in real-world scenarios, providing a final measure of its effectiveness. Although the term evaluation is commonly referred to as the final step before the model is applied in, for example, clinical settings, where its performance is tested on a final large test dataset, I will here use the term evaluation when we test the model on the test dataset. Thus, I will use the term validation when the model is validated on the validation data and the term evaluation to determine the final performance of the validated model. Without proper validation and evaluation, a model may overfit, underperform, or provide misleading results when applied to real-world scenarios. Suppose that you would do an exam. We here assume that you do not "train" on the course material before you do the exam. Your teacher may then evaluate your knowledge by using an exam with 100 questions. However, suppose that you have access to all the 100 questions with the correct answers before you do the exam. You then memorize all the correct answers before you take the exam. You would then probably get a full score on the exam. This would be referred to as overfitting because you get a full score on the exam without knowing the general content of the course. If you would take a new exam with questions that you have previously not seen, you will likely not pass the exam. To evaluate how well you know the content of the course, you should of course not see the exam before you take it. This relates to ML models, because some models, such as decision trees, can split the data so that they always result in 100% accuracy, but they will fail to predict new unseen data because they have just memorized the data without understanding general patterns. However, some models, such as LDA and logistic regression, are less prone to overfitting since they rely on a single cutoff value in comparison to, for example, decision trees. Figure 11.1 illustrates the most basic process in training an ML model. For example, suppose that you have measured variables, or features, like blood pressure, weight, sex, and concentrations of different proteins in the blood of 300 individuals (n=300). Of these individuals, 150 are known to have a certain disease, while 150 are known to be healthy. Then you train your model on all data, which means that you will optimize the parameters of the model so that the model learns how to predict if a person has the disease based on the variables in your dataset. Then you use the same data to evaluate the performance of the model. Suppose that the model correctly predicts 90% of the 300

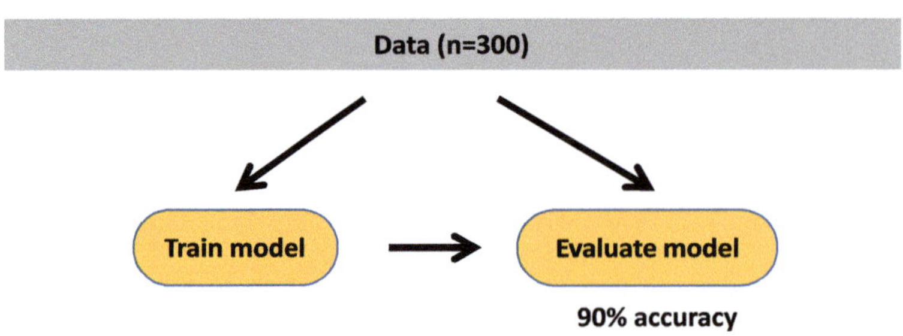

Fig. 11.1 An illustration of an example where all data is used to train a model and where the same data is used to evaluate the model

individuals as being healthy or having the disease. The accuracy of the model is therefore 90%.

This type of evaluation would be the same as the example with the exam, where the model has seen the correct answers on the exam and is evaluated on the same questions. The problem with this approach is that the model usually overfits, which means that it performs very well on the data it has been trained on but will perform worse on new unseen data. We will therefore overestimate the true performance of the model. This type of approach is common in exploratory studies where simple models, such as logistic regression, are based on a few variables because simple models are less prone to overfit. These kinds of studies require follow-up studies to evaluate the results in order to confirm if the model is useful in real-world applications.

11.1.1 The Hold-Out Method

The hold-out method is a simple and widely used technique for evaluating ML models. It involves splitting the dataset into training data and test data (Fig. 11.2). For example, our dataset with 300 individuals might be split into a training dataset with 200 individuals and a test dataset with 100 individuals. Thus, we use two-thirds of the original data to train the model, and one-third of the original data to see how well the trained model can predict if the persons in the test dataset are healthy or have the disease. Usually, one uses stratified sampling so that we get an equal proportion of healthy and diseased individuals in the training and test datasets. Suppose that 85 out of the 100 individuals in the test dataset were correctly predicted by the trained model. This will give us an accuracy of 85%.

This accuracy should reflect how well the model will perform on future data. However, only 100 individuals were used to determine the "true" performance of

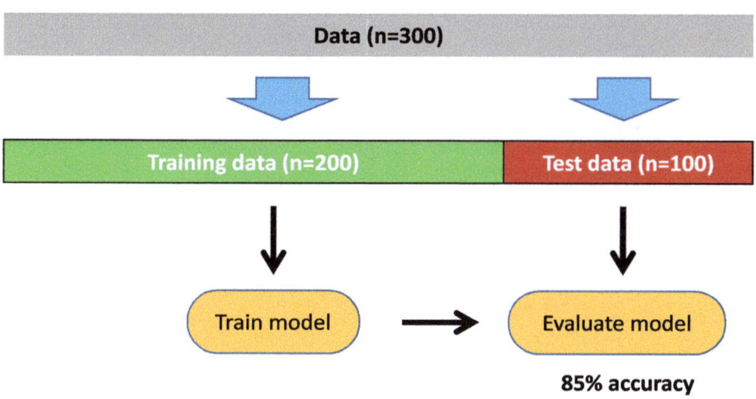

Fig. 11.2 An illustration of the hold-out method where two-thirds of the data is used to train the model and one-third is used to evaluate the model

the model. The larger the sample size we use, the better estimate of its true performance we will obtain. There is, however, a trade-off between the sample size in the two datasets. A larger sample size of the training data will allow the model to learn better, whereas a larger sample size of the test data will provide a better estimate of how well the model performs. If you have a large dataset, for example, 10,000 individuals, you might think that it is enough to use only 2000 individuals for the test dataset because that might give you a good estimate of the "true" performance. In such a case, you might use a split of 80:20. However, what do we do if we have, for example, just 100 data points (100 individuals) in our dataset? Using 20 individuals for our test data is generally too few to evaluate the model. Due to chance, the 20 individuals might differ from the individuals in the training data which might result in a very high or low accuracy. When we deal with small datasets, we should therefore consider using cross-validation.

11.1.2 k-fold Cross-Validation

k-fold cross-validation is an alternative method used to evaluate the performance of an ML model by splitting the dataset into multiple subsets (folds). Unlike the hold-out method, which uses a fixed train-test split, cross-validation iteratively trains and tests the model on different subsets of the data. In Fig. 11.3, a 3-fold cross-validation is shown because the data is divided into three subsets. The first subset is the same as the one shown in Fig. 11.2. For this subset, the model is trained based on the 200 individuals in the training data and is then evaluated based on the 100 individuals in the test data. Since the individuals in the two datasets are the same as in the hold-out method (Fig. 11.2), the accuracy, 85%, will be identical to the hold-out method.

After the accuracy has been calculated, a new subset of data is created. Half of the individuals that were used as training data in the first subset are now instead used in the test dataset, whereas the 100 individuals in the previous test dataset are now used in the training dataset together with the 100 individuals that were previously used in the training dataset. The model is now trained on the 200 individuals

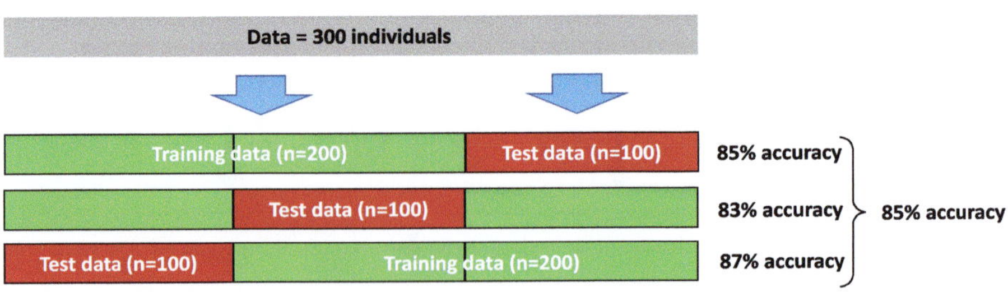

Fig. 11.3 An illustration of a 3-fold cross-validation where three subsets of data are created. Two-thirds of the data is used to train the model, and one-third is used to evaluate the model in each of the three subsets

in the training data and evaluated based on the new test dataset. Suppose that the model now results in an accuracy of 83%. Finally, the 100 individuals that were included in the training data in the first two subsets are now used in the test data, whereas the other individuals are used in the training data. Suppose that the trained model now results in an accuracy of 87%. To estimate the overall performance of the model, we can then calculate the average of the three different accuracies. The advantage of cross-validation is that we make use of all the data for both training and testing, which should give a better estimate of the accuracy of the model since it is less sensitive to which individuals that happen to end up in the test dataset, in comparison to the hold-out method, and that we use more data to estimate the performance. The disadvantage is that we will end up with three models with different estimates of their parameters. So which one should we use? One way is to retrain the model on the entire dataset to create a single final model but then we have no test data to evaluate such a model. Thus, using k-fold cross-validation on small datasets is usually only used for exploratory studies where the aim is to identify a good model that can be tested once a new larger dataset has been collected. Note that the example explained here used a 3-fold cross-validation because we have created three subsets of data. It is more common to use a 5-fold or a 10-fold cross-validation. For example, a 10-fold cross-validation means that we will create 10 subsets, where 30 individuals are used in the test dataset in each of the subsets. The mean of the accuracies from the 10 folds is then calculated. A larger fold is commonly used for smaller datasets. A special case of k-fold cross-validation that is commonly used for small datasets, typically less than 50 samples, is the leave leave-one-out cross-validation (LOOCV). Based on our example data, this would mean that we will create 300 subsets, where only one data point is used in the test dataset in each of these subsets.

11.1.3 Validation

In the previous examples, only one model has been trained based on the training data. Often, we usually like to try a range of different models and select the one that performs best. Although it is tempting to select the model that performs best based on the test data, that may actually result in misleading results. Suppose that you would train 1000 different models based on the training data. Then, just by chance, one of these models might perform very well on the test data. This is related to overfitting because we perform model selection based on the test dataset. Generally, the test data should only be used once we have found the best model that we like to evaluate and should not be used during the training process. To compare different models, one should instead use a so-called validation dataset. So, what do I mean with different models? Well, in this chapter you will learn about different ML models, such as LDA, logistic regression, and decision trees. We could, for example, train these different ML models on the same training data and select the one that performs best on the validation data. Finally, we evaluate this best model based on the test dataset. We may also have different models based on the same ML method. Generally, a model that is trained on many variables in the training data will result in a better training performance than a model based on fewer variables. However, a model based on fewer variables that actually are meaningful to predict the outcome may perform better on the validation data compared to a model trained on many variables because such a model may have picked up more noise from redundant variables in the dataset. For example, we may create two models with logistic regression, model 1 and model 2 (Fig. 11.4). These two models are then trained on the 100 individuals in the training data. Model 1 may include all variables in the training dataset, whereas model 2 may include fewer variables that were selected based on how well they separated the groups from, for example, a univariate analysis. We then use the validation data to validate these two competing models. Suppose that model 1 results in an accuracy of 79%, whereas model 2 results in an accuracy of 86%.

Since model 2 shows a higher accuracy in discriminating healthy individuals from individuals with the disease based on the validation data, we select model 2. We then retrain model 2, the best model, on the final training data that merges the previous training data with the validation data. The retrained best model is then evaluated based on the test data, which here happens to result in an accuracy of 85%. One problem with this method is that the split of the data into training and validation data may result in a bias when we have a small sample size. Due to chance, the individuals that are randomly assigned to the validation data may differ a lot from the ones that are assigned to the training data. It is therefore common to

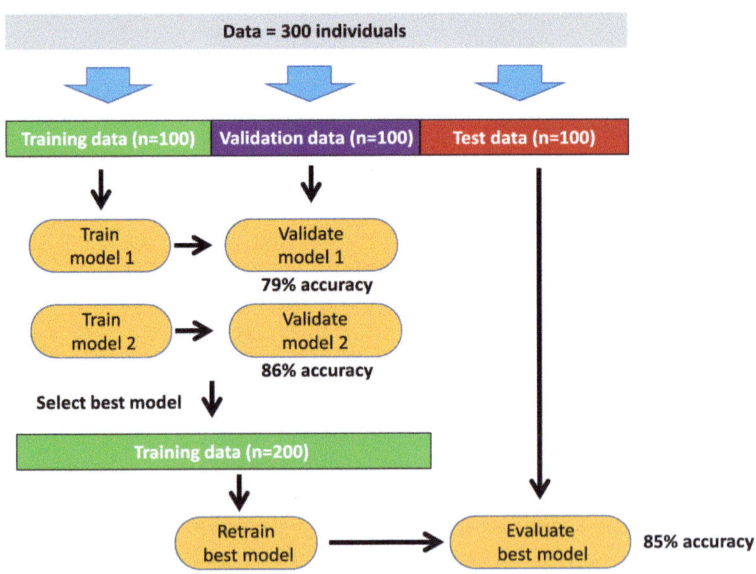

Fig. 11.4 An illustration of how to compare different models using validation data where the model that performs best on the validation data is selected to be retrained on the full training data and then evaluated based on the test data

instead perform k-fold cross-validation of the training data and the validation data (Fig. 11.5). To illustrate how this works, we will here use a 2-fold cross-validation although a 5-fold or a 10-fold cross-validation is more commonly used.

Models 1 and 2 are here validated based on two subsets of data. For example, the average accuracy of model 1 based on the two validation datasets is 80% ((0.79+0.81)/2), whereas model 2 results in an average accuracy of 85% ((0.86+0.84)/2). Since model 2 performs best, it is selected as the best model and retrained on the training data with 200 individuals—the combination of the validation data and the training data. The retrained best model is then evaluated based on the test data, which here happens to result in an accuracy of 85%.

Another common reason why we like to use validation data is when we use ML models that include hyperparameters. Hyperparameters are parameters that are not automatically optimized by the ML model during the training process. Instead, these hyperparameters need to be set by the user before the internal parameters are optimized. For example, we will later use an ML method called random forest. This method includes, for example, the hyperparameter "mtry", which is the number of variables or features a decision tree uses to consider a split in the tree. This hyperparameter needs to be set by the user before the training starts. We can, for example, set mtry to 2 (model 1) and train the random forest and then set mtry to 3 and train a second random forest (model 2). After we have trained these two models, we can use the validation dataset to see which of these two models that performs best. We may even try 10 models with different values of the hyperparameters.

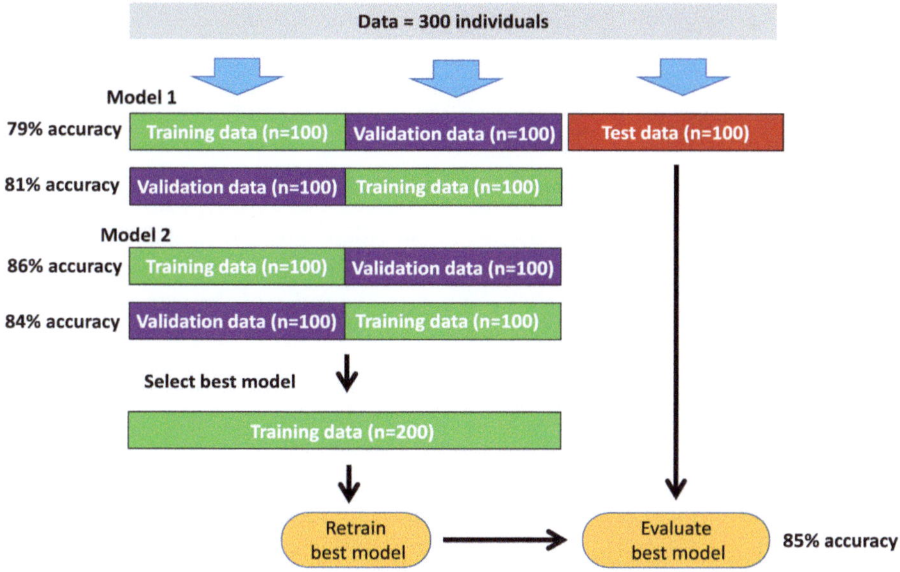

Fig. 11.5 An illustration of how to compare different models using a 2-fold cross-validation. The model that performs best on the cross-validation is selected to be retrained on the full training data and then evaluated based on the test data

This is called hyperparameter tuning, or just tuning, because we tune the parameter to find its optimal value. Once we have found the optimal value of the hyperparameter that results in the best performance on the validation data, we can retrain the model with its optimized value of the hyperparameter on the full training data with 200 individuals and then evaluate this trained model on the test data. So basically, we can try a number of different ML models, and try to optimize their parameters or the number of variables they use in the training data, and select the best model based on the validation data. Our best model is then finally evaluated based on the test data.

11.2 Linear Discriminant Analysis

The first supervised ML model that we will learn is linear discriminant analysis (LDA). LDA is one of the oldest and simplest supervised ML methods. Due to its simplicity, and relation to PCA, it is still widely used. Although the method is simple, it performs surprisingly well on biological data in comparison to modern more advanced ML models. In Chap. 7, we discussed the details of how LDA combined variables to maximize the separation between two or more groups. We will here see how linear discriminant analysis can be used for classification to predict if a person has a viral or bacterial infection. Watch the video below to see how LDA can be used as an ML model.

11.2.1 Video

https://youtu.be/A1t61bzTpw0
www.tilestats.com/ml/

We will here use the same dataset as in the video, where we calculated the discriminant scores based on body temperature and CRP level. In this example, we set the category "virus" as our baseline. However, the order of the categories in this example is arbitrary since both categories are associated with a disease. Note that, since "Virus" is our baseline (the first category) in this example, "Bacteria" detection will be considered as a positive result.

```
Temp=c(36.0, 37.2, 36.5, 39.4, 39.6, 40.7,37.6, 42.2, 38.5,
39.4, 38.6, 42.7)
CRP=c(40.0, 11.1, 30.0, 21.4, 10.7, 3.4,42.0, 31.1, 50.0,
60.4, 45.7, 17.3)
Group=factor(c(rep("Virus",6),rep("Bacteria",6)),
levels=c("Virus","Bacteria"))
df=data.frame(CRP,Temp,Group)
```

```
par(mfrow=c(1,2))
stripchart(CRP~Group,data=df,ylim=c(0,80),ylab="CRP (mg/L)",
vertical = TRUE,xlim=c(0.5,2.5))
stripchart(Temp~Group,data=df,ylim=c(35,43),ylab="Temp (C)",
vertical = TRUE,xlim=c(0.5,2.5))
```

Using either the CRP or the body temperature alone as biomarkers for viral or bacterial infection, it is not possible to find a clear cutoff that can be used to separate the groups (Fig. 11.6). However, when we combined the variables by using LDA as we did in Chap. 7:

$$D = 0.11 \cdot CRP + 0.70 \cdot Temp$$

we will obtain a really good separation between the groups (Fig. 11.7). The code below computes and plots the discriminant scores.

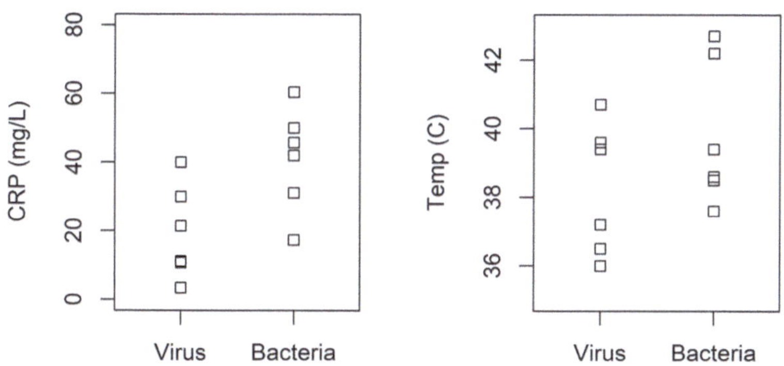

Fig. 11.6 One-dimensional scatter plots of the CRP (left) and body temperature (right) separated based on the type of infection

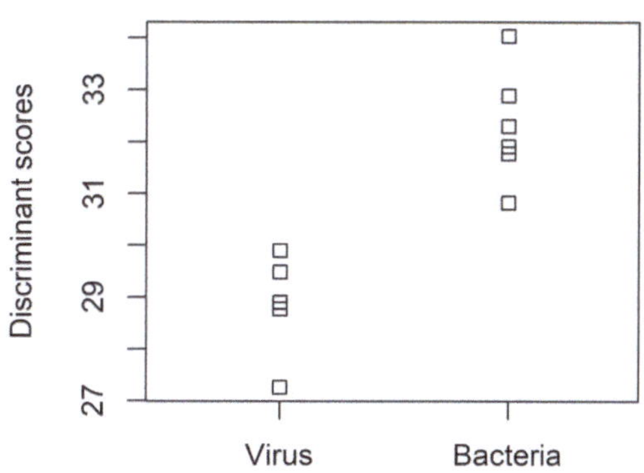

Fig. 11.7 A one-dimensional scatter plot of the discriminant scores separated based on the type of infection

```
library(MASS)
fit = lda(Group ~ CRP + Temp, data=df)
alfa1= coef(fit)[1]  # Weight for CRP
alfa2= coef(fit)[2]  # Weight for Temp
D=alfa1*CRP+alfa2*Temp
df2=cbind(df,D)
stripchart(D~Group,data=df2,ylab="Discriminant scores",
vertical = TRUE,xlim=c(0.5,2.5))
```

A reasonable cutoff value is the mean of the mean discriminant scores of the two groups:

```
Mean1=tapply(df2$D,df2$Group,mean)
 Virus        Bacteria
28.86792    32.28663
cut=mean(Mean1) # Cutoff value
abline(h=cut,col="red",lty=2)
```

We see that such a cutoff separates the groups completely (Fig. 11.8). We could also use the centered discriminant scores, which have a mean of zero:

$$D = 0.11\left(CRP - \overline{CRP}\right) + 0.70\left(Temp - \overline{Temp}\right)$$

A reasonable cutoff value for centered discriminant scores, when we have two groups, is therefore zero. The centered discriminant scores can be computed with the "predict" function:

```
# Compute centered discriminant scores
D_norm=as.numeric(predict(fit)$x)
```

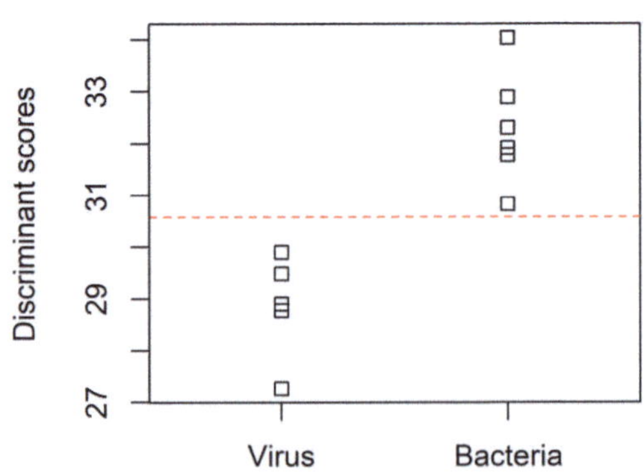

Fig. 11.8 A one-dimensional scatter plot of the discriminant scores separated based on the type of infection with a cutoff line at 30.58

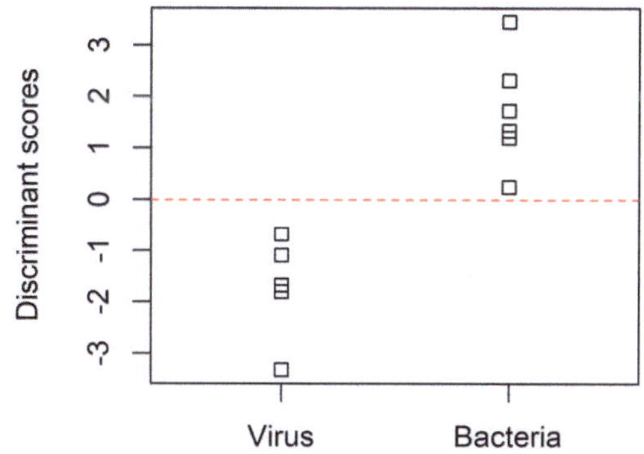

Fig. 11.9 A one-dimensional scatter plot of the centered discriminant scores separated based on the type of infection with a cutoff line at zero

Let's create a new data frame with the original data and the centered discriminant scores and make a plot of the scores:

```
df3=cbind(df,D_norm)
stripchart(D_norm~Group,data=df3,ylab="Discriminant scores",
vertical = TRUE, xlim=c(0.5,2.5))
abline(h=0,col="red",lty=2)
```

We see that the model separates the two classes completely since the discriminant scores of the bacteria group are all positive, whereas the discriminant scores of the virus group are negative (Fig. 11.9).

11.2.2 Accuracy

Once we have established the discriminant function and a cutoff value, we can compute the accuracy of our model. In our previous example, we used all our data to estimate the discriminant function. This data is known as our training set where we know the group membership from a previous study. As we discussed at the beginning of this chapter, it is not recommended to use the same data to train and evaluate the model unless we use a simple model for exploratory purposes. However, to learn how LDA works, we will for simplicity use the same data for training and testing and later see how to use a test dataset. Let's set bacteria to be the positive prediction. Hence, a positive result (centered discriminant scores greater than zero) indicates a bacterial infection, whereas a negative result indicates a viral infection. Given our cutoff value, we can see that all patients with a bacterial infection have actually been classified as having a bacterial infection (Fig. 11.10). Thus, the sensitivity in our case is 100%. The same accounts for the specificity since all patients with viral infection are below the cutoff line (they do not have a bacterial infection):

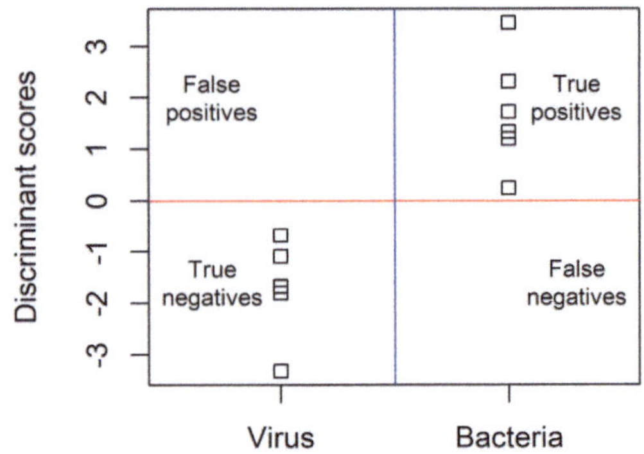

Fig. 11.10 A one-dimensional scatter plot of the centered discriminant scores with a horizontal cutoff line at zero. Patients with bacterial infection above the cutoff line are defined as true positives, whereas patients with a viral infection below the cutoff line are defined as true negatives

$$\text{Sensitivity} = \frac{\text{TP}}{\text{TP}+\text{FN}} = \frac{6}{6+0} = 1 = 100\%$$

$$\text{Specificity} = \frac{\text{TN}}{\text{TN}+\text{FP}} = \frac{6}{6+0} = 1 = 100\%$$

Since we have no false positives or false negatives, we have 100% sensitivity and 100% specificity. We can compute these measures in R and generate the confusion matrix by:

```
# Predict class based on our LDA model
pred=predict(fit,df)$class
CT = table(pred, df$Group)
CT # Print table
pred          Virus    Bacteria
  Virus         6           0
  Bacteria      0           6
```

The rows in the above table represent the predicted class, whereas the columns represent the actual class. We can calculate the accuracy by:

$$\text{Accuracy} = \frac{\text{TP}+\text{TN}}{\text{TP}+\text{TN}+\text{FP}+\text{FN}} = \frac{6+6}{6+6+0+0} = 1 = 100\%$$

To generate more performance metrics, we can use the “confusionMatrix” function in the **caret** package:

```
library(caret)
confusionMatrix(data=pred,reference=df$Group,
positive="Bacteria")
```

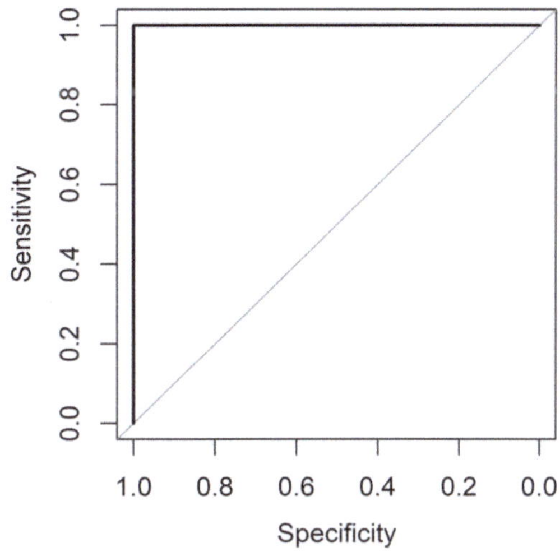

Fig. 11.11 An ROC curve illustrating the performance of the LDA model to discriminate between patients with a bacterial and viral infection

11.2.3 ROC Curve

We can use our centered discriminant scores to generate an ROC curve. However, since we in this example have 100% sensitivity and specificity, the "curve" will reach the top-left corner (Fig. 11.11).

```
library(pROC)
roc1=roc(df3$Group, df3$D_norm)
plot(roc1)
```

11.2.4 Changing the Cutoff Value

By default, the "predict" function uses the cutoff value of zero for the discriminant scores, which is, in this case, the optimal value to get a good accuracy. However, sometimes we might want to change the cutoff value to increase the sensitivity or the specificity. In our example, it does not make sense to change the cutoff value since we already have 100% sensitivity and specificity. However, we will here test another cutoff value for illustrative purposes. Let's use a cutoff value of 0.3 for the discriminant score. Hence, a discriminant score greater than 0.3 will be classified as a bacterial infection:

```
Score=predict(fit,df)$x  # Extract discriminant scores
# Use cutoff value of 0.3
pred=ifelse(Score<0.3,"Virus","Bacteria")
# Use Virus as the first category (baseline)
pred=factor(pred,levels=c("Virus","Bacteria"))
```

```
CT=table(pred, df$Group)
CT # Print classification table
pred          Virus    Bacteria
  Virus       6            1
  Bacteria    0            5
sum(diag(CT))/sum(CT) # Calculate accuracy
0.9166667
```

Changing the cutoff value to 0.3 will change the accuracy from 100% to 91.6% because one person with a bacterial infection is now incorrectly predicted to have a viral infection.

11.2.5 Probabilities

If we assume that the discriminant scores are normally distributed, we can calculate the probability that a certain observation belongs to one of the classes. Using the "predict" function, we will get the probability that the observations in our training data belong to the virus or the bacterial group.

```
predict(fit)
...
$posterior
        Virus            Bacteria
1   9.767371e-01   2.326290e-02
2   9.999881e-01   1.185019e-05
3   9.979046e-01   2.095383e-03
4   9.116596e-01   8.834043e-02
5   9.967815e-01   3.218540e-03
6   9.968169e-01   3.183099e-03
7   3.050983e-01   6.949017e-01
8   3.722569e-04   9.996277e-01
9   2.781452e-03   9.972185e-01
10 7.419850e-06   9.999926e-01
11 1.033257e-02   9.896674e-01
12 1.648440e-02   9.835156e-01
```

For example, the probability that the first person has a viral infection is 97.67%, whereas the probability of bacterial infection is 2.33%. We can extract the probability for the class bacteria by:

```
Prob=predict(fit)$posterior[,2]
```

and make a nice output of these together with the discriminant scores:

```
data.frame(df,D=round(D,1),Dnomr=round(D_norm,1),
Prob=round(Prob,3))
     CRP    Temp    Group      D     Dnomr    Prob
1    40.0   36.0    Virus      29.5  -1.1     0.023
2    11.1   37.2    Virus      27.3  -3.3     0.000
3    30.0   36.5    Virus      28.8  -1.8     0.002
4    21.4   39.4    Virus      29.9  -0.7     0.088
5    10.7   39.6    Virus      28.9  -1.7     0.003
6    3.4    40.7    Virus      28.9  -1.7     0.003
7    42.0   37.6    Bacteria   30.8   0.2     0.695
8    31.1   42.2    Bacteria   32.9   2.3     1.000
9    50.0   38.5    Bacteria   32.3   1.7     0.997
10   60.4   39.4    Bacteria   34.0   3.5     1.000
11   45.7   38.6    Bacteria   31.9   1.3     0.990
12   17.3   42.7    Bacteria   31.8   1.2     0.984
```

For example, we see that the probability that the first patient has a bacterial infection is only 2.3%.

11.2.6 Predict with LDA

Once we have determined an appropriate cutoff value that can separate the groups, we can use this cutoff value to predict group membership of new data. For example, let's say that a patient has a body temperature of 40° C and a CRP concentration of 70 mg/L, then we calculate its discriminant score by:

$$D = 0.11 \cdot CRP + 0.70 \cdot Temp = 0.11 \cdot 70 + 0.70 \cdot 40 = 35.7$$

The discriminant score is greater than the cutoff of 30.58 we determined earlier when we used all data as our training data (Fig. 11.8). Hence, the patient is predicted to have a bacterial infection. We can do the same calculations based on the centered discriminant score by:

$$\begin{aligned} D &= 0.11\left(CRP - \overline{CRP}\right) + 0.70\left(Temp - \overline{Temp}\right) \\ &= 0.11 \cdot \left(70 - 30.26\right) + 0.70 \cdot \left(40 - 39.03\right) = 5.05 \end{aligned}$$

Instead of calculating this manually, we can use the function "predict". The function takes the previous output ("fit") from the "lda" function and predicts the group membership of a new observation that is stored as a data frame:

```
new=data.frame(CRP=70,Temp=40)
predict(fit, new)
$class
[1] Bacteria
Levels: Virus Bacteria

$posterior
       Virus          Bacteria
1   5.415312e-08    0.9999999
$x
            LD1
1   4.894077
```

We see that the model predicts the class bacteria for a CRP of 70 and a body temperature of 40. Also, we can see, under "$posterior", that the model predicts that we are more than 99% sure that the observation is classified as a bacterial infection. Under the row "$x", we see the discriminant score 4.894, which is a bit different from our previous calculations (5.05). The difference is due to rounding effects because we used rounded values of the weights when we calculated the discriminant score by hand. Let's say that we have another patient with a CRP of 24 and a body temperature of 40:

```
new=data.frame(CRP=24,Temp=40)
predict(fit, new)
$class
[1] Bacteria
Levels: Virus Bacteria

$posterior
   Virus        Bacteria
1 0.488223    0.511777
$x
   LD1
1 0.01378205
```

We see that the observation is still classified as bacterial infection (its centered discriminant score is greater than zero). However, the probability that the observation belongs to the bacteria group is only 51%. The reason for this uncertainty is that the observation has a discriminant score that is very close to the cutoff value. Note that the discriminant score, 0.013, is close to zero.

11.2.7 Validation of LDA

The problem with the above calculations is that we used the same data for both training and testing the model, which will overestimate how well our classifier performs. Let's say that we would collect CRP and body temperature on 12 new patients with bacterial and viral infections and use our discriminant function to see if these new observations would be correctly classified. Would we then still get 100% accuracy? Probably not since our discriminant function has been optimized based on our training data. There are two common approaches to validating a classifier: the hold-out method and k-fold cross-validation as we discussed at the beginning of this chapter.

11.2.8 The Hold-Out Method

Although our sample size is way too small to be validated by the hold-out method, we will here use it just to learn how it works. Let's use one-third of the data points as our test set and the other two-thirds as our training set. To split the data into training data and a test data, we will here generate random numbers with the function "createDataPartition" in the **caret** package:

```
library(caret)
set.seed(1) #For reproducibility
train_ind=createDataPartition(y=df$Group, p=2/3, list=FALSE)
train_ind
     Resample1
[1,]         1
[2,]         3
[3,]         4
[4,]         6
[5,]         8
[6,]         9
[7,]        10
[8,]        11
```

The numbers that you see in the printout are the row numbers we will use to extract the training data from the original data. If you happen to get other random values than the ones above, although you use the same seed, it is probably due to that you use a different R-version. Remember that you might then get different results compared to the ones below. Let's extract the training data:

```
train_data=df[train_ind,]
train_data # Print test data
      CRP    Temp   Group
1     40.0   36.0   Virus
3     30.0   36.5   Virus
4     21.4   39.4   Virus
6     3.4    40.7   Virus
8     31.1   42.2   Bacteria
9     50.0   38.5   Bacteria
10    60.4   39.4   Bacteria
11    45.7   38.6   Bacteria
```

Note that individuals 1, 3, 4, 6, 8, 9, 10, and 11 were randomly selected to be used as the training data and that we have four individuals from each group. We will now create the test data, which is simply the rest of the individuals:

```
test_data=df[-train_ind,]
test_data
      CRP     Temp    Group
2     11.1    37.2    Virus
5     10.7    39.6    Virus
7     42.0    37.6    Bacteria
12    17.3    42.7    Bacteria
```

We will now use the training data to train the model:

```
fit=lda(Group ~ CRP + Temp, data=train_data)
```

Next, we use the test data in the "predict" function to see how well the model predicts these individuals with known class:

```
pred=predict(fit, test_data)$class
tab=table(pred, test_data$Group)
tab

pred            Virus   Bacteria
  Virus           2          1
  Bacteria        0          1
```

The columns represent the actual classes or labels, whereas the rows represent the predicted classes or labels. The two patients with a viral infection were correctly predicted as having a viral infection. Out of the two individuals with bacterial infection, one was incorrectly predicted to have a viral infection, whereas one was correctly predicted to have a bacterial infection. We see that we now get 75% accuracy by using the hold-out method because three out of four individuals were correctly predicted. More metrics can be computed with the "confusionMatrix" function in the **caret** package:

```
library(caret)
confusionMatrix(data=pred,reference=test_data$Group,positive=
"Bacteria")
...
               Accuracy : 0.75
                 95% CI : (0.1941, 0.9937)
    No Information Rate : 0.5
    P-Value [Acc > NIR] : 0.3125...
```

We see that although we get an accuracy of 75%, this accuracy is not significantly different from 50%, since 0.5 is included in the confidence interval. This is simply due to that we have too few data points to draw any conclusion about the accuracy. The fewer data points we have, the wider our confidence interval will be. The computed p-value is also greater than the general significance level of 0.05.

11.2.9 k-fold Cross-Validation

A more appropriate validation method to use when we have a small sample size is to use the k-fold cross-validation. The function "lda" includes the method LOOCV, which can be used if we set the argument "CV" to "TRUE":

```
fit=lda(Group ~  CRP + Temp ,data=df, CV=TRUE)
```

The predictions based on LOOCV can be printed by:

```
fit$class
Virus     Virus     Virus     Virus     Virus     Virus     Virus
Bacteria  Bacteria  Bacteria  Bacteria  Bacteria
Levels: Virus Bacteria
```

To generate the confusion matrix, we type:

```
CT=table(pred=fit$class, df$Group)
CT
pred          Virus    Bacteria
  Virus         6          1
  Bacteria      0          5
Accuracy=sum(diag(CT))/sum(CT)
Accuracy
0.9166667
```

By using the LOOCV, we see that the accuracy is now approximately 91.6%.

11.2.10 LDA on More Than Two Groups

Linear discriminant analysis can be used to discriminate between more than two groups. We will here use the Iris dataset to see how well we can classify the three different Iris species. Note that "Species ~ ." below means that we want to predict the Species based on all (".") the other variables in the data frame. If we only want to predict based on certain variables, we need to instead put the corresponding column names to the right-hand side of the ~ sign, for example:

Species ~ Sepal.Length + Sepal.Width.

```
library(MASS)
(fit = lda(Species ~., data=iris))
Prior probabilities of groups:
 setosa     versicolor    virginica
 0.3333333  0.3333333     0.3333333
….
Coefficients of linear discriminants:
                    LD1           LD2
Sepal.Length    0.8293776     0.02410215
Sepal.Width     1.5344731     2.16452123
Petal.Length   -2.2012117    -0.93192121
Petal.Width    -2.8104603     2.83918785

Proportion of trace:
   LD1         LD2
0.9912      0.0088
```

Note that the prior probabilities have been set according to the proportion of the species in the data. Since there are 50 flowers of each species in the dataset, there will be an equal prior probability for the different groups. We see that we now have two discriminant functions (LD1 and LD2) because we have three groups. The "proportion of trace" tells us the proportion of separation achieved by the two discriminant functions. We can use both discriminant functions to predict the class of new observations. However, if we plot the two discriminant functions:

```
D1=predict(fit)$x[,1] # Discriminant function 1
D2=predict(fit)$x[,2] # Discriminant function 2
plot(D1,D2,col=iris$Species)
legend("topright", legend=levels(iris$Species),pch=1,
col=1:3)
```

we see that only discriminant function 1 (D1) is useful for separating the groups because two vertical lines in Fig. 11.12 can separate the three groups, whereas that is not possible if we use horizontal lines. However, if both LD1 and LD2 would

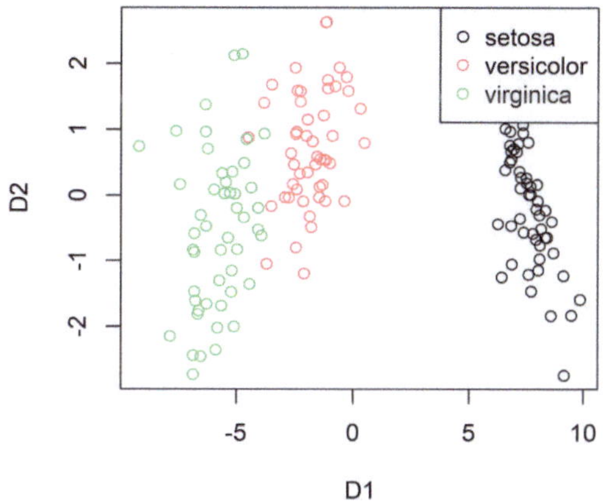

Fig. 11.12 A linear discriminant analysis (LDA) plot of the Iris dataset showing the separation of the species (Setosa, Versicolor, and Virginica) along the two linear discriminants (LD1 and LD2). Each point represents an individual flower, colored according to its species

contribute to a good separation, diagonal lines can be used to better separate the groups if we use both discriminate functions to predict. To simplify our model, we will here only use D1 for further classification and validations because the second discriminant function barely improves our model. Let's see how well the first discriminant function can be used as a classifier based on the training data. In the "predict" function, we set the argument "dimen" equal to 1 in order to use only the first discriminant function:

```
# Predict based on the LDA model
pred=predict(fit,iris,dimen=1)$class
CT=table(pred, iris$Species) # Predicted class vs true class
CT

pred          setosa    versicolor    virginica
  setosa        50          0             0
  versicolor     0         48             0
  virginica      0          2            50

accuracy=sum(diag(CT))/sum(CT)
accuracy
0.9866667
```

We see that only 2 out of 150 (1.3%) flowers are incorrectly classified. The accuracy is more than 98% when we use the same data to both train and predict. Since we have more than two groups, we can no longer estimate sensitivity and specificity as these metrics are constrained to only two groups.

11.2.11 Predict a New Flower

Similar to what we have done before, we can use the "predict" function to predict the class of a new observation. Let's predict the species of an Iris flower with a sepal length of 5 cm, a sepal width of 4 cm, a petal length of 3 cm, and a petal width of 1 cm. To predict, we here only use the first discriminant function (dimen=1) to be consistent with our previous model:

```
new=data.frame(Sepal.Length=5,Sepal.Width=4,Petal.Length=3,
Petal.Width=1)
predict(fit,new,dimen=1)
$class
[1] setosa
Levels: setosa versicolor virginica

$posterior
   setosa        versicolor      virginica
 1 0.6893782      0.3106218     6.918416e-13

$x
         LD1
1   2.975792
```

We see that the flower has been predicted to be of class Setosa. The posterior probability for class Setosa is 69%, and the discriminant score has been calculated to 2.97. Study Fig. 11.12 and try to understand why a discriminant score of 2.97 results in this prediction.

11.2.12 Using the Caret Package for Validation

We will here use the **caret** package to validate an LDA model based on the Iris dataset. First, we split the Iris data into training data (70%) and test data (30%) by:

```
set.seed(15) #For reproducibility
library(caret)
index=createDataPartition(y=iris$Species, p=0.7, list=FALSE)
train=iris[index,]
test=iris[-index,]
```

We are now ready to train the model. Before we train the model, we can run the "modelLookup" function to get some metadata about the lda method implemented in the **caret** package:

```
modelLookup("lda")
  model parameter  label      forReg  forClass  probModel
1 lda   parameter  parameter  FALSE   TRUE      TRUE
```

The output shows that the model we will use is “lda”. The column ”parameter” normally lists tunable hyperparameters for the model. In the case of LDA, this column simply shows ”parameter” as the “lda” function does not have hyperparameters to tune. The column ”label” describes the hyperparameter(s). The last three columns show if the model can perform regression or classification tasks and if the model can produce class probabilities as part of its output.

The general code to train an ML model with the **caret** package by using a 10-fold cross-validation is as follows:

```
fit = train(Species ~ ., data=train, method="lda",
                trControl = trainControl(method = "cv"))
```

The argument “trainControl” is here set to cross-validation (cv), which can be used by some ML models to find optimal values of the hyperparameters. However, since we have no hyperparameters in our simple LDA model, the cross-validation will have no effect here.

The trained model with its weights can be printed if we run the following code:

```
fit$finalModel
...
Coefficients of linear discriminants:
                    LD1        LD2
Sepal.Length  0.8860029 -0.8587254
Sepal.Width   1.3718683 -1.7419350
Petal.Length -2.0749777  1.6295429
Petal.Width  -2.8563718  -3.6010122

Proportion of trace:
 LD1       LD2
0.9882   0.0118
```

This output will be exactly the same as if we use the “lda” function on the training data:

```
lda(Species ~. ,data=train)
```

After we have trained the model, we will use the test dataset to see how well it predicts. Note that, similar to before, we here use only the first discriminant function:

```
pred=predict(fit, test,dimen=1)
Tab=table(pred, test$Species)
Tab
pred          setosa   versicolor    virginica
  setosa          15            0            0
  versicolor       0           15            0
  virginica        0            0           15
sum(diag(Tab))/sum(Tab)
1
```

Our LDA model performs very well because the accuracy of the test data is 100%. However, the accuracy is quite sensitive to the split of the data into training and test data. Try to run the code above with a different seed (change it from 15 to another number) and note that the accuracies may vary quite much from the different runs. This is due to that we have quite few data points. The smaller the datasets we have, the larger the variation in the accuracies we will get. For small datasets, it might therefore be better to use cross-validation.

11.2.13 k-fold Cross-Validation

To instead perform k-fold cross-validation, which is appropriate to use for small datasets, we can use the same lines of code as above but where we now include all 150 flowers (data=iris instead of data=train):

```
set.seed(15) #For reproducibility
fit = train(Species ~ ., data=iris, method="lda",
        trControl = trainControl(method = "cv"))
fit$resample
     Accuracy    Kappa      Resample
1    1.0000000    1.0        Fold01
2    1.0000000    1.0        Fold02
3    1.0000000    1.0        Fold03
4    1.0000000    1.0        Fold04
5    0.9333333    0.9        Fold05
6    1.0000000    1.0        Fold06
7    1.0000000    1.0        Fold07
8    0.9333333    0.9        Fold08
9    1.0000000    1.0        Fold09
10   0.9333333    0.9        Fold10
```

We can see that the method has performed a 10-fold cross-validation because we have results from 10 subsets. The average accuracy and the standard deviation of these accuracies can be found by:

```
fit$results
  parameter   Accuracy   Kappa    AccuracySD       KappaSD
1     none       0.98     0.97    0.03220306    0.04830459
```

Note that it says "none" in the column "parameter" because we have no hyperparameter to tune in the LDA model. The average accuracy from the 10 folds is here 98%.

If we instead run LOOCV, it is possible to generate a confusion matrix since every iteration will then determine if a single observation is correctly classified or not:

```
fit=train(Species ~ ., data=iris, method="lda",
                trControl = trainControl(method = "LOOCV"))
pred= predict(fit,dimen=1)
Tab=table(pred, iris$Species)
Tab
 pred            setosa    versicolor     virginica
  setosa             50             0             0
  versicolor          0            48             1
  virginica           0             2            49
```

We see that one Virginica flower is incorrectly predicted as a Versicolor and that two Versicolors are incorrectly predicted as Virginica. The accuracy from the LOOCV is 98%:

```
sum(diag(Tab))/sum(Tab)
0.98
```

We will get the same result if we use the "lda" function and set the argument CV to TRUE as we did previously to compute the LOOCV. However, note that the "lda" function uses both discriminant functions to predict, whereas we only used the first function in our previous predictions (predict(fit,dimen=1)).

11.3 Exercises

1. Combine the numerical variables in the Crab dataset by using LDA on all data to classify male and female crabs. Create an ROC curve of the discriminant scores.
2. Calculate the accuracy, sensitivity, and specificity using the default cutoff value of 0 in the "predict" function. Use the category "female" as the baseline.
3. Suppose that you find a crab and would like to know the sex of the crab with the following measurements: FL = 8.0, RW = 6.7, CL = 16.2, CW = 18.9, BD = 7.0. Use your LDA model to compute the probability that the crab is a female.

4. Build an LDA model based on the Crab dataset to classify male and female crabs. Use the hold-out method to validate your model. Use 70% of the data to train your model and 30% to test your model. Report the accuracy of your model based on the test data.

11.4 Logistic Regression

Logistic regression is a regression technique to estimate the parameters of a logistic model. However, we will here only use logistic regression as a classifier. We will therefore not discuss the biological interpretation of its estimated parameters. Watch the videos below to understand how logistic regression works and how it can be used for classification.

11.4.1 Videos

https://youtu.be/WCvj-kzMXoY
https://youtu.be/Da_VQoRhR3k
www.tilestats.com/ml/

To learn how binary logistic regression can be used to predict the probability of an outcome, we will first start with only one independent variable. Note that independent variables are also called explanatory variables or predictor variables. We will use the same dataset as shown in the video. In this dataset, one has measured the PSA level in 14 subjects, where we know that seven of these subjects are healthy, whereas the other seven subjects have prostate cancer. The PSA levels are shown in Table 11.1.

Table 11.1 PSA levels in the 14 subjects

Prostate cancer	NO	NO	NO	NO	NO	NO	NO	YES	YES	YES	YES	YES	YES	YES
PSA level (μg/L)	2.5	2.0	1.7	1.4	1.2	0.9	0.8	3.8	3.4	2.9	2.8	2.7	2.1	1.6

Let's first enter the data:

```
rm(list=ls()) # Clear environment
PSA=c(3.8, 3.4, 2.9, 2.8, 2.7, 2.1, 1.6,2.5, 2.0, 1.7, 1.4,
1.2, 0.9, 0.8)
Group=factor(rep(c("Cancer","Healthy"),c(7,7)),
levels=c("Healthy","Cancer"))
df=data.frame(Group,PSA)
```

For logistic regression, it is important to decide, which of the two binary outcomes that should be coded as "0" or "1" because the model will be used to predict the probability of the category coded as "1". Usually, we want to code the disease state as "1" since we then can predict the probability of having the disease given the values of the independent variables (predictors). This is the reason why we here set "healthy" as the first level (=0) and "Cancer" as the second level (=1) in the argument "levels" for the variable "Group" in the above code. Generally, we should code the baseline category as the first level. Next, we plot the data where we place the group variable on the y-axis coded as 0 = healthy and 1 = cancer:

```
# Recode to Cancer -> 1, Healthy -> 0
state=ifelse(Group=="Cancer",1,0)
plot(PSA,state,col=Group,xlab="PSA µg/L",ylab="Probability",
xlim=c(0,5))
legend("bottomright",levels(Group),col=1:2,pch=1)
```

The next step is to fit an S-shaped curve that takes values between zero and one, which can be done with the logistic function:

$$p = \frac{1}{1 + e^{-(a + b \cdot x)}}$$

This function may result in an S-shaped (sigmoid) curve that takes values between zero and one. We will now fit this function to the data (in Table 11.1), meaning that we will find the values of the parameters "*a*" and "*b*" that generate a curve that fits the data as well as possible (Fig. 11.13). To fit the logistic function to the data, we use the "glm" function for generalized linear models where we set the argument "family" to "binomial":

```
fit = glm(Group~PSA,data=df,family=binomial)
fit # Print output
Coefficients:
(Intercept)          PSA
   -5.754          2.747
…
```

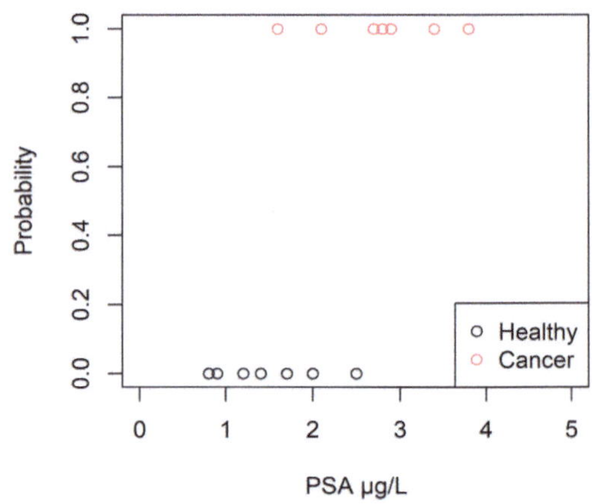

Fig. 11.13 A one-dimensional scatter plot of the PSA levels of the 14 individuals

We see that the function has estimated "*a*" (the intercept) to -5.75 and "*b*" (PSA) to 2.75. Now, let's plot the predicted probabilities as a function of x (the PSA values) using the estimated coefficients. To plot a smooth curve, we generate a range of possible x-values between zero and five with a step size of 0.1, which will give us a reasonable range of PSA values based on our data:

```
a=coef(fit)[1] # Estimated value of a
b=coef(fit)[2] # Estimated value of b
x=seq(0,5,0.1) # To generate a smooth curve
p=1/(1 + exp(-(a+b*x)))
lines(x,p,col="blue")
```

Based on the fitted curve, we can now predict the probability of having prostate cancer given a certain PSA level. For example, a PSA level of 2 µg/L generates a probability of about 40%, whereas a PSA level of 4 µg/L results in almost 100% probability according to the plot (Fig. 11.14). To predict the probability of having prostate cancer, given a PSA level of 2 µg/L we can either calculate this manually:

```
x=2 # PSA level
p=1/(1 + exp(-(a+b*x)))
as.numeric(p) # Print predicted value of p
0.4352234
```

or use the "predict" function:

```
new=data.frame(PSA=2)
predict(fit, new,type="response")
0.4352234
```

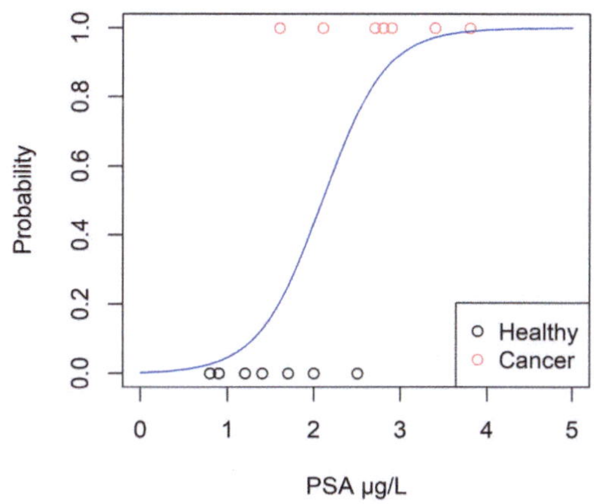

Fig. 11.14 A one-dimensional scatter plot of the PSA levels of the 14 individuals. The blue curve represents the predicted values by the logistic regression model

11.4.2 Classifying

We can now use the fitted logistic function to determine the class (healthy or cancer) based on a given PSA value. To classify, we first need to determine a cutoff value that can distinguish between cancer and healthy subjects. An appropriate threshold value is to use the probability of 0.5. Hence, if a given PSA value results in a probability greater than 0.5, the subject is classified as having prostate cancer, whereas a probability lower than 0.5 will predict the subject as being healthy. Let's add a threshold line at 0.5 in the figure:

```
abline(h=0.5)
```

From Fig. 11.15, we can see that the healthy subject with a PSA value of 2.5 is predicted to have prostate cancer with a probability of about 0.75, which is above the cutoff value of 0.5. Thus, this subject will result in a false positive case since we know that the subject is healthy. To calculate an x-value for a given probability, we can solve the equation:

$$p = \frac{1}{1 + e^{-(a + b \cdot x)}}$$

for x:

$$x = \frac{\log\left(\frac{1}{p} - 1\right) + a}{-b}$$

The corresponding PSA value given a cutoff value of p=0.5 can now be calculated:

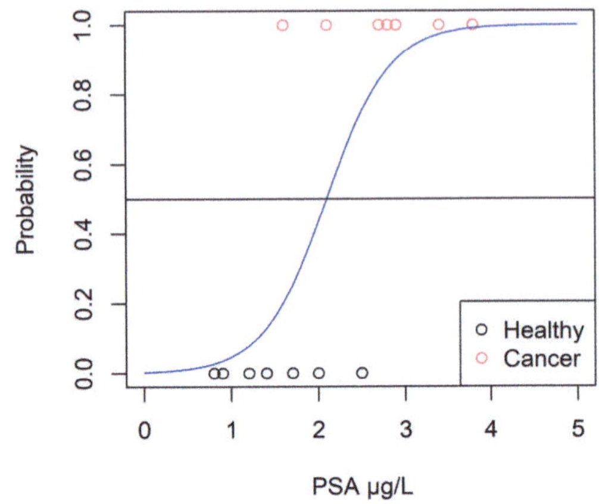

Fig. 11.15 A one-dimensional scatter plot of the PSA levels of the 14 individuals. The blue curve represents the predicted values by the logistic regression model. A cutoff line is shown at 0.5

```
cutoff=0.5
PSA_threshold=(log(1/cutoff-1)+a)/-b
as.numeric(PSA_threshold) # Print cutoff for PSA
2.09486
```

This means that all subjects with a PSA level greater than 2.09486 will be predicted to have prostate cancer. Let's place a vertical line at the corresponding cutoff value of PSA and define the squares as true positive (TP), true negative (TN), false positive (FP), and false negative (FN):

```
abline(v=PSA_threshold)
text(1,0.8,"FN",cex=2)
text(4,0.8,"TP",cex=2)
text(1,0.26,"TN",cex=2)
text(4,0.26,"FP",cex=2)
```

Figure 11.16 tells us that six out of the seven prostate cancer patients will be correctly classified as having prostate cancer with a cutoff value of 0.5. Using this cutoff value generates a sensitivity and specificity of:

$$\text{Sensitivity} = \frac{\text{TP}}{\text{TP}+\text{FN}} = \frac{6}{6+1} = 86\%$$

$$\text{Specificity} = \frac{\text{TN}}{\text{TN}+\text{FP}} = \frac{6}{6+1} = 86\%$$

We can use the "predict" function to compute the probability of each subject in the dataset for having prostate cancer (if no new data is supplied, the "predict" function will predict the probability of our training data):

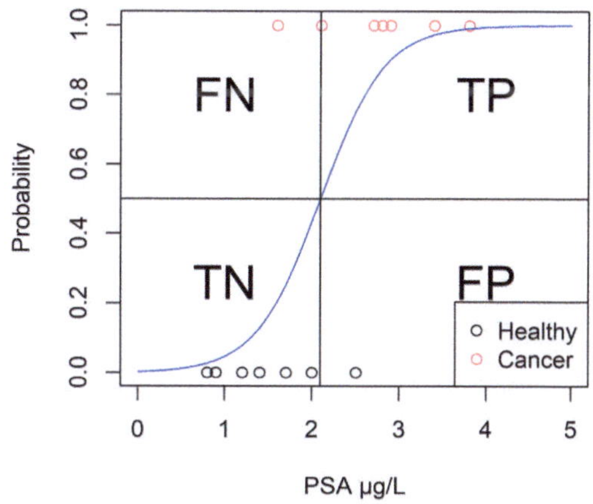

Fig. 11.16 A one-dimensional scatter plot of the PSA levels of the 14 individuals. The blue curve represents the predicted values by the logistic regression model. A horizontal cutoff line is shown at a probability of 0.5, whereas the vertical cutoff line, based on the corresponding PSA level, is shown at 2.09486. The squares define if the prediction will result in a true positive (TP), true negative (TN), false positive (FP), or false negative (FN) result

```
pred_prob=predict(fit,type="response")
round(pred_prob,2)
   1    2    3    4    5    6    7    8    9   10   11   12   13   14
0.99 0.97 0.90 0.87 0.84 0.50 0.20 0.75 0.44 0.25 0.13 0.08 0.04 0.03
```

The output tells us the predicted probability for each individual to have prostate cancer. The ones who have a probability greater than 0.5 will be classified as having prostate cancer. We can use the "ifelse" function to predict the class of each subject:

```
pred_class=ifelse(pred_prob<=0.5,"Healthy","Cancer")
pred_class
        1         2         3         4         5         6         7         8
 "Cancer"  "Cancer"  "Cancer"  "Cancer"  "Cancer"  "Cancer" "Healthy"  "Cancer"
        9        10        11        12        13        14
"Healthy" "Healthy" "Healthy" "Healthy" "Healthy" "Healthy"
```

Before we move on to generate the confusion matrix, we first need to set the level of "pred_class" to correspond to our variable "Group", which means that "Healthy" should be set as the first category:

```
pred_class=factor(pred_class,levels=c("Healthy","Cancer"))
```

Finally, we generate the confusion matrix:

```
CT=table(pred_class, Group)
CT
           Group
pred_class   Healthy   Cancer
   Healthy         6        1
   Cancer          1        6
```

11.4.3 Changing the Cutoff Value

If we like to increase specificity or sensitivity, we can simply change the cutoff value. For example, a cutoff value of 0.2 will generate 100% sensitivity and 57% specificity (Fig. 11.17).

To change the cutoff value, we simply change the threshold in the function "ifelse" to 0.2:

```
pred_class=ifelse(pred_prob<=0.2,"Healthy","Cancer")
pred_class=factor(pred_class,levels=c("Healthy","Cancer"))
CT=table(pred_class, Group)
CT
            Group
pred_class  Healthy   Cancer
   Healthy        4        0
   Cancer         3        7
```

By using a lower cutoff value, all patients with prostate cancer are now correctly predicted to have prostate cancer, whereas three healthy individuals are now incorrectly predicted to have prostate cancer.

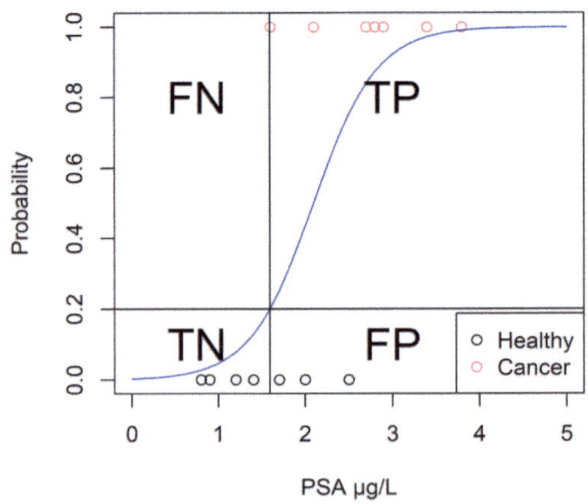

Fig. 11.17 Same as Fig. 11.16 but where the horizontal cutoff line is set at 0.2

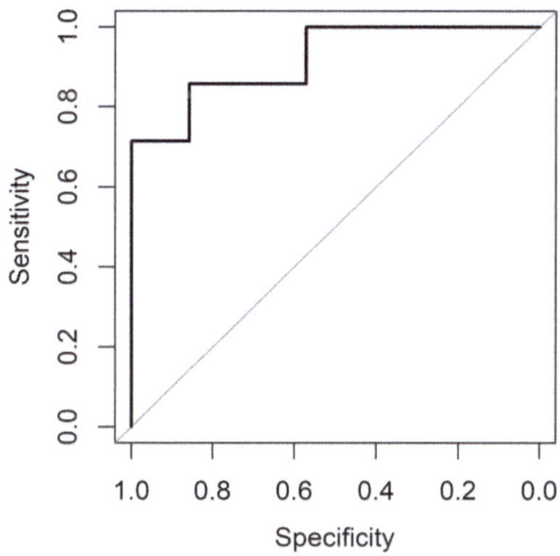

Fig. 11.18 An ROC curve illustrating the performance of the logistic regression model to discriminate between the healthy controls and the patients with prostate cancer

11.4.4 ROC

To find other cutoff values that can generate a certain sensitivity or specificity, we can use an ROC plot (Fig. 11.18):

```
library(pROC)
roc1=roc(df$Group, pred_prob)
plot(roc1)
```

We then use the output from the "roc" function to create a data frame of sensitivities and specificities for different cutoff values.

```
data.frame(roc1$thresholds,roc1$sensitivities,
roc1$specificities)
   roc1.thresholds roc1.sensitivities roc1.specificities
1             -Inf          1.0000000          0.0000000
2       0.03196263          1.0000000          0.1428571
3       0.05751843          1.0000000          0.2857143
4       0.10398712          1.0000000          0.4285714
5       0.16673720          1.0000000          0.5714286
6       0.22848874          0.8571429          0.5714286
7       0.34392600          0.8571429          0.7142857
8       0.46937660          0.8571429          0.8571429
9       0.62809780          0.7142857          0.8571429
10      0.79660356          0.7142857          1.0000000
11      0.85727911          0.5714286          1.0000000
12      0.88765349          0.4285714          1.0000000
13      0.93715223          0.2857143          1.0000000
14      0.98192785          0.1428571          1.0000000
15             Inf          0.0000000          1.0000000
```

For example, if we use a cutoff value of about 0.469, we will get a sensitivity and specificity of about 86%.

11.4.5 Multiple Logistic Regression

In the previous example, we used only one independent variable in order to illustrate how the method works. Using two independent variables would require a three-dimensional plot to see the relationship between two independent variables and the computed probabilities. To illustrate how to use logistic regression with two independent variables, we will here use the same example data as we used for the LDA model where we used the CRP and body temperature to predict the type of infection:

```
rm(list=ls()) # Clear environment
Temp=c(36.0, 37.2, 36.5, 39.4, 39.6, 40.7,37.6, 42.2, 38.5,
39.4, 38.6, 42.7)
CRP=c(40.0, 11.1, 30.0, 21.4, 10.7, 3.4,42.0, 31.1, 50.0,
60.4, 45.7, 17.3)
Group=factor(c(rep("Virus",6),rep("Bacteria",6)),
levels=c("Virus","Bacteria"))
df=data.frame(CRP,Temp,Group)
```

Adding more than one variable in the "glm" function is straightforward:

```
fit=glm(Group~Temp+CRP,data=df,family=binomial)
Warning message:
glm.fit: fitted probabilities numerically 0 or 1 occurred
fit
Coefficients:
(Intercept)          Temp          CRP
  -1043.567        23.519        4.338
```

Note that a warning message is generated when you run this code because we have achieved a perfect separation between the groups. This is not a big problem when we use logistic regression as a classifier. However, the predicted coefficients of the model will be unreliable if we have perfect separation but we do not need to worry about this here since we do not draw any conclusions of the estimated parameters. We will now generate the confusion matrix:

```
pred_prob=predict(fit,type="response")
pred_class=ifelse(pred_prob<0.5,"Virus","Bacteria")
pred_class=factor(pred_class,levels=c("Virus","Bacteria"))
table(pred_class, Group) # Print confusion matrix
```

```
              Group
pred_class    Virus    Bacteria
  Virus         6         0
  Bacteria      0         6
```

We see that the model makes a good job of separating the groups because we get 100% sensitivity and 100% specificity. Thus, by using a cutoff value of 0.5, all patients in the virus group are separated from the patients in the bacteria group. Remember that the LDA also achieved perfect separation of the discriminant scores of the same dataset when the variables were combined.

11.4.6 Using Logistic Regression to Simplify the Model

We will here illustrate how to reduce the number of variables of the Iris dataset. Since we use binary logistic regression, we need to eliminate one category from the Iris dataset so that we only have two categories. We will here eliminate all Setosa flowers from the dataset and use logistic regression to compute the probability of a flower being of type Versicolor or Virginica. Note that we set "Versicolor" as our baseline category in this example:

```
rm(list=ls()) # Clear environment
df_iris=iris[(iris$Species !="setosa"),] # Remove Setosa
df_iris$Species=factor(df_iris$Species,levels=c("versicolor",
"virginica"))
```

Let's first use the full model, including all four numeric variables:

```
fit = glm(Species~.,data=df_iris,family=binomial)
summary(fit)
….
Coefficients:
              Estimate    Std.Error   z value    Pr(>|z|)
(Intercept)   -42.638     25.707      -1.659     0.0972 .
Sepal.Length   -2.465      2.394      -1.030     0.3032
Sepal.Width    -6.681      4.480      -1.491     0.1359
Petal.Length    9.429      4.737       1.991     0.0465 *
Petal.Width    18.286      9.743       1.877     0.0605 .
….
```

$$p = \frac{1}{1 + e^{-(-42.64 - 2.47S_L - 6.68S_W + 9.43P_L + 18.29P_W)}}$$

The p-values tell us the importance of each variable in discriminating between the two classes. We see that the petal length has the lowest p-value, which suggests that it is the best variable to separate the Versicolors from the Virginicas in this model. If we would like to reduce the model, we could start by removing the variable with the highest p-value. Another alternative is to use automatic elimination in R. We will here use backward elimination to find a model with the lowest Akaike information criterion (AIC). The model with the lowest AIC value is usually selected as the most likely model, given the data. Note that the full model usually predicts the training data best but may perform equally well or worse on the test data compared to a reduced model. Thus, the elimination procedure aims to remove irrelevant variables that do not, or only marginally, reduce the accuracy of the model. Running the code:

```
fit2=step(fit,direction="backward")
```

will generate the following output:

```
Start:  AIC=21.9
Species ~ Sepal.Length + Sepal.Width + Petal.Length +
Petal.Width

                 Df     Deviance       AIC
- Sepal.Length   1       13.266       21.266
 <none>                  11.899       21.899
- Sepal.Width    1       15.492       23.492
- Petal.Width    1       23.772       31.772
- Petal.Length   1       25.902       33.902
```

The AIC value of the full model (<none>) is 21.899. The algorithm then removes each variable from the full model and calculates the AIC value. The removal of sepal length is the only variable that generates a lower AIC value (21.266) compared to the full model. The next part of the output shows the model where the sepal length has been removed:

```
Step:  AIC=21.27
Species ~ Sepal.Width + Petal.Length + Petal.Width

                Df     Deviance       AIC
 <none>                 13.266       21.266
- Sepal.Width   1       20.564       26.564
- Petal.Length  1       27.399       33.399
- Petal.Width   1       31.512       37.512
```

The AIC value of this reduced model is 21.266. When the algorithm now removes each variable from this reduced model, none of the reduced models will generate lower AIC values than the current model. Hence, the algorithm stops and reports the model “Species ~ Sepal.Width + Petal.Length + Petal.Width” as the most likely model. Let’s check the summary output of the reduced model:

```
summary(fit2)
...

               Estimate    Std. Error    z value    Pr(>|z|)
(Intercept)    -50.527     23.995        -2.106     0.0352 *
Sepal.Width     -8.376      4.761        -1.759     0.0785 .
Petal.Length     7.875      3.841         2.050     0.0403 *
Petal.Width     21.430     10.707         2.001     0.0453 *
...
```

The estimated coefficients for petal length and petal width are now significantly different from zero because their associated p-values are now less than 0.05. Let’s check how well the reduced model performs compared to the full model by computing the area under the ROC curve:

```
library(pROC)
pred_prob_full=predict(fit,type = "response")
roc(df_iris$Species, pred_prob_full)$auc
Area under the curve: 0.9972
pred_prob_reduced=predict(fit2,type = "response")
roc(df_iris$Species, pred_prob_reduced)$auc
Area under the curve: 0.9972
```

We see that both models generate the same AUC, which suggests that the reduced model predicts as well as the full model. In such a case, one should always select the simpler model because variables that do not contribute to the prediction are redundant.

11.4.7 Validation

We will here see how to validate a logistic regression model by using the **caret** package.

11.4.8 The Hold-Out Method

We will here validate the logistic regression model based on the Iris dataset, using the hold-out method, where we set aside 30% of the data points as test data. For simplicity, we here use a full model with all variables in the Iris dataset.

```
set.seed(15) #For reproducibility
library(caret)
df_iris=iris[(iris$Species !="setosa"),] # Remove Setosa
df_iris$Species=factor(df_iris$Species,levels=c("versicolor",
"virginica")) # Set to two levels
index = createDataPartition(y=df_iris$Species, p=0.7, list=FALSE)
train = df_iris[index,]
test = df_iris[-index,]
modelLookup("glm")
    model   parameter  label       forReg   forClass    probModel
1   glm     parameter  parameter   TRUE     TRUE        TRUE
```

We see that, similar to the LDA model, the logistic regression model does not have any hyperparameters to tune. The output tells us that the model can be used for both regression and classification tasks and that it provides probabilities. We will now train the model based on the training dataset by using the "train" function in the **caret** package:

```
fit = train(Species ~ ., data=train, method="glm",
family="binomial",
      trControl = trainControl(method = "cv"))
fit$finalModel
 Coefficients:
 (Intercept) Sepal.Length Sepal.Width Petal.Length Petal.Width
  -45.943       -1.611        -5.261       9.189        15.274

 Degrees of Freedom: 69 Total (i.e. Null);  65 Residual
 Null Deviance:     97.04
 Residual Deviance: 10.85    AIC: 20.85
```

Since the training process in this case only involves estimating the parameters of the model, without tuning any hyperparameters, we will get the same results as with "glm" function

```
# To compare with
#fit2 = glm(Species~.,data=train,family=binomial)
#summary(fit2)
```

Next, we compute how well the model can predict the test data:

```
pred= predict(fit, test)
Tab=table(pred, test$Species)
Tab
pred             versicolor   virginica
  versicolor         15           0
  virginica           0          15
sum(diag(Tab))/sum(Tab)
1
```

We see that 100% of the flowers in the test dataset were correctly classified. However, the accuracy is quite sensitive to the split of the training and test data as we discussed when we validated the LDA model. Try to run the code above with a different seed (change it from 15 to another number) and note that the accuracies may vary quite much from the different runs. Thus, for smaller datasets, it is more appropriate to use cross-validation.

By using the following code, we can compare the ROC curves based on the training data and the test data:

```
library(pROC)
# Train model on the training data
fit = glm(Species~.,data=train,family=binomial)
# Use trained model to predict the training data
pred_train=predict(fit,train,type="response")
# Use trained model to predict the test data
pred_test=predict(fit,test,type="response")

# Compute ROC based on training data
roc_train=roc(train$Species, pred_train)
# Compute ROC based on test data
roc_test=roc(test$Species, pred_test)

plot(roc_train)
lines(roc_test,col="red")
legend("bottomright",c("Training data",
"Test data"),col=1:2,lty=1,lwd=2)
```

Note that test data generates a larger AUC compared to the training data in this example (Fig. 11.19). This is normally not the case, because the model usually performs worse on the test data compared to the training data.

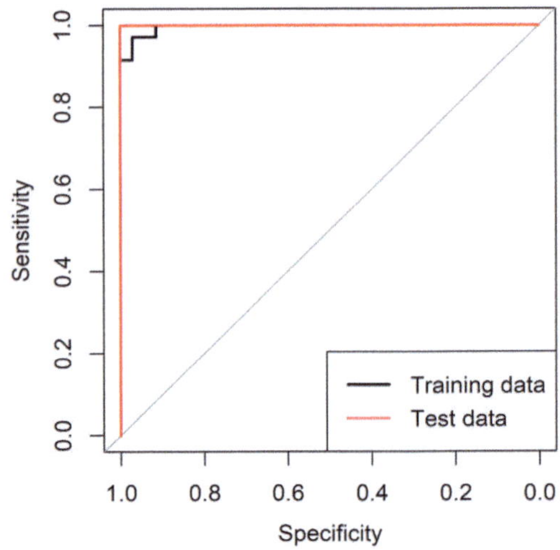

Fig. 11.19 ROC curves that show the performance of the logistic regression model to predict the Versicolors and Virginicas in the Iris dataset based on the training data and test data

11.4.9 *k-fold Cross-Validation*

To instead perform a 10-fold cross-validation, we can use the same lines of code as above but where we now include all data and study the output in the "fit$results"

```
set.seed(15) #For reproducibility
fit = train(Species ~ ., data=df_iris, method="glm",
family="binomial",
                trControl = trainControl(method = "cv"))
fit$resample
fit$results
   parameter    Accuracy    Kappa    AccuracySD     KappaSD
1      none       0.96       0.92    0.06992059    0.1398412
```

We see that the 10-fold cross-validation has resulted in an average accuracy of 96%. Let's also try the LOOCV:

```
fit = train(Species ~ ., data=df_iris, method="glm",
family="binomial",
            trControl = trainControl(method = "LOOCV"))
pred= predict(fit)
Tab=table(pred, df_iris$Species)
Tab
pred            versicolor    virginica
  versicolor       49             1
  virginica         1            49
sum(diag(Tab))/sum(Tab)
0.98
```

The LOOCV results in an accuracy of 98%.

11.5 Exercises

1. Combine the numerical variables in the Crab dataset by using logistic regression on all data. Create an ROC curve based on the computed probabilities to classify male and female crabs and report the AUC value.
2. Simplify the logistic model by using the "step" function with backward selection. Which variables were included in the simplified model?
3. Calculate the accuracy of your simplified model versus the full model using a cutoff value of 0.5.
4. Suppose that you find a crab and would like to know the sex of the crab with the following measurements: FL = 8.0, RW = 6.7, CL = 16.2, CW = 18.9, BD = 7.0. Use your simplified logistic regression model to compute the probability that the crab is a female.
5. Use the hold-out method to validate your simplified model. Use 70% of the data as your training data and 30% as your test data. Then calculate the accuracy of the model based on the test dataset. Note, as we discussed at the beginning of this chapter, we should perform model selection on a validation data and not on all data as in this example. We will discuss such approach in the next section.

11.6 Decision Trees

A decision tree is a graphical illustration where a node represents a choice between alternatives based on the value of the measured variable. Leaf nodes represent the decision. A decision tree where the target variable has a categorical scale, such as yes or no, is called a classification tree. If the target variable is on a continuous scale, the tree is called a regression tree. In this book, we will only discuss classification trees. Watch the video below to learn how decision trees can be used for classification and to understand the concept of the Gini index.

11.6.1 Video

https://youtu.be/XFafaKsnSuM
www.tilestats.com/ml/

We will here start with a very simple example, as shown in the video, to learn how to manually construct a decision tree. In this case, we have only one variable, the PSA level, of four healthy individuals and five individuals with prostate cancer (Table 11.2).

Table 11.2 PSA levels in the nine subjects

Prostate cancer	NO	NO	NO	YES	NO	YES	YES	YES	YES
PSA level (µg/L)	2.2	2.5	2.7	3.1	3.5	4.0	4.2	4.5	4.8

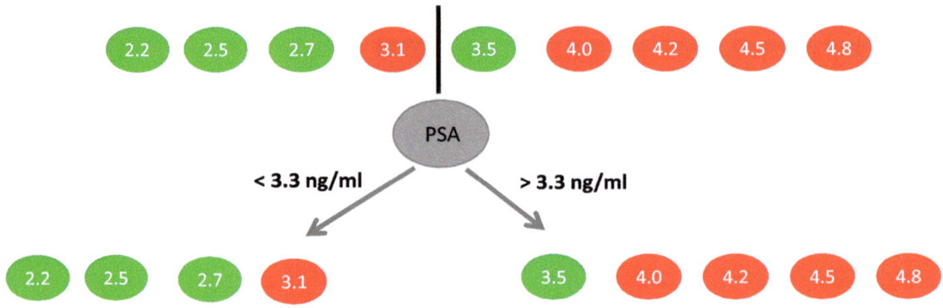

Fig. 11.20 An illustration of how to separate healthy controls (green) from patients with prostate cancer (red) based on their PSA levels with a cutoff value of 3.3

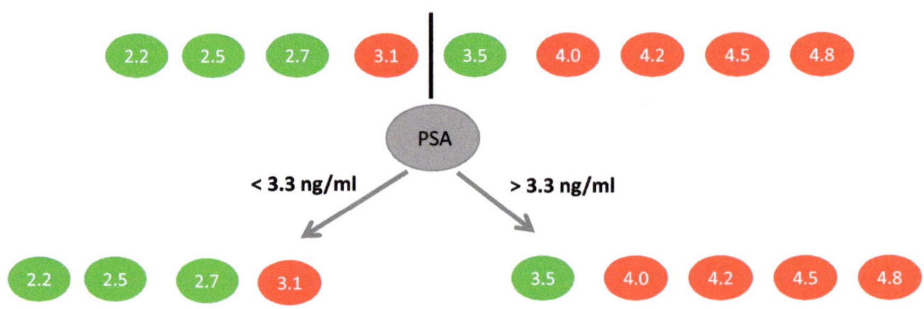

$$\text{Gini}(T_1) = 1 - \sum_{j=1}^{n} p_j^2 = 1 - \left((3/4)^2 + (1/4)^2\right) = 0.375 \qquad \text{Gini}(T_2) = 1 - \sum_{j=1}^{n} p_j^2 = 1 - \left((1/5)^2 + (4/5)^2\right) = 0.32$$

$$\text{Gini}(T) = \frac{n_1}{N}\text{Gini}(T_1) + \frac{n_2}{N}\text{Gini}(T_2) = \frac{4}{9}\cdot 0.375 + \frac{5}{9}\cdot 0.32 = \boxed{0.34}$$

Fig. 11.21 An illustration of how to calculate the Gini index based on a cutoff value of 3.3 to separate healthy controls (green) from patients with prostate cancer (red) based on their PSA levels

To manually create a decision tree, we first begin to sort the individuals based on their PSA values. Next, we should find a good cutoff value that separates the two groups. Suppose that we would use a cutoff value of 3.3 (Fig. 11.20).

However, how do we know that this is the best split? There are many types of metrics to define the "best" split. Generally, the metrics are often based on how well the spit generates purity (or impurity) of the groups. The Gini index is one metric that measures the impurity of the cutoffs. From the video, we know that the Gini index for a cutoff value of 3.3 can be calculated as in Fig. 11.21.

We see that such a split will result in a Gini index of about 0.34 (Fig. 11.21). The lower the value is, the more pure the groups are. To compute the Gini index for all possible splits, we can use the R code below. Note that the PSA values have already been ordered here:

```
rm(list=ls()) # Clear environment
PSA=c(2.2,2.5,2.7,3.1,3.5,4.0,4.2,4.5,4.8)
Group=factor(c("NO","NO","NO","YES","NO","YES","YES",
"YES","YES"))
df=data.frame(PSA,Group)
Gini=NULL
N=nrow(df) # Total number of data points
for (i in 1:(N-1)){
  #Split data frame into two groups
  df1=df[1:i,]
  df2=df[(i+1):N,]
  # Check the size of the groups
  n1= nrow(df1)
  n2= nrow(df2)
  # Sum numb of NO and YES in each data frame
  n_NO_1=sum(df1$Group=="NO")
  n_YES_1=sum(df1$Group=="YES")
  n_NO_2=sum(df2$Group=="NO")
  n_YES_2=sum(df2$Group=="YES")
  # Calc Gini
  GiniT1=1-((n_NO_1/n1)^2+(n_YES_1/n1)^2)
  GiniT2=1-((n_NO_2/n2)^2+(n_YES_2/n2)^2)
  Gini[i]=(n1/N)*GiniT1+(n2/N)*GiniT2
}
round(Gini,2) # Print Gini
0.42  0.32  0.19  0.34  0.18  0.30  0.38  0.44
```

Let's summarize our Gini calculations in a table.

Calculating the Gini index for all possible splits shows that a cutoff value of 3.75 results in the lowest Gini index (Table 11.3). We have now identified where to split the data for the root node in order to minimize the Gini index (Fig. 11.22).

To split the remaining group with four NOs and one YES, we just repeat the same process as we did above. The complete splitting process can be summarized with the following steps:

1. Sort the data based on the values that are used for the decision tree.
2. Split the data into two groups.
3. Calculate the Gini index for the split.
4. Repeat steps 2–3 for all possible splits.
5. Find the lowest Gini index.
6. Split the data based on the minimum Gini index and use the mean value of the two values on each side of the split as the cutoff value.
7. Repeat steps 2–6 until the tree is fully split into pure groups.

The final decision tree is shown in Fig. 11.23.

Table 11.3 Gini indexes for different cutoff values

Prostate cancer	NO	NO	NO	YES	NO	YES	YES	YES	YES
PSA	2.2	2.5	2.7	3.1	3.5	4.0	4.2	4.5	4.8
Cutoff value (mean)	2.35	2.6	2.9	3.3	3.75	4.1	4.35	4.65	
Gini index	0.42	0.32	0.19	0.34	**0.18**	0.30	0.38	0.44	

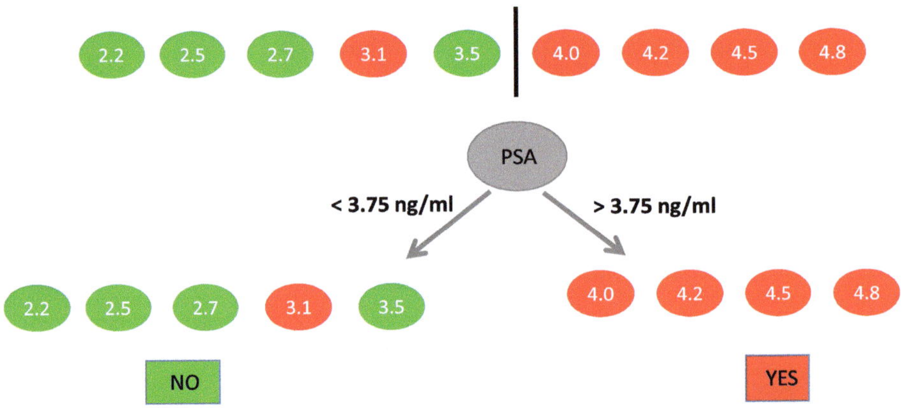

Fig. 11.22 An illustration of how a cutoff value of 3.75 results in the lowest Gini index to separate healthy controls (green) from patients with prostate cancer (red) based on their PSA levels. If a person has a PSA level greater than 3.75, it will be classified as having prostate cancer

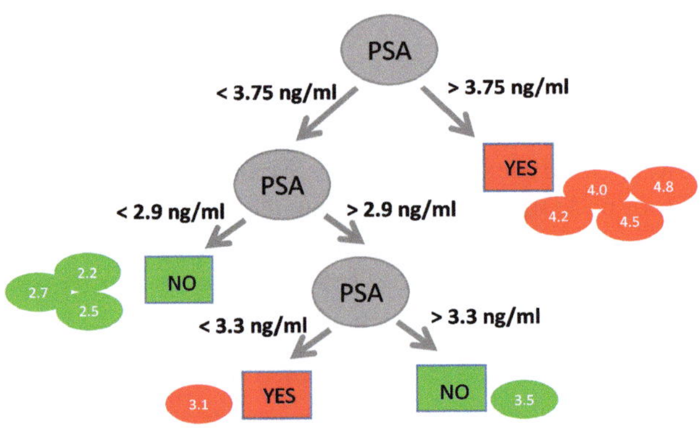

Fig. 11.23 An illustration of how a decision tree separates healthy controls (green) from patients with prostate cancer (red) based on their PSA levels. If a person has a PSA level greater than 3.75, it will be classified as having prostate cancer. If a person has a PSA level less than 3.75 but in the range of 2.9–3.3, it will also be classified as having prostate cancer

11.6.2 The Final Gini Indexes

Once we have built our tree, we can compute the Gini indexes for the different splits. The Gini index at the root node can be calculated by:

$$Gini_{\text{root}} = 1 - \left(\left(\frac{4}{9} \right)^2 + \left(\frac{5}{9} \right)^2 \right) = 0.494$$

The Gini index after the first split, at 3.75, is:

$$Gini(T_1) = 1 - \left(\left(\frac{4}{5} \right)^2 + \left(\frac{1}{5} \right)^2 \right) = 0.32$$

$$Gini(T_2) = 1 - \left(\left(\frac{0}{4} \right)^2 + \left(\frac{4}{4} \right)^2 \right) = 0$$

$$Gini(T) = \left(\frac{n_1}{N} \right) Gini(T_1) + \left(\frac{n_2}{N} \right) Gini(T_2) = \left(\frac{5}{9} \right) 0.32 + \left(\frac{4}{9} \right) 0 = 0.178$$

The Gini index after the second split, at 2.9, is:

$$Gini(T_1) = 1 - \left(\left(\frac{3}{3} \right)^2 + \left(\frac{0}{3} \right)^2 \right) = 0$$

$$Gini(T_2) = 1 - \left(\left(\frac{1}{2} \right)^2 + \left(\frac{1}{2} \right)^2 \right) = 0.5$$

$$Gini(T) = \left(\frac{n_1}{N} \right) Gini(T_1) + \left(\frac{n_2}{N} \right) Gini(T_2) = \left(\frac{3}{5} \right) 0 + \left(\frac{2}{5} \right) 0.5 = 0.2$$

Note that the Gini index did not reduce at this split, it actually increased the impurity.

The Gini index after the third split, at 3.3, is:

$$Gini(T_1) = 1 - \left(\left(\frac{1}{1} \right)^2 + \left(\frac{0}{0} \right)^2 \right) = 0$$

$$Gini(T_2) = 1 - \left(\left(\frac{0}{0} \right)^2 + \left(\frac{1}{1} \right)^2 \right) = 0$$

$$Gini(T) = \left(\frac{n_1}{N}\right) Gini(T_1) + \left(\frac{n_2}{N}\right) Gini(T_2) = \left(\frac{1}{2}\right)0 + \left(\frac{1}{2}\right)0 = 0$$

We see that if we continue to spit the tree, the impurity will finally be zero.

11.6.3 The rpart Package

We can build the same decision tree using the function "rpart" in the **rpart** package, which uses the CART decision tree algorithm. The function "rpart" can generate both regression and classification trees. Since we will generate a classification tree, we set the argument "method" to class. Per default, the function will not split the data unless the node includes at least 20 observations (minsplit = 20). Hence, to generate a fully split decision tree we will need to reduce this parameter since we only have 10 observations. Finally, we set the splitting method to Gini to be consistent with our earlier calculations. Note that we do not have to sort the data before we use the "rpart" function.

```
rm(list=ls()) # Clear environment
PSA=c(2.2,2.5,2.7,3.1,3.5,4.0,4.2,4.5,4.8)
Group=factor(c("Healthy","Healthy","Healthy","Cancer",
"Healthy","Cancer","Cancer","Cancer","Cancer"),
levels=c("Healthy","Cancer"))
df=data.frame(PSA,Group)
library(rpart)
fit=rpart(Group~PSA,data=df,method="class",minsplit=1,
parms = list(split = "gini"))
```

We can now plot the tree by using the **rpart.plot** package:

```
library(rpart.plot)
rpart.plot(fit,extra=1,digits=3)
```

This tree is exactly the same as we generated by manual calculations. The values that are shown within each node are the number of healthy individuals and cancer patients at each node (Fig. 11.24). The labels of each node (Cancer or Healthy) indicate the majority class in that node. For example, the node at the right-hand side is "Cancer 0 4", which means that if the PSA level is greater than 3.75, a person will be predicted as having "Cancer". When the tree predicts the training data, "4" cancer patients, and "0" healthy individuals, had a PSA level that was greater than 3.75. Let's see how well the tree predicts:

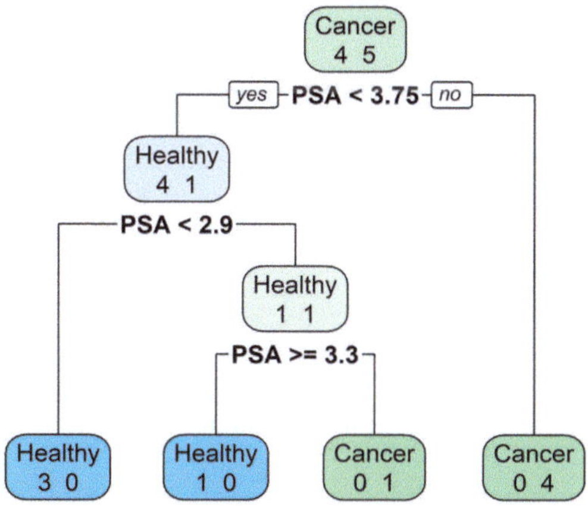

Fig. 11.24 A decision tree that separates healthy controls from patients with prostate cancer based on their PSA levels. If a person has a PSA level greater than 3.75, it will be classified as having prostate cancer. If a person has a PSA level less than 3.75 but in the range of 2.9–3.3, it will also be classified as having prostate cancer. The values that are shown within each node are the number of healthy individuals and cancer patients at each node, respectively. The labels of each node (Cancer or Healthy) indicate the majority class in each node

```
pred = predict(fit, type="class")
table(pred, Group)
           Group
pred          Healthy   Cancer
  Healthy        4         0
  Cancer         0         5
```

We see that the tree classifies with 100% accuracy. If a decision tree is allowed to grow without any restrictions (e.g., no limit on depth, no minimum samples per leaf, or no minimum samples per split), it will achieve 100% accuracy on the training data. This happens because the tree keeps splitting until it perfectly classifies all training data. As we discussed at the beginning of this chapter, the model then just memorizes the training data and will therefore cause overfitting.

11.6.4 Pruning to Prevent Overfitting

To avoid overfitting when building a decision tree, we can prune the tree based on the so-called complexity parameter (cp). The cp parameter controls how the decision tree is pruned to balance the trade-off between model complexity (tree size) and predictive accuracy. The calculation of the cp parameter is somewhat technical and will not be discussed here. For each value of the cp, cross-validation is computed to estimate the relative error for a given tree size. To compute this, we can run the following code:

```
plotcp(fit,las=1)
```

Note that the relative error has been computed versus different values of cp (Fig. 11.25). A certain value of cp corresponds to a certain tree size (number of leaf nodes in the tree shown at the top of the plot). Note that the plot does not show a cp value for 3 leaf nodes because the split at a cutoff of 2.9 does not increase the accuracy of the tree. Remember that the Gini index increased at a split of 2.9 compared to the previous split at 3.75 when we calculated the final Gini index of the tree by hand. According to the reference manual for the **rpart** package, an appropriate value of the cp parameter is often the leftmost value for which the error is below the horizontal reference line. Hence, in our case (Fig. 11.25), we would set the cp value to 0.31, which corresponds to a tree with two leaf nodes:

```
pt=prune(fit,cp=0.31)
rpart.plot(pt,extra=1,digits=3)
```

Let's check how well the pruned tree (Fig. 11.26) predicts:

```
pred = predict(pt, type="class")
table(pred, Group)
                  Group
pred          Healthy   Cancer
  Healthy         4         1
  Cancer          0         4
```

We see that the tree now incorrectly classifies one cancer patient as being healthy.

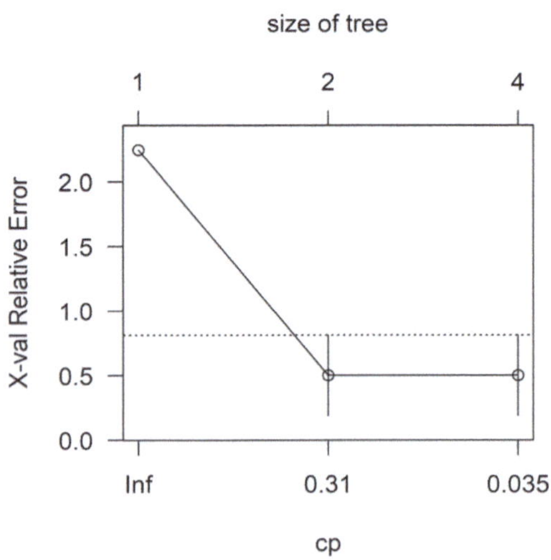

Fig. 11.25 A plot showing the cross-validated relative error versus the complexity parameter (cp) values for different tree sizes of the decision tree. The size of the tree is indicated at the top of the plot. The dashed line represents the baseline relative error, while open circles correspond to the relative errors at specific cp values

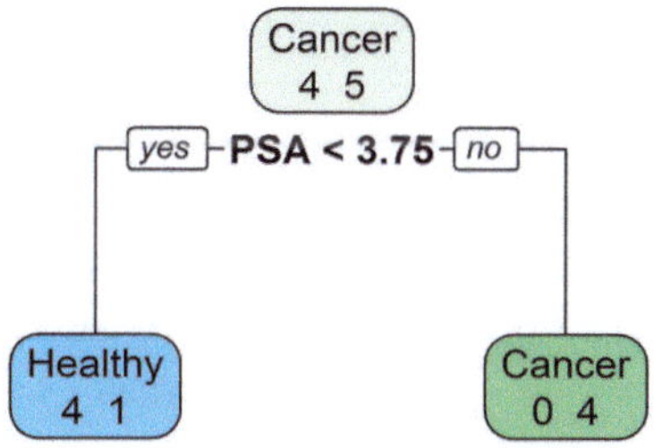

Fig. 11.26 A pruned decision tree that separates healthy controls from patients with prostate cancer based on a cutoff value of 3.75. If a person has a PSA level greater than 3.75, it will be classified as having prostate cancer. The values that are shown within each node are the number of healthy individuals and cancer patients at each node, respectively. The labels of each node (Cancer or Healthy) indicate the majority class in each node

11.6.5 Predict New Cases

We can now use our pruned tree to predict if an individual has prostate cancer or not. Let's say that a person has a PSA level of 3.0. If we follow the tree structure (Fig. 11.26), we see that the person should be predicted as being healthy. We can use the function "predict" to make the same prediction in R:

```
new=data.frame(PSA=3.0)
predict(pt, new, type="class")
          1
Healthy
Levels: Healthy Cancer
```

We see that the tree predicts that the person is healthy.

11.6.6 Use the Iris Data

We will now use the Iris dataset to construct a decision tree. To initially generate a fully split tree, we set the cp parameter to zero:

```
library(rpart)
fit=rpart(Species~.,data=iris,method="class",minsplit=1,
parms = list(split = "gini"),cp=0)
rpart.plot(fit,extra=1,digits=3)
```

This tree (Fig. 11.27) predicts the training data with 100% accuracy since no flower is incorrectly predicted. Thus, the tree clearly overfits because it has learned to split the training data perfectly.

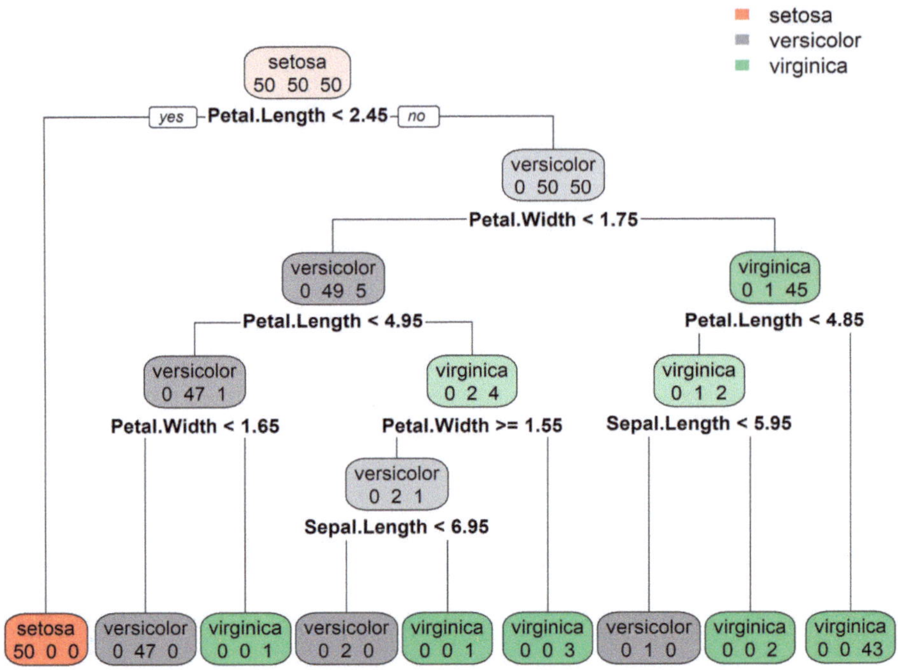

Fig. 11.27 A decision tree that fully separates the three species in the Iris dataset. The values that are shown within each node are the number of flowers of type Setosa, Versicolor, and Virginica. The labels of each node indicate the majority class in each node

To avoid overfitting, we will therefore prune this tree, where we plot how the relative error changes with different cp values (or with different sizes of the tree) by:

```
plotcp(fit,las=1)
```

From Fig. 11.28, we see that we should prune the tree by setting the cp value to 0.094 so that we generate a tree with three leaf nodes:

```
pt=prune(fit,cp=0.094)
rpart.plot(pt,extra=1,digits=3)
```

We see that our pruned tree makes six incorrect predictions (Fig. 11.29). Five Virginicas are incorrectly predicted as Versicolors (0 49 **5**) and one Versicolor (0 **1** 45) is incorrectly predicted as Virginica.

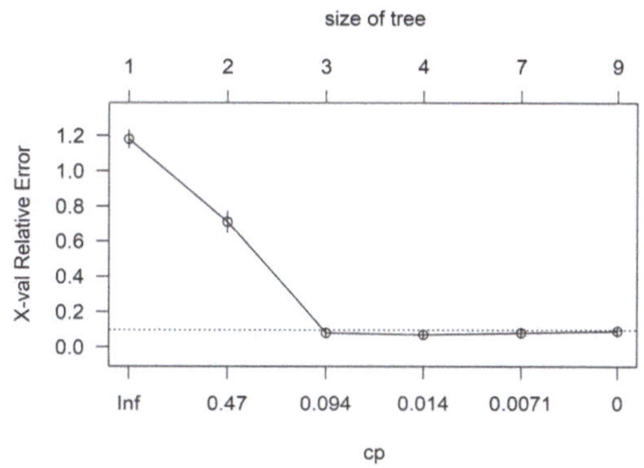

Fig. 11.28 A plot showing the cross-validated relative error versus the complexity parameter (cp) values for different tree sizes of the decision tree based on the Iris data. The size of the tree is indicated at the top of the plot. The dashed line represents the baseline relative error, while open circles correspond to the relative errors at specific cp values

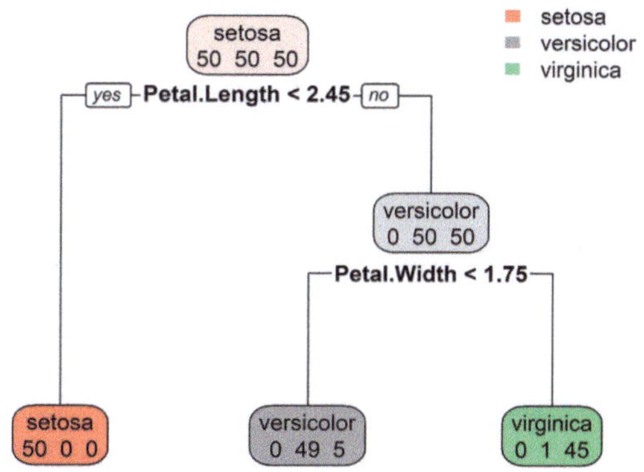

Fig. 11.29 A pruned decision tree that separates the three species in the Iris dataset based on the petal length and the petal width. The values that are shown within each node are the number of flowers of type Setosa, Versicolor, and Virginica. The labels of each node indicate the majority class in each node

11.6.7 Validation with the Hold-Out Method

We will here see how to validate a decision tree by using the hold-out method based on the Iris dataset. We therefore first split the dataset into a test set and a training set:

```
set.seed(10) #For reproducibility
library(caret)
index = createDataPartition(y=iris$Species, p=0.7,
list=FALSE) # 70% as training data
train = iris[index,]
test = iris[-index,]
```

Next, we create a decision tree based on the training data and check how to prune this tree:

```
fit=rpart(Species~.,data=train,method="class",minsplit=1,
parms = list(split = "gini"),cp=0)
plotcp(fit,las=1)
```

According to Fig. 11.30, we prune the tree by setting the cp value to 0.08, which will result in a tree with three leaf nodes.

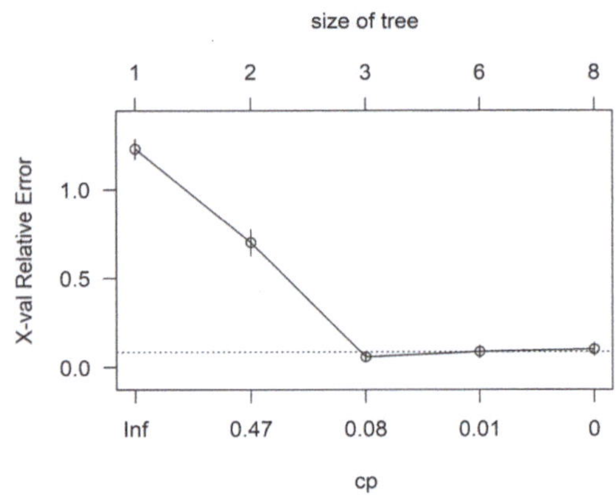

Fig. 11.30 A plot showing the cross-validated relative error versus the complexity parameter (cp) values for different tree sizes of the decision tree based on the training data. The size of the tree is indicated at the top of the plot. The dashed line represents the baseline relative error, while open circles correspond to the relative errors at specific cp values

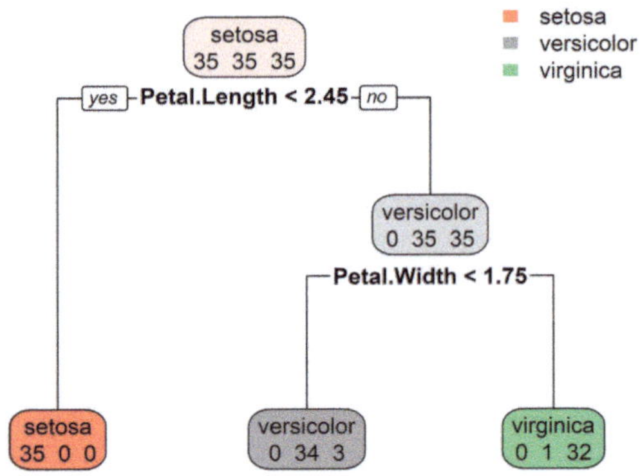

Fig. 11.31 A pruned decision tree that separates the three species in the Iris dataset based on the training data. The values that are shown within each node are the number of flowers of type Setosa, Versicolor, and Virginica. The labels of each node indicate the majority class in each node

```
pt=prune(fit,cp=0.08)
library(rpart.plot)
rpart.plot(pt,extra=1,digits=3)
```

Our pruned tree based on the training data is shown in Fig. 11.31.

Next, we validate our pruned tree (Fig. 11.31) by using the test dataset:

```
pred=predict(pt, test, type="class")
(tab1=table(pred, test$Species))
pred          setosa    versicolor    virginica
  setosa        15          0             0
  versicolor     0         15             2
  virginica      0          0            13
```

We see that two Virginicas are incorrectly predicted as Versicolors,

```
(accuracy=sum(diag(tab1))/sum(tab1))
0.9555556
```

and that the accuracy is about 95.5%.

11.6.8 Hyperparameter Tuning with the Caret Package

Previously, we have used a plot to identify an appropriate value of the parameter cp based on the training data. Another method to find the "best" value of the parameter is to use cross-validation of the training data with the **caret** package. Let's first use the function "modelLookup" to see which parameters we can tune:

```
library(caret)
modelLookup("rpart")
  model    parameter label                 forReg forClass probModel
1 rpart    cp        Complexity Parameter  TRUE   TRUE     TRUE
```

The rpart model has only one hyperparameter to tune, which is the cp parameter. We can now create a sequence of values of the cp parameter. Based on the plot of the different cp values we previously generated (Fig. 11.30), the values 0.47, 0.08, 0.01, and 0 result in trees with different sizes. We can use the function "expand. grid", which creates a data frame of the cp values:

```
cp_grid=expand.grid(cp = c(0.47,0.08,0.01,0))
cp_grid
    cp
1 0.47
2 0.08
3 0.01
4 0.00
```

This means that we will try these four different values of the parameter cp. Each value will be used to create a decision tree based on the training data and the performance of such tree will be calculated based on the validation data in the cross-validation. We will here use a 10-fold cross-validation, which means that each cp value will be validated on 10 subsets and the mean performance of these 10 subsets will be calculated. Then the process starts over with a new value of the cp parameter.

```
set.seed(12) #For reproducibility
fit_train=train(Species ~ ., data=train,
method="rpart",minsplit=1,
parms = list(split = "gini"),cp=0,
trControl=trainControl(method = "cv"), tuneGrid = cp_grid)
fit_train
CART

105 samples
  4 predictor
  3 classes: 'setosa', 'versicolor', 'virginica'

No pre-processing
Resampling: Cross-Validated (10 fold)
Summary of sample sizes: 93, 96, 95, 96, 96, 95, ...
Resampling results across tuning parameters:

   cp      Accuracy    Kappa
  0.00     0.9353535  0.9027426
  0.01     0.9353535  0.9027426
  0.08     0.9353535  0.9027426
  0.47     0.6472727  0.4809524

Accuracy was used to select the optimal model using the
largest value.
The final value used for the model was cp = 0.08.
```

We see that the "train" function has performed a 10-fold cross-validation on four different values of the cp parameter. It has selected the model with the highest mean accuracy based on the cross-validations, which is a model with a cp value of 0.08. However, note that the cp parameters 0, 0.01, and 0.08 all result in the same accuracy. When we have ties like this, one usually selects the simplest model, which is a model with a larger cp parameter because such a model will result in a smaller tree. We now retrain the model based on all training data where we set the cp parameter to 0.08:

```
fit=rpart(Species~.,data=train,method="class",minsplit=1,
parms = list(split = "gini"),cp=0.08)
```

The generated tree will be identical to the tree we plotted before (Fig. 11.31) because the cross-validation proposed the same value of the cp parameter as when we pruned the tree based on the plot in Fig. 11.30.

Finally, we evaluate this tree with the test dataset:

```
pred=predict(fit, test, type="class")
Tab=table(pred, test$Species)
Tab
```

```
pred            setosa   versicolor   virginica
  setosa            15            0           0
  versicolor         0           15           2
  virginica          0            0          13
```

We see that two Virginicas have incorrectly been predicted as Versicolors.

11.7 Exercises

1. Use a decision tree to classify female and male crabs of the Crab dataset (you can use all numerical variables as well as the categorical variable species in the dataset to classify). Use all data to create the tree. To avoid overfitting, set the argument minsplit to 80.
2. Calculate the accuracy of your tree.
3. Suppose that you find a crab and would like to know the sex of the crab with the following measurements: RW = 6.7, BD = 7.0. Use your tree to compute if the crab is a male or a female. Also, explain in words how the tree makes this prediction.
4. Use a decision tree to classify female and male crabs of the Crab dataset (you can use all numerical variables as well as the categorical variable species in the dataset to classify). Use the hold-out method to evaluate your tree. Use 70% of the data to build your tree (to find an appropriate value of the cp parameter) and 30% of the data to test your tree.

11.8 Random Forest

A random forest is simply a method that generates a large number of decision trees that form a "forest". Each tree in the forest is trained on a random subset of the data and a random selection of features/variables. This randomness ensures diversity among the trees, making the method more robust to noise and overfitting compared to a single decision tree. The predicted class of a new observation is determined by each tree in the forest. Its final prediction is based on the majority vote from all trees. Watch the video to learn how the method works.

11.8.1 Video

https://youtu.be/013hWEugXQ8
www.tilestats.com/ml/

We will here use the package **randomForest** to construct a random forest with 100 trees based on the Iris dataset:

```
rm(list=ls()) # Clear environment
library(randomForest)
set.seed(1980) #For reproducibility
iris_RF = randomForest(Species~.,data=iris, ntree=100)
```

11.8.2 Predict a New Observation

Once we have generated a random forest, we can use it to predict the class of a new observation. Suppose that we want to predict the class of an Iris flower with an unknown class based on the following measures:

```
new=data.frame(Sepal.Length=5.5,Sepal.Width=2,Petal.Length=3,
Petal.Width=1.6)
predict(iris_RF,new)
versicolor
Levels: setosa versicolor virginica
```

The iris flower was predicted to be of class Versicolor. Hence, the majority of the 100 trees classified the flower as a Versicolor.

11.8.3 The OOB Error

One advantage of a random forest is that it internally estimates the error during the computation. Let's have a look at the out-of-bag (OOB) error for our random forest:

```
plot(iris_RF)
legend("topright",c("Average","Setosa","Versicolor",
"Virginic "),lty=1:4,col=1:4)
```

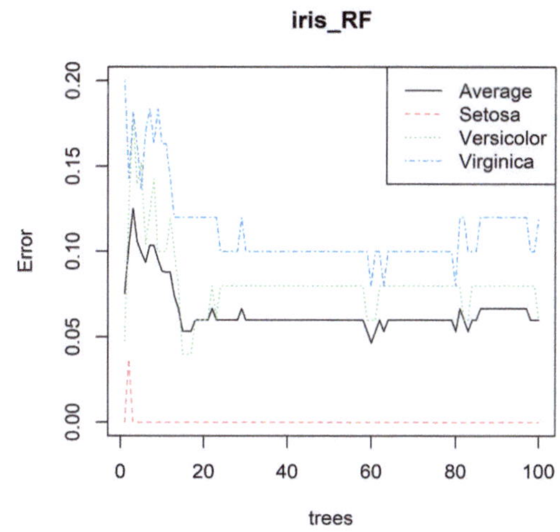

Fig. 11.32 Error rate plot for the random forest model applied to the Iris dataset. The x-axis represents the number of trees in the forest, and the y-axis shows the error rate. The black line indicates the average error across all classes, whereas the dashed lines represent the error rates for individual species (Setosa, Versicolor, and Virginica)

We see that the mean error (the black line) decreases when the forest grows in size (Fig. 11.32). Note that almost all trees in the forest predict Setosa with 100% accuracy since the error for Setosa is zero during the growth of the forest. However, the average error does not seem to stabilize when the forest keeps growing.

11.8.4 Selecting the Number of Trees

From Fig. 11.32, we see that the error keeps changing for different numbers of trees in the forest. We should therefore use a larger number of trees in our forest so that the error stabilizes. There is no disadvantage to using a very big forest other than it will require a long time to compute. Let's generate a forest with 1000 trees and plot how the OOB error changes:

```
set.seed(1980) #For reproducibility
iris_RF = randomForest(Species~.,data=iris, ntree=1000)
plot(iris_RF)
```

We see that the OOB error stabilizes after about 500 trees (Fig. 11.33). A reasonable number of trees for our forest is therefore around 500.

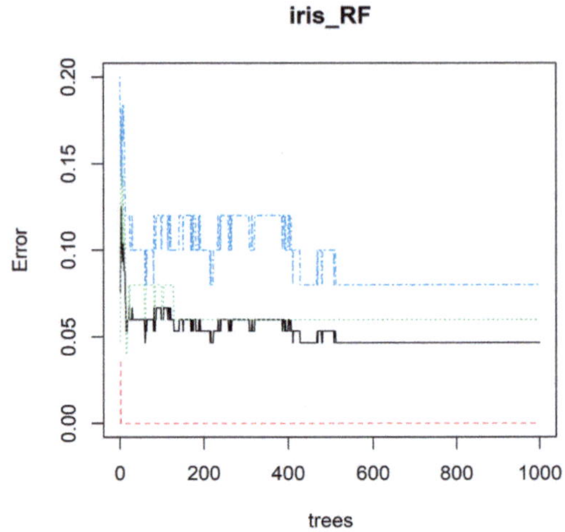

Fig. 11.33 Error rate plot for the random forest model applied to the Iris dataset. The x-axis represents the number of trees in the forest, and the y-axis shows the error rate. The black line indicates the average error across all classes, whereas the dashed lines represent the error rates for individual species (Setosa, Versicolor, and Virginica). The plot demonstrates how the error rate stabilizes as the number of trees increases, indicating the convergence of the random forest model

11.8.5 Confusion Matrix

We can generate the confusion matrix from the random forest, which is based on the OOB portion as explained in the video:

```
tab=iris_RF$confusion
tab
           setosa  versicolor  virginica  class.error
setosa         50           0          0         0.00
versicolor      0          47          3         0.06
virginica       0           4         46         0.08
```

Note that the output also shows the class error rate in the last column. For example, three out of 50 (6%) Versicolors were misclassified. The total accuracy is:

```
Accuracy=sum(diag(tab[,-4]))/sum(tab[,-4])
Accuracy
0.9533333
```

The average error rate is simply just one minus the accuracy:

```
error_rate=1-Accuracy
error_rate
0.04666667
```

Note that this error rate is the same error as the mean OOB error with 1000 trees in the previous plot (black line). This error rate can be extracted by:

```
iris_RF$err.rate[1000,1]
       OOB
0.04666667
```

Since a random forest internally estimates the OOB error during the computation through bootstrapping, the accuracy of 95.3% we calculated above can be seen as the accuracy from using a validation method.

11.8.6 Variable Importance

One nice feature of random forests is that they predict the importance of the input variables (features). For each split that is made in the trees, the Gini index decreases. Thus, a variable that decreases the Gini index more than the other variables in the forest can be seen as more important for separating the groups. To compute importance, we need to run the random forest again and set the importance argument to true:

```
set.seed(1980) #For reproducibility
iris_RF = randomForest(Species~.,data=iris, ntree=1000,
importance=TRUE)
```

With the function "varImpPlot", we can plot the importance:

```
varImpPlot(iris_RF)
```

The mean decrease in accuracy (MDA) is computed as follows: for each tree, the accuracy based on the out-of-bag portion of the data is recorded. Then the same is done after permuting each feature (randomly shuffle its values). The difference between the original and permuted accuracies is averaged across all trees and normalized by the standard deviation of these differences. The mean decrease in Gini (MDG) is the total decrease in node impurities from splitting the variable, averaged over all trees. This basically means that the features with higher MDA or MDG are more important for the model to separate the groups. We see that the petal length and petal width are the most important variables/features to separate the Iris species (Fig. 11.34).

For the Iris dataset, we only have four variables. However, if we have hundreds of variables, the random forest can be used to select a certain number of variables that are the most important for the classification based on the training data. Thus, a random forest can also be used as a method for feature selection to create a simpler model with only the most important features.

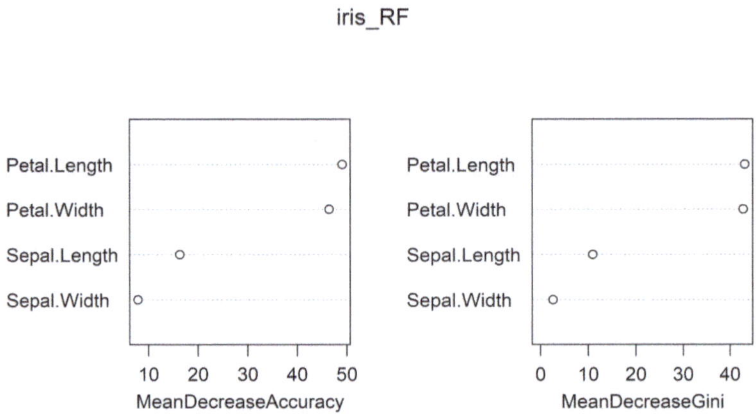

Fig. 11.34 Variable importance plot for the random forest model applied to the Iris dataset, based on the Mean Decrease in Accuracy (left) and Mean Decrease in Gini index (right). The y-axis shows the features (petal length, petal width, sepal length, and sepal width). Features with higher mean decrease in accuracy or Gini values are more important for the model to separate the species

11.8.7 Validation with the Hold-Out Method

We will here see how to validate a random forest model with the hold-out method by using the Iris dataset. To validate the random forest with the hold-out method, we can split the data into a training and a test set:

```
set.seed(10) #For reproducibility
library(caret)
index = createDataPartition(y=iris$Species, p=0.7,
list=FALSE)
train = iris[index,]
test = iris[-index,]
```

Then we generate a forest with, for example, 1000 trees based on the training data and let the forest predict based on the test data:

```
iris_RF = randomForest(Species~.,data=train, ntree=1000)
pred=predict(iris_RF,test)
(tab1=table(pred, test$Species))

pred            setosa  versicolor  virginica
  setosa          15         0           0
  versicolor       0        15           1
  virginica        0         0          14
(accuracy=sum(diag(tab1))/sum(tab1))
0.9777778
```

We see that only one Virginica was incorrectly predicted as a Versicolor.

11.8.8 Hyperparameter Tuning with the Caret Package

We will now perform hyperparameter tuning by using the **caret** package. To see which parameters we can tune, we can use the function "modelLookup"

```
modelLookup("rf")
  model parameter label                          forReg  forClass  probModel
1 rf    mtry      #Randomly Selected Predictors  TRUE    TRUE      TRUE
```

We see that the only parameter to tune is the parameter called "mtry", which is the number of variables or features that are randomly selected as candidates at each split to build a tree. We first split the data into training data and test data:

```
set.seed(10) #For reproducibility
library(caret)
index = createDataPartition(y=iris$Species, p=0.7,
list=FALSE)
train = iris[index,]
test = iris[-index,]
```

Since we have four numeric variables in the Iris dataset that are used to create the trees, we can try three different values of the mtry parameter:

```
mtry_grid=expand.grid(mtry = c(1,2,3))
```

We now use the "train" function, which will use a 10-fold cross-validation to test the performance of using three different values of the mtry parameter:

```
fit_train = train(Species ~ ., data=train, method="rf",
ntree=1000,
trControl = trainControl(method = "cv"),tuneGrid = mtry_grid)
fit_train
....
Resampling: Cross-Validated (10 fold)
Summary of sample sizes: 93, 95, 94, 95, 94, 96, ...
Resampling results across tuning parameters:

  mtry  Accuracy   Kappa
  1     0.9551515  0.9329141
  2     0.9349495  0.9024975
  3     0.9460606  0.9191641

Accuracy was used to select the optimal model using the
largest value.
The final value used for the model was mtry = 1.
```

From the output, we see that the value of mtry that results in the highest accuracy is 1. Let's retrain the model by using the optimal value of the mtry parameter and evaluate its performance on the test data:

```
iris_RF = randomForest(Species~.,data=train,
ntree=1000, mtry=1)
pred=predict(iris_RF,test)
(tabl=table(pred, test$Species))
pred               setosa   versicolor   virginica
  setosa             15          0            0
  versicolor          0         15            2
  virginica           0          1           13
(accuracy=sum(diag(tabl))/sum(tabl))
0.9555556
```

Note that the accuracy, 95.5%, of a model with the mtry parameter set to 1 is now lower compared to when we used the default setting in the hold-out method where we did not perform hyperparameter tuning, which was then 97.78%. The default value of the mtry parameter is the square root of the number of features. In our case, the default value is therefore 2. Since we have a small dataset, random effects may have a large impact on identifying the optimal values of the hyperparameters. If you try other seeds in the above code, you will see that the different values of the parameter mtry will be considered optimal. One way is to try a range of different seeds so that we can compute many accuracies for each mtry parameter. We could then calculate the mean of these accuracies and select the value of mtry that results in the largest mean accuracy. We will have a look at repeated cross-validation at the end of this chapter.

11.9 Exercises

1. Create a random forest with 2000 trees to classify female and male crabs of the Crab dataset (you can use all numerical variables as well as the categorical variable species in the dataset to classify). Use all data to create the forest.
2. Calculate the accuracy of your forest based on the OOB error.
3. Suppose that you find a blue crab (sp="B") and would like to know the sex of the crab with the following measurements: FL = 8.0, RW = 6.7, CL = 16.2, CW = 18.9, BD = 7.0. Use your forest to predict if it is a male or a female crab.
4. Use a random forest with 1000 trees to classify female and male crabs of the Crab dataset (you can use all numerical variables as well as the categorical variable species in the dataset to classify). Use the hold-out method to evaluate your forest. Use 70% of the data to build your model and 30% of the data to test your model.
5. Use all numeric variables and the variable species (sp) in the Crab dataset to find the most important variable to predict the sex of the crabs.

11.10 k-Nearest Neighbors

Depending on the distribution of your data, certain ML models might be more appropriate to use than others. We will here learn about the k-nearest neighbors (KNN) algorithm, which is a very simple and straightforward method to use. The method does not use any model to fit data. Instead, it simply calculates the distances from the data points with known group membership to the new observation with unknown membership. The majority of the *k*-nearest neighbors decide the class of the new observation.

11.10.1 Video

https://youtu.be/KHA1fDFW-Ig
www.tilestats.com/ml/

Let's consider the same example data as in the video where we have data on patients that have either a viral or bacterial infection. In this dataset, we have 12 individuals. The CRP and PCT of each individual have been measured from blood samples. We also know if they have bacterial or viral infections. This dataset constitutes our training data with known group membership:

```
rm(list=ls()) # Clear environment
PCT=c(36, 30, 45, 55, 47, 40, 59, 67, 50, 65, 55, 68)
CRP=c(40, 30, 32, 37, 40, 52, 48, 60, 68, 40,  55, 58)
Group=factor(c(rep("Virus",6),rep("Bacteria",6)),
levels=c("Virus","Bacteria"))
df=data.frame(CRP,PCT,Group)
```

Let's say that we have a new observation, an individual with a CRP of 42 and a PCT of 60, and want to predict if this individual has a bacterial or viral infection:

```
new=data.frame(CRP=42,PCT=60)
```

If we plot the data and the new observation:

```
plot(PCT,CRP,col=Group)
legend("topleft",levels(Group),col=1:2,pch=1)
# Add new observation
points(new$PCT,new$CRP,pch=17,col="blue",cex=1.5)
```

we see that the new observation (the blue triangle) seems to be closer to the data points belonging to the group bacteria (Fig. 11.35). In order to determine the class membership of a new observation, KNN performs the following steps:

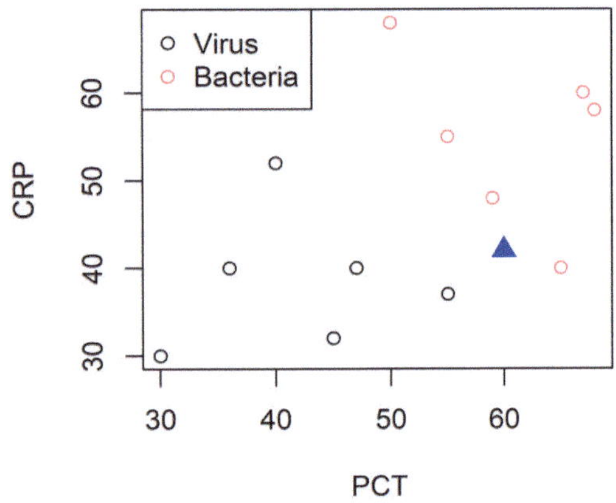

Fig. 11.35 A scatter plot of CRP and PCT levels from 12 individuals that have either a bacterial infection (red circles) or a viral infection (black circles). The blue triangle represents a new patient with an unknown infection type that will be predicted by the KNN model

1. Determine the Euclidean distance between the new observation and all data points in the dataset.
2. Sort the distances.
3. Select the *k*-nearest neighbors.
4. Determine the class of the new observation based on the group majority of the *k*-nearest neighbors.

Let's compute these steps with R:

1. **Calculate the Euclidean distances**
We first calculate the Euclidean distances between the new observation (PCT = 60, CRP = 42) and all the data:

```
# Calculate distances
D=sqrt((new$PCT-df$PCT)^2+(new$CRP- df$CRP)^2)
```

2. **Sort the distances**
Next, we create a new data frame that combines the distances with our old data frame. The rows of the new data frame are then sorted based on the distances:

```
df2=data.frame(df,D)
df2=df2[order(df2$D),]
df2
     CRP   PCT    Group       D
10   40    65   Bacteria    5.385165
7    48    59   Bacteria    6.082763
4    37    55     Virus     7.071068
5    40    47     Virus    13.152946
11   55    55   Bacteria   13.928388
12   58    68   Bacteria   17.888544
3    32    45     Virus    18.027756
8    60    67   Bacteria   19.313208
```

```
6     52    40      Virus     22.360680
1     40    36      Virus     24.083189
9     68    50    Bacteria    27.856777
2     30    30      Virus     32.310989
```

We see that the new observation has the closest distance to the person at row number 10 who has a bacterial infection.

3. **Select the *k*-nearest neighbors**
   As in the video, we will here set *k* to 5, which means that we select the five nearest neighbors. The five nearest neighbors are simply the first five individuals in the sorted data frame we computed earlier:

```
      CRP   PCT     Group          D
10    40    65    Bacteria     5.385165
7     48    59    Bacteria     6.082763
4     37    55      Virus      7.071068
5     40    47      Virus     13.152946
11    55    55    Bacteria    13.928388
12    58    68    Bacteria    17.888544
3     32    45      Virus     18.027756
8     60    67    Bacteria    19.313208
6     52    40      Virus     22.360680
1     40    36      Virus     24.083189
9     68    50    Bacteria    27.856777
2     30    30      Virus     32.310989
```

4. **Determine the class of the new observation**
   Since the majority of the *k*-nearest neighbors are of class "bacteria", we classify the new observation as bacteria, which means that we predict that the patient has a bacterial infection.

11.10.2 Using the "knn" Function

With the "knn" function in the **class** package, we can determine the class membership simply by:

```
library(class)
data1=df[,1:2] # Features of the training data
# Class membership of training data (bacteria or virus)
class1=df[,3]
knn(data1, new, class1, k = 5)
[1] Bacteria
Levels: Virus Bacteria
```

The output from the "knn" function tells us that the new observation is predicted as bacteria.

11.10.3 Validation and Hyperparameter Tuning

We will here see how to validate a KNN model by using the Iris dataset with the **caret** package. We will first use the hold-out method where we use the training data to perform hyperparameter tuning by changing the value of *k*. The optimal value of *k* will then be used to evaluate the model with the test data. To see which hyperparameter we can tune, we can use the "modelLookup" function:

```
library(caret)
modelLookup("knn")
    model parameter   label       forReg   forClass   probModel
1   knn   k           #Neighbors  TRUE     TRUE       TRUE
```

We see that the only hyperparameter to tune is the parameter *k*.

11.10.4 The Hold-Out Method

To validate the KNN with the hold-out method, we first split the data into a training and a test set:

```
set.seed(10) #For reproducibility
library(caret)
index = createDataPartition(y=iris$Species, p=0.7,
list=FALSE)
train = iris[index,]
test = iris[-index,]
```

Then we compute a 10-fold cross-validation on the training data with many different *k*'s (1, 3, 5, ..., 29):

```
tune = expand.grid(k = seq(1,29,2))
fit_train = train(Species ~ ., data=train, method="knn",
     trControl = trainControl(method = "cv"),tuneGrid = tune)
fit_train
...
  k     Accuracy     Kappa
   1   0.9540404   0.9311728
   3   0.9540404   0.9311728
```

```
   5   0.9631313   0.9447531
   7   0.9631313   0.9447531
   9   0.9520202   0.9280864
  11   0.9451515   0.9175365
  13   0.9451515   0.9175365
  15   0.9340404   0.9008698
  17   0.9440404   0.9157882
  19   0.9340404   0.9008698
  21   0.9138384   0.8709541
  23   0.9249495   0.8876208
  25   0.9360606   0.9042875
  27   0.9443939   0.9167875
  29   0.9340404   0.9008698

Accuracy was used to select the optimal model using the
largest value.
The final value used for the model was k = 7.
```

From this output, we can see that the optimal value of *k* is 5 or 7 because both these values result in the highest accuracy. The "train" function has selected a value of 7.

We can also plot the performance for different values of *k* by:

```
plot(fit_train)
```

We can see that if we set *k* to 5 or 7 (Fig. 11.36), we get the highest accuracy. According to the output from the "train" function, the optimal value of *k* is set to 7. Our final model based on the training process will therefore check the 7 nearest neighbors. We will now see how well the KNN performs on the test data:

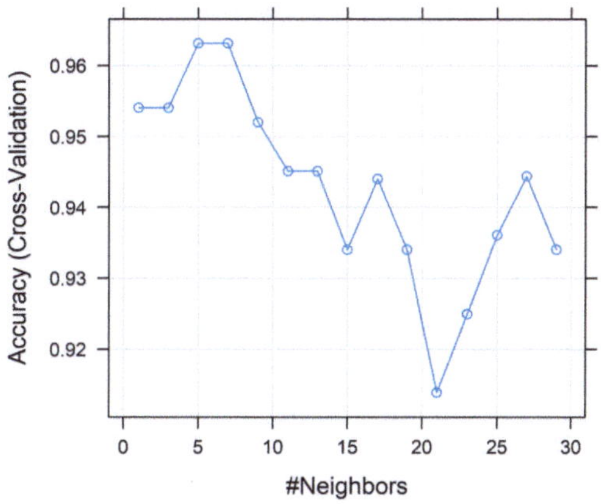

Fig. 11.36 A plot showing the accuracy based on the 10-fold cross-validation for different values of *k*

```
library(class)
data1=train[,1:4] # Extract features
class1=train$Species # Class membership of training data
pred=knn(data1, test[,1:4], class1, k = 7) # Predict
tab=table(pred, test$Species)
pred            setosa    versicolor    virginica
  setosa          15          0             0
  versicolor       0         15             1
  virginica        0          0            14
```

We see that only one Virginica is incorrectly predicted as a Versicolor.

Note that when KNN is based on the Euclidean distances, variables with large values will dominate the distance and therefore the prediction. One should therefore consider standardizing the variables to ensure that all variables contribute equally to the distance metric.

11.11 Exercises

1. Suppose that you find a crab and would like to know the sex of the crab with the following measurements: FL = 8.0, RW = 6.7, CL = 16.2, CW = 18.9, BD = 7.0. Use KNN, where you set k to 5, to predict if it is a male or female crab based on the numeric variables in the Crab dataset.
2. Use KNN to classify female and male crabs of the Crab dataset based on all numeric variables in the dataset. Use the hold-out method to validate your KNN. Use 70% of the data to train your KNN to find an optimal value of k and 30% of the data to test your classifier.

11.12 Gaussian Naive Bayes

Naive Bayes (NB) is one of the simplest and fastest ML models. A Gaussian naive Bayes model is based on continuous variables that are assumed to have a Gaussian (or normal) distribution. Watch the video to learn how the method works.

11.12.1 Video

https://youtu.be/YgGVmnYb0_c
www.tilestats.com/ml/

We will here use the same dataset as shown in the video where one has measured the prostate-specific antigen (PSA) concentration from a blood sample in seven patients with prostate cancer and seven healthy controls (Table 11.4).

Let's plot this data in the same way as shown in the video:

```
rm(list=ls()) # Clear environment
PSA=c(4.1, 3.4, 2.9, 2.8, 2.7, 2.1, 1.6,2.5, 2.0, 1.7, 1.4,
1.2, 0.9, 0.8) # PSA
Group=factor(rep(c("Cancer","Healthy"),c(7,7)),
levels=c("Healthy","Cancer"))
df=data.frame(Group,PSA)
y=rep(0,14) # 14 y-coordinates of zero
plot(PSA,y,ylim=c(0,0.8),xlim=c(0,4.5),
pch=16,col=c(rep("orange",7),rep("green",7)),cex=1.6,las=1)
```

We will now place two Gaussian curves (normal distribution curves) above each of the two groups in Fig. 11.37. We therefore first begin to calculate the mean and the sample standard deviation of the two groups:

Table 11.4 PSA levels in the 14 subjects

Prostate cancer	YES	YES	YES	YES	YES	YES	YES	NO	NO	NO	NO	NO	NO	NO
PSA level (μg/L)	4.1	3.4	2.9	2.8	2.7	2.1	1.6	2.5	2.0	1.7	1.4	1.2	0.9	0.8

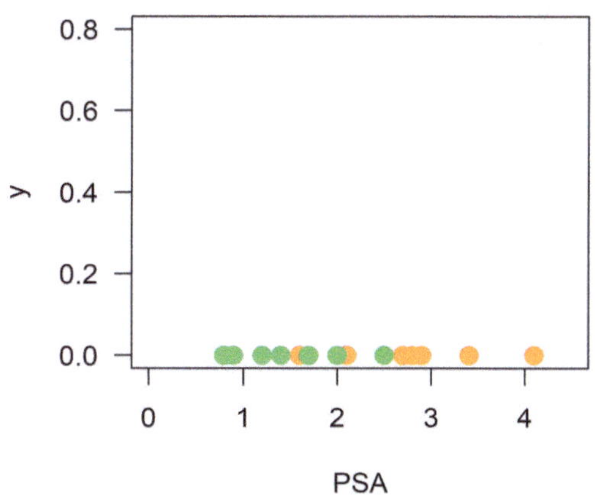

Fig. 11.37 A plot showing the PSA values of the healthy controls (green) and the prostate cancer patients (orange)

```
(means=tapply(PSA,Group,mean))
Healthy    Cancer
   1.5        2.8
(SD=tapply(PSA,Group,sd))
Healthy        Cancer
0.6110101      0.8164966
```

Then we compute the heights of the Gaussian curves by the function "dnorm" over a range of values between zero and five, which is a reasonable range for this data (Fig. 11.37), and draw these two curves in the plot:

```
x=seq(0,5,0.1)
height_H=dnorm(x,means[1],SD[1])
height_C=dnorm(x,means[2],SD[2])
lines(x,height_H,col="green")
lines(x,height_C,col="orange")
```

We now simply use the curves in Fig. 11.38 to predict the class of a new observation. Suppose that we like to predict if a person with a PSA level of 2.6 has prostate cancer or not. We can then calculate the probability that the person has prostate cancer based on the following equation:

$$\text{posterior}(\text{Cancer}) = \frac{\text{p}(\text{Cancer})\text{p}(\text{PSA}|\text{Cancer})}{\text{p}(\text{Healthy})\text{p}(\text{PSA}|\text{Healthy}) + \text{p}(\text{Cancer})\text{p}(\text{PSA}|\text{Cancer})}$$

where p(Cancer) is the prevalence of prostate cancer (or prior probability) which is here taken to be the proportion of patients with prostate cancer in our sample:

```
psa=2.6 # Predict based on a PSA level of 2.6
pC=0.5  # Prevalence/proportion of prostate cancer
pH=1-pC # Proportion of healthy individuals
```

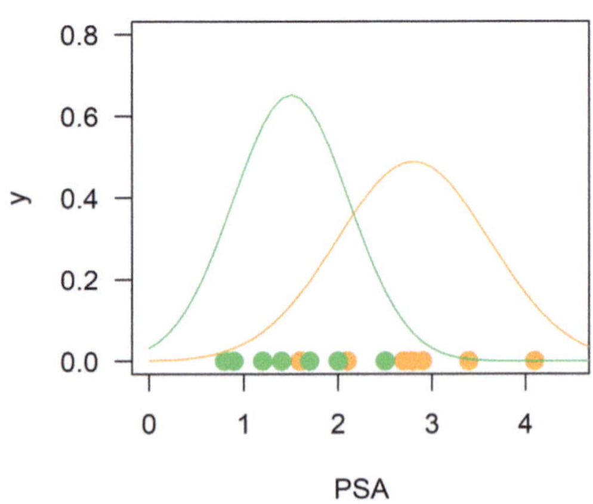

Fig. 11.38 A plot showing the PSA values of the healthy controls (green) and the prostate cancer patients (orange). The corresponding Gaussian curves are shown for each group

The term p(PSA|Healthy) is simply the height of the Gaussian curve for the healthy individuals, whereas p(PSA|Cancer) is the height of the curve associated with the prostate cancer patients:

```
pPSA_H=dnorm(psa,means[1],SD[1])
pPSA_C=dnorm(psa,means[2],SD[2])
```

We can now compute the probability that the person with a PSA level of 2.6 has prostate cancer by:

```
(pC*pPSA_C)/(pH*pPSA_H+pC*pPSA_C)
0.7859404
```

We see that the probability is about 78.6%.

We can compute the same thing if we use the function "naive_bayes" in the **naivebayes** package:

```
library(naivebayes)
model=naive_bayes(Group~.,df)
predict(model,data.frame(PSA=psa),type="prob")
  Healthy          Cancer
  0.2140596        0.7859404
```

By using this function, we can also specify if we instead like to use a kernel density estimation by:

```
fit=naive_bayes(Group~.,df, usekernel = TRUE)
predict(fit,data.frame(PSA=psa),type="prob")
  Healthy            Cancer
  0.2914822        0.7085178
```

For continuous data, the standard approach is to model each feature's likelihood using the Gaussian distribution. However, when the data does not follow a known distribution, kernel density estimation provides a non-parametric way to estimate the probability density function.

11.12.2 Validation and Hyperparameter Tuning

We will here see how to tune hyperparameters of the NB model by using the Iris dataset using the hold-out method. To see which hyperparameter we can tune, we can use the "modelLookup" function:

```
modelLookup("naive_bayes")
  model       parameter label                forReg forClass probModel
1 naive_bayes laplace   Laplace Correction   FALSE  TRUE     TRUE
2 naive_bayes usekernel Distribution Type    FALSE  TRUE     TRUE
3 naive_bayes adjust    Bandwidth Adjustment FALSE  TRUE     TRUE
```

We see that we have three hyperparameters to tune. The Laplace parameter is typically applied to categorical features, which we do not have in this data since all features are numeric. Laplace correction adds a small constant to each observed frequency to ensure that no probability is zero. This prevents the model from assigning a zero probability to unseen feature-class combinations, which could otherwise cause the entire classification to fail. The parameter usekernal can be set to TRUE if the feature data does not follow a Gaussian distribution. By using kernel density estimation, the model can estimate the probability distribution of the features without assuming a Gaussian form that might improve the performance of the model when the data is non-Gaussian. By using kernel density estimation, the "adjust" parameter allows us to fine-tune the flexibility in estimating the feature distributions. A larger value of this parameter leads to a smoother distribution.

11.12.3 The Hold-Out Method

To evaluate the NB model with the hold-out method, we can split the data into a training and a test set:

```
set.seed(10) #For reproducibility
library(caret)
index = createDataPartition(y=iris$Species, p=0.7,
list=FALSE)
train = iris[index,]
test = iris[-index,]
```

Then we define a grid with different parameter values. Since we have no categorical features in our dataset, the laplace parameter can be fixed to zero.

```
tune_grid = expand.grid(
  laplace = 0,
  # Try both kernel density estimate and Gaussian distribution
  usekernel = c(TRUE, FALSE),
  adjust = c(0.5, 1, 2)
)
tune_grid
```

```
     laplace      usekernel    adjust
1       0            TRUE        0.5
2       0            FALSE       0.5
3       0            TRUE        1.0
4       0            FALSE       1.0
5       0            TRUE        2.0
6       0            FALSE       2.0
```

Since the parameter "adjust" is only used when the parameter "usekernel" is TRUE, we can set the parameter "adjust" to NA when "usekernel" is FALSE:

```
tune_grid$adjust[tune_grid$usekernel == FALSE] = NA
```

Note that we will here try three different values of the parameter adjust when we use a kernel and then a model without using a kernel. We will therefore validate four different models. To validate these four models, we compute a 10-fold cross-validation on the training data:

```
fit_train = train(Species ~ ., data=train,
method="naive_bayes",
trControl = trainControl(method = "cv"),tuneGrid = tune_grid)
fit_train
Naive Bayes

105 samples
  4 predictor
  3 classes: 'setosa', 'versicolor', 'virginica'

No pre-processing
Resampling: Cross-Validated (10 fold)
Summary of sample sizes: 93, 95, 94, 95, 94, 96, ...
Resampling results across tuning parameters:

  usekernel   adjust     Accuracy     Kappa
    FALSE       NA       0.9634848   0.9454141
     TRUE       0.5      0.9460606   0.9193339
     TRUE       1.0      0.9551515   0.9329141
     TRUE       2.0      0.9634848   0.9454141

Tuning parameter 'laplace' was held constant at a value of 0
Accuracy was used to select the optimal model using the
largest value.
The final values used for the model were laplace = 0,
usekernel = FALSE
 and adjust = NA.
```

We see that the highest accuracy, 96.3%, is obtained from a model without using a kernel and a model by using a kernel where the parameter "adjust" is set to 2.0. The "train" function has selected a model without using a kernel (usekernel = FALSE).

Finally, we retrain the model with the optimal hyperparameters and evaluate how well it performs on the test data:

```
library(naivebayes)
fit=naive_bayes(Species~ .,train, usekernel = FALSE)
# Predict based on the numeric variables in the test data
pred=predict(fit, test[,-5])
Tab=table(pred, test$Species)
Tab
pred              setosa    versicolor    virginica
  setosa            15          0             0
  versicolor         0         15             2
  virginica          0          0            13
```

We see that 43 out of the 45 flowers have been correctly predicted.

11.13 Exercises

1. Use Naive Bayes to classify female and male crabs, using all numeric variables of the Crab dataset, and calculate its accuracy. Use the default settings in the "naive_bayes" function.
2. Suppose that you find a crab and would like to know the sex of the crab with the following measurements: FL = 8.0, RW = 6.7, CL = 16.2, CW = 18.9, BD = 7.0. Use your NB model to predict if it is a male or female crab based on the numeric variables.
3. Use Naive Bayes to classify female and male crabs, using all numeric variables of the Crab dataset. Use the hold-out method to validate your model. Use 70% of the data to build and tune the hyperparameters of your model and 30% of the data to test your model.

11.14 Comparing ML Models with Repeated Cross-Validation

As we have seen previously, the random split into training and validation data in the cross-validation may lead to certain estimates due to chance. A better way is to try a range of different random splits to smooth out randomness and give a more robust estimate of the error. We will here have a look at how to compare ML models by using the Crab dataset. We will use all the numerical variables in this dataset to see how well different models can predict the sex of the crabs. Suppose that we like to compare an LDA model with a logistic regression model based on a 10-fold cross-validation. We can then use the "train" function in the **caret** package:

```
rm(list=ls()) # Clear environment
set.seed(1) #For reproducibility
library(caret)
library(MASS) # To get access to the Crab dataset
# sex will be predicted based on all numeric variables
model=sex ~ FL+RW+CL+CW+BD
# Use a 10-fold cross-validation
cv_control = trainControl(method = "cv", number = 10)
lda_model = train(model, data = crabs, method = "lda",
trControl = cv_control)
# Print the average accuracy of the LDA model
lda_model$results
LR_model = train(model, data = crabs,
method="glm",family="binomial", trControl = cv_control)
# Print the average accuracy of the logistic regression model
LR_model$results
```

Run the above code several times with different seeds (change "set.seed(1)" to, for example, "set.seed(2)") and note that the average accuracy is changing every time you use a new seed. This is due to that a new seed will result in new random subsets every time you run the code. Sometimes the LDA model performs best, and sometimes the logistic regression model performs best. Thus, the model that performs best depends on which seed is used. It would therefore be fair to use many different seeds when we compare models. This can be done with repeated cross-validation where we set "method" to "repeatedcv" and decide how many repeats we like to use with the argument "repeats". We will here try repeated cross-validation on the LDA model with 50 repeats.

```
rm(list=ls()) # Clear environment
model=sex ~ FL+RW+CL+CW+BD
cv_control = trainControl(method = "repeatedcv", number = 10,
repeats = 50)
lda_model = train(model, data = crabs, method = "lda",
trControl = cv_control)
lda_model$resample # Print all accuracies
```

If you run the above code, note that 500 accuracies have been calculated because each 10-fold cross-validation results in 10 accuracies, which is repeated 50 times with different seeds. Let's make a boxplot of the 500 accuracies and Kappa values:

```
boxplot(lda_model$resample$Accuracy,
lda_model$resample$Kappa,horizontal =TRUE,names=c("Accuracy",
"Kappa"))
```

From this plot (Fig. 11.39), we can see that one validation dataset, out of the 500, resulted in only 80% accuracy. However, the majority of the 500 validation datasets resulted in an accuracy of around 95%.

Let's compare the ML models: LDA, logistic regression, Naive Bayes, and KNN on the Crab dataset. We will here standardize the data for the KNN model and illustrate, for simplicity, how to perform hyperparameter tuning only when we use the KNN model:

```
rm(list=ls()) # Clear environment
set.seed(1) #For reproducibility
model=sex ~ FL+RW+CL+CW+BD
cv_control = trainControl(method = "repeatedcv", number = 10,
repeats = 50)
# Define the hyperparameter grid for k in KNN
knn_grid = expand.grid(k = c(1 ,3, 5, 9))
# Standardize variables for KNN
crabs_scaled=data.frame(sex=crabs$sex,scale(crabs[,4:8]))
# Train the models
NB_model =  train(model, data = crabs, method = "naive_bayes",
trControl = cv_control)
knn_model = train(model, data = crabs_scaled, method = "knn",
trControl = cv_control, tuneGrid = knn_grid)
lda_model = train(model, data = crabs, method = "lda",
trControl = cv_control)
LR_model = train(model, data=crabs, method="glm",
family="binomial",trControl = cv_control)
# Collect data for plotting
results = resamples(list(Naive_Bayes= NB_model,
KNN = knn_model, LDA=lda_model, LR=LR_model))
# Boxplot to visualize performance comparison
bwplot(results)
```

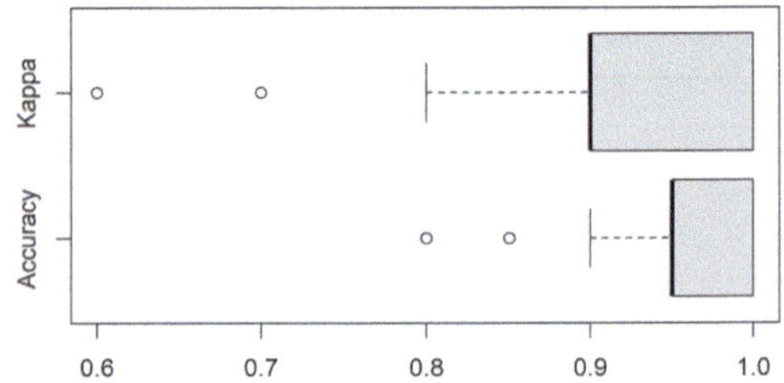

Fig. 11.39 A boxplot showing the accuracy and Kappa from 50 repeats of a 10-fold cross-validation, using an LDA model to predict the sex of the crabs in the Crab dataset

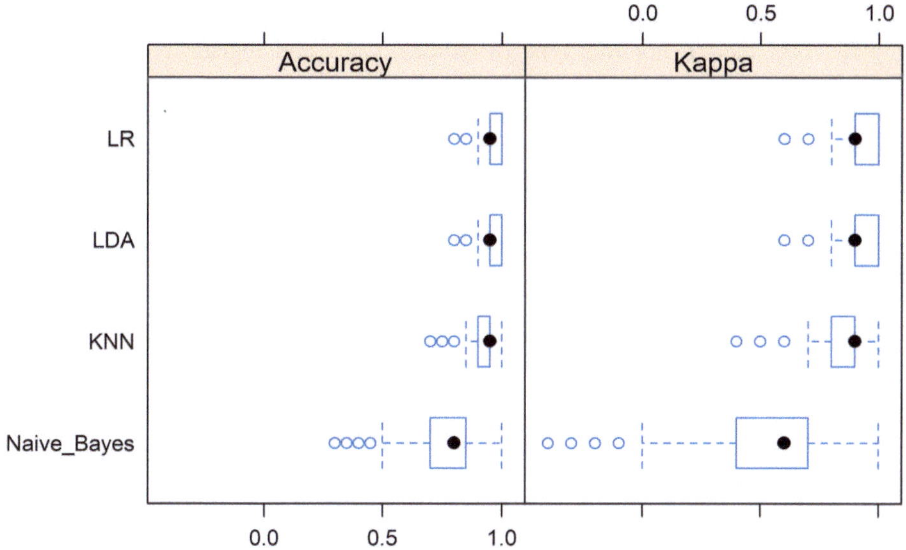

Fig. 11.40 Boxplot showing the accuracy and Kappa from 50 repeats of a 10-fold cross-validation, using different ML models to predict the sex of the crabs in the Crab dataset

We can now compare the models. The black points inside the boxes represent the median accuracy (or Kappa) of the models (Fig. 11.40). We can see that logistic regression and LDA perform equally well. Although KNN has the same median accuracy as logistic regression and LDA, it has a larger spread compared to the other two models. Naive Bayes is clearly the worst model for this type of data. To extract the values behind this plot, we can use the "summary" function that will also show the mean accuracies:

```
summary(results)
Call:
summary.resamples(object = results)

Models: Naive_Bayes, KNN, LDA, LR
Number of resamples: 500

Accuracy
              Min.   1st Qu.   Median   Mean     3rd Qu.   Max.   NA's
Naive_Bayes   0.3    0.70      0.80     0.7744   0.85      1      0
KNN           0.7    0.90      0.95     0.9324   0.95      1      0
LDA           0.8    0.95      0.95     0.9568   1.00      1      0
LR            0.8    0.95      0.95     0.9589   1.00      1      0
 ...
```

By comparing the models like this, we get a better overall measure for choosing the best model. For this type of dataset, LDA and logistic regression perform best.

Instead of comparing models by using the accuracy, we can also compare them by the AUC values from ROC analyses. The "train" function will create models based on the training data and compute predicted values of the validation data in the cross-validation process. It will then use these predicted values to compute an ROC curve and calculate the AUC. Since creating a robust ROC curve requires more data, we will here compute an ROC curve based on a 5-fold cross-validation:

```
rm(list=ls()) # Clear environment
set.seed(1) #For reproducibility
model=sex ~ FL+RW+CL+CW+BD
cv_control = trainControl(method = "repeatedcv", number = 5,
repeats = 50 ,classProbs = TRUE,summaryFunction = twoClassSummary)
# Define the hyperparameter grid for k in KNN
knn_grid = expand.grid(k = c(1 ,3, 5, 9))
# Standardize variables for KNN
crabs_scaled=data.frame(sex=crabs$sex,scale(crabs[,4:8]))
# Train the models
NB_model =  train(model, data = crabs, method =
"naive_bayes",  trControl = cv_control,metric = "ROC")
knn_model = train(model, data = crabs_scaled, method = "knn",
trControl = cv_control, tuneGrid = knn_grid,metric = "ROC")
lda_model = train(model, data = crabs, method = "lda",
trControl = cv_control,metric = "ROC")
LR_model = train(model, data=crabs, method="glm",family=
"binomial",trControl = cv_control,metric = "ROC")
# Collect data for plotting
results = resamples(list(Naive_Bayes= NB_model, KNN =
knn_model, LDA=lda_model, LR=LR_model))
# Boxplot to visualize performance comparison
bwplot(results)
summary(results)
ROC
              Min.    1st Qu.  Median   Mean      3rd Qu.   Max.   NA's
Naive_Bayes   0.3675  0.7175   0.8225   0.799420  0.90250   1      0
KNN           0.8450  0.9700   0.9825   0.977435  0.99125   1      0
LDA           0.9700  0.9925   0.9975   0.995180  1.00000   1      0
LR            0.8750  0.9925   0.9975   0.988720  1.00000   1      0
```

By using the AUC to find the best model for this dataset, LDA now seems to perform best because it has the highest mean AUC values. Try to run the code a few times with different seeds and folds for the cross-valuation and note that LDA generally results in the highest mean AUC. Using repeated cross-validation is therefore a great way to select an appropriate ML based on the training data before it is applied to the test data.

11.15 The Problem with Imbalanced Datasets in ML

All our examples have so far included an equal sample size in the groups. However, unequal sample sizes across the groups in the data may cause problems in supervised ML. Imbalanced datasets can lead to biased model training, where the model focuses too much on the majority class and therefore performs poorly on the minority class. Standard accuracy metrics may therefore give a misleading impression of model performance, as high accuracy can often be achieved by simply predicting the majority class. Features and patterns specific to the minority class may therefore not be learned by the model, which will reduce its performance in real-world applications. Different ML models are more sensitive to imbalanced datasets than others. For example, the KNN model is highly sensitive to imbalanced datasets since it predicts the class based on the majority class of the closest neighbors. If one class is overrepresented, it will likely predict the new unknown observation as the majority class because there are simply more data points of this class. In contrast, by using models like LDA and logistic regression, that has a single cutoff value for a binary outcome, we can easily change the cutoff value manually so that the model favors the minority class when it predicts. However, for more advanced models like decision trees, KNN, and random forests where we do not have a single cutoff value to change, an imbalanced dataset may cause problems. One simple way to deal with imbalanced datasets is to use under-sampling where the number of samples in the majority class is reduced to match the size of the minority class. However, the model will then have less data to train on. Another strategy is to use oversampling where the number of samples in the minority class is commonly increased by generating synthetic samples using methods such as the synthetic minority oversampling technique (SMOTE), which is implemented in the "SMOTE" function from the **DMwR** package. However, we will here try the "ROSE" (random oversampling examples) function in the **ROSE** package, which is very simple to use for binary classification problems. We first load the package:

```
library(ROSE)
```

Let's create an example of an imbalanced dataset where we extract the 50 Versicolors and 20 Virginicas from the Iris dataset:

```
# Exclude Setosa
imbalanced_data = iris[iris$Species != "setosa",]
# Set to two levels
imbalanced_data$Species = factor(imbalanced_data$Species)
# Select the first 70 flowers
```

```
imbalanced_data = imbalanced_data[1:70, ]

# Inspect the imbalanced class distribution
table(imbalanced_data$Species)
versicolor           virginica
        50                  20
```

We now split the data into training data and test data:

```
# Split the data into training and test sets
set.seed(123) #For reproducibility
library(caret)
train_index=createDataPartition(y=imbalanced_data$Species,
p=0.7, list=FALSE)
train_data = imbalanced_data[train_index, ]
test_data = imbalanced_data[-train_index, ]
# Inspect the class distribution in the two dataset
table(train_data$Species)
versicolor     virginica
     35             14
table(test_data$Species)
versicolor     virginica
     15            6
```

Next, we generate synthetic samples based on the original distribution of the training data by using the “ROSE” function:

```
# Apply ROSE to balance the training dataset
balanced_train_data = ROSE(Species ~ ., data = train_data,
seed = 123)$data

# Inspect the balanced class distribution
table(balanced_train_data$Species)
versicolor     virginica
      25           24
```

Note that the function has generated a new dataset with 49 samples, which is equal to the original sample size of the training dataset. The difference is that the dataset is now balanced and has been synthetically generated to reflect the distribution of the original data. We can now train a model on this new balanced dataset. As an example, we will here train a random forest:

```
library(randomForest)
model = randomForest(Species ~ ., data = balanced_train_data)
```

Finally, we evaluate the trained model on the test dataset. Note that we use the original test dataset when we evaluate the model although it is imbalanced. Thus, we only use synthetic data to train the model and "real" data to test the model.

```
pred = predict(model, test_data)
table(Pred = pred, test_data$Species)
Predicted        versicolor       virginica
  versicolor         13              0
  virginica           2              6
```

We see that the model correctly predicts all Virginicas as Virginica and that two Versicolor flowers are incorrectly predicted as Virginica. When we deal with imbalanced datasets, it might be misleading to report accuracy. If we would always guess the majority class in this example, we will be correct in about 15/21 = 71.43% of the cases since we have 15 Versicolors out of the 21 flowers in the test dataset. An accuracy of 71% would therefore not be better than chance if we always predict the majority class. For imbalanced datasets, it is recommended to also report measures like Kappa as we discussed in Chap. 10. Such additional measures can be computed by the "confusionMatrix" function in the **caret** package:

```
library(caret)
confusionMatrix(data=pred,reference=test_data$Species)
Confusion Matrix and Statistics


            Reference
Prediction      versicolor       virginica
  versicolor        13              0
  virginica          2              6


               Accuracy : 0.9048
                 95% CI : (0.6962, 0.9883)
    No Information Rate : 0.7143
    P-Value [Acc > NIR] : 0.03671

                  Kappa : 0.7879
...
```

Chapter 12
Clustering

Clustering is an unsupervised ML method that is used to identify hidden structures in data without relying on predefined labels. By grouping similar observations into clusters, clustering may reveal patterns and groups in the dataset. In this chapter, we will explore two widely used clustering methods: hierarchical clustering and K-means clustering. We will also discuss heatmaps, a graphical tool, that use hierarchical clustering to provide a visual representation of patterns in the data. Heatmaps integrate color gradients to highlight relationships within the dataset, which makes it easier to detect patterns in the data and to understand why objects cluster.

12.1 Hierarchical Clustering

Hierarchical clustering is a common method to use to identify clusters or groups in a dataset. We will here study agglomerative hierarchical clustering. This is a bottom-up method, which is the most common method. The method starts by agglomerating (merging) the closest pair, according to a given distance method, into a cluster. Similar pairs of clusters are then joined to form bigger clusters. The procedure is repeated until all data has formed one big cluster. Watch the video to learn how hierarchical clustering works and how different distance measures and linkage functions affect the clustering process.

12.1.1 Video

https://youtu.be/x4eHoCm1dA8
www.tilestats.com/ml/

A. Tilevik, *Multivariate Statistics and Machine Learning in R For Beginners*,
https://doi.org/10.1007/978-3-032-01851-9_12

Table 12.1 Example data to be used for hierarchical clustering

	A	B	C	D	E
Diastolic BP (mmHg)	70	86	78	60	75
Systolic BP (mmHg)	130	147	137	121	134
Weight (kg)	100	90	100	90	106
Height (cm)	180	170	181	171	185
Total cholesterol (mg/dL)	190	215	192	215	200

We will here use the same dataset (Table 12.1) as in the video where the variables diastolic (DBP) and systolic blood pressure (SBP), weight, height, and total cholesterol level have been measured on five individuals (A-E).

To get a first feeling of the similarity between the variables, we can generate a profile plot:

```
rm(list=ls()) # Clear environment
A=c(70,130  ,100 ,180, 190)
B=c(86,147  ,90 ,170,215)
C=c(78, 137 ,100, 181, 192)
D=c(60, 121 ,90 ,171 ,215)
E=c(75,134  ,106 , 185, 200)
df=data.frame(A,B,C,D,E)
variables=c("DBP","SBP","Weight","Height","Cholesterol")
# So that R does not rearrange the order
variables=factor(variables,levels=variables)
rownames(df)=variables

library(GGally)
df2=cbind(df,variables)
ggparcoord(df2, columns=1:5, groupColumn=6,
scale="globalminmax")
```

From this plot (Fig. 12.1), it is clear that, for example, the cholesterol level and height have similar values. In addition, the diastolic blood pressure (DBP) and the weight have similar values.

We will now calculate the distances between the variables. There are several distance metrics to use, such as Euclidean, Mahalanobis, and correlation. We will here first use the Euclidean distance. We can use the “dist” function to calculate the Euclidean distances:

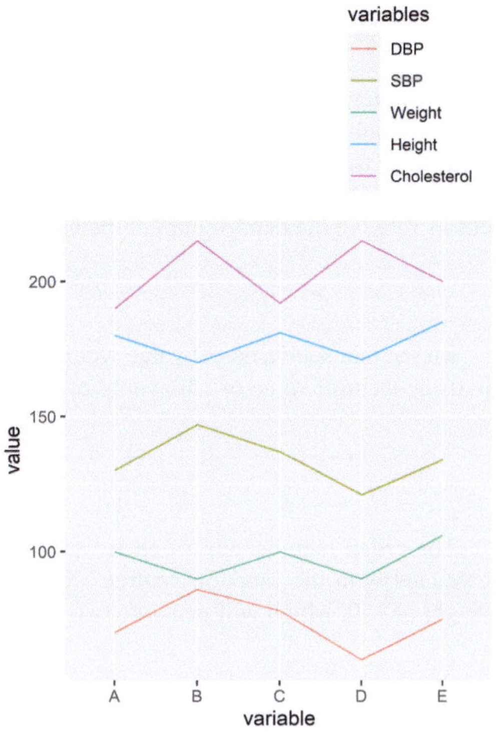

Fig. 12.1 A profile plot showing the values of the five variables for each individual (A-E) in the dataset

```
(h=dist(df, method = "euclidean"))
             DBP          SBP          Weight       Height
SBP          134.17898
Weight        57.10517     85.22324
Height       232.77887    100.32946    179.34046
Cholesterol  289.28705    156.33618    238.01260    66.38524
```

We then generate the clusters with the "hclust" function using the average (mean) distances between clusters:

```
hp=hclust(h,method="average")
```

The average distances between the clusters can be extracted by:

```
hp$height
57.10517   66.38524   109.70111   199.34744
```

Finally, we plot the dendrogram:

```
plot(hp,ylab="Euclidean distance")
```

12.1.2 *Identify Clusters*

Once, we have generated a dendrogram (Fig. 12.2), we usually want to identify a certain number of clusters or groups. From the dendrogram in Fig. 12.2, it seems reasonable to define three groups, where group 1 consists of Height and Cholesterol, group 2 of DBP and Weight, whereas group 3 only includes the SBP. If we place a cutoff value in the dendrogram at the height of 100:

```
abline(h=100,lty="dashed")
```

we see that such a cutoff value would generate three groups (Fig. 12.3). In comparison, a cutoff value of 150 would produce only two groups (Fig. 12.4):

```
plot(hp,ylab="Euclidean distance")
abline(h=150,lty="dashed")
```

The group membership of each variable for a given cutoff value can easily be extracted with the function "cutree". If we set h to 150, the tree will be cut at a height of 150, which will generate two groups:

```
cutree(hp, h=150)
        DBP    SBP    Weight    Height    Cholesterol
         1      1       1         2            2
```

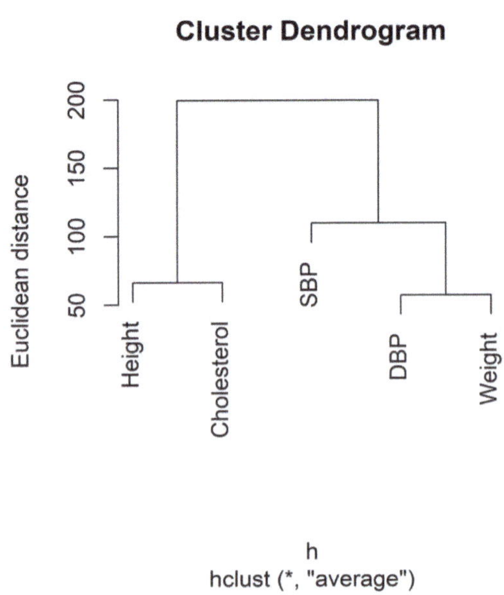

Fig. 12.2 A dendrogram showing how the variables cluster based on the raw data, using Euclidean distance and the average linkage function

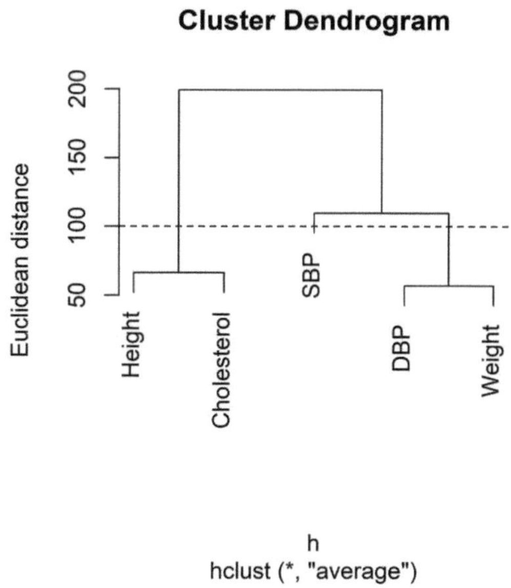

Fig. 12.3 A dendrogram showing how the variables cluster based on the raw data, using Euclidean distance and the average linkage function. The dashed line shows how the dendrogram can be cut to identify three clusters

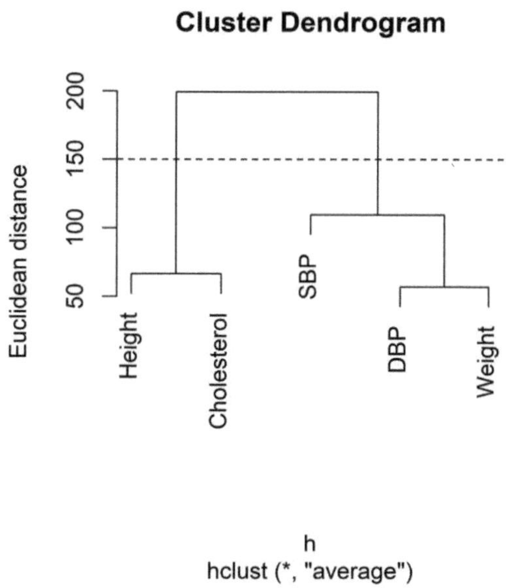

Fig. 12.4 A dendrogram showing how the variables cluster based on the raw data, using Euclidean distance and the average linkage function. The dashed line shows how the dendrogram can be cut to identify two clusters

The output shows that the DBP, SBP and Weight belong to cluster 1, whereas Cholesterol and Height belong to cluster 2. We can also set the number of groups we want to identify with the argument k. If we set k to, for example, 3, the function will find an appropriate cutoff value to identify three clusters:

```
cutree(hp, k=3) # cut tree into 3 clusters
        DBP         SBP       Weight       Height    Cholesterol
         1           2           1            3            3
```

We can also illustrate the groups in the dendrogram with the function "rect. hclust", which draws rectangles around the clusters (Fig. 12.5):

```
plot(hp)
rect.hclust(hp, k=3, border="red")
```

12.1.3 Use Different Linkage Functions

There are many different linkage functions to choose between as discussed in the video. We have previously used the average linkage function. For example, let's generate a dendrogram based on the complete linkage function:

```
h_complete=hclust(h,method="complete")
plot(h_complete)
```

Using the complete linkage function generates a similar dendrogram as before (Fig. 12.5) but where the height of the dendrogram now represents the maximum distance between the clusters (Fig. 12.6). The complete linkage function defines the distance between two clusters as the maximum distance between any pair of data

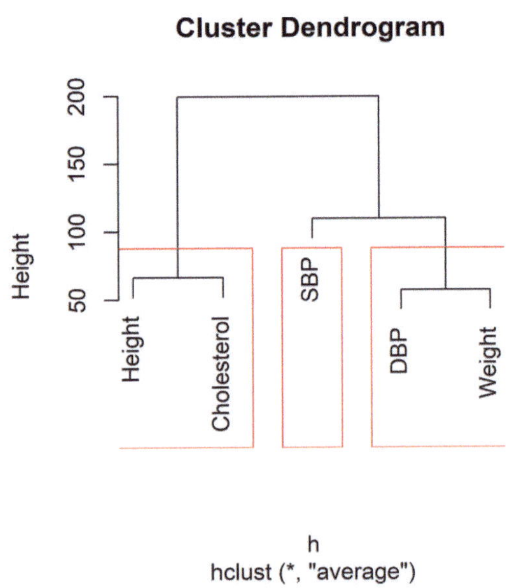

Fig. 12.5 A dendrogram showing how the variables cluster based on the raw data, using Euclidean distance and the average linkage function. The red boxes illustrate the identification of three clusters

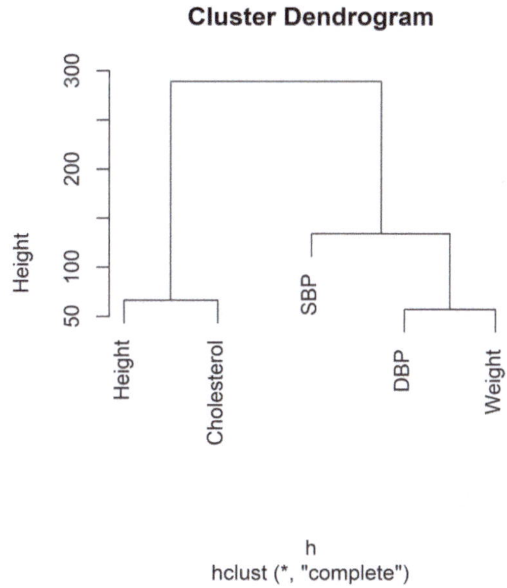

Fig. 12.6 A dendrogram showing how the variables cluster based on the raw data, using Euclidean distance and the complete linkage function

points. This method, which is the default method in the "hclust" function, tends to create compact and tightly bound clusters. Later, we will see how to evaluate different linkage functions.

12.1.4 Use Different Distance Metrics

In addition to different linkage functions, it is important to select an appropriate distance metric that reflects how we define similarity. In the previous example, we grouped the variables that had similar values. However, it makes more sense to instead group variables that have similar patterns across the individuals. One way to group the variables based on similarity in their pattern, or profile, is to first standardize the variables so that all variables have a mean of zero and a standard deviation of one. We can standardize our variables with the function "scale". Per default, this function standardizes the columns but since we instead like to standardize the rows (the variables), we standardize the transposed data frame and then transpose it back so that we again have the variables on the rows:

```
sdf=t(scale(t(df)))
```

Then we compute the distance matrix and generate the dendrogram by:

```
(h=dist(sdf, method = "euclidean"))
hp=hclust(h,method="average")
plot(hp)
```

This dendrogram now makes more sense because the variables that are expected to correlate are now grouped (Fig. 12.7). For example, it makes more sense that the two blood pressure variables form a cluster, and that Weight and Height cluster. Another way to group variables with a similar pattern is to use a distance metric based on correlation coefficients. For example, we can calculate the Pearson correlation between each pair of variables and generate a correlation matrix by:

```
round(cor(t(df)),2)
              DBP     SBP    Weight   Height    Cholesterol
DBP           1.00    0.99    0.09     0.05       -0.04
SBP           0.99    1.00   -0.01    -0.05        0.04
Weight        0.09   -0.01    1.00     0.99       -0.78
Height        0.05   -0.05    0.99     1.00       -0.82
Cholesterol  -0.04    0.04   -0.78    -0.82        1.00
```

For example, we can see that the SBP and DBP have a strong positive correlation. It would therefore make sense to cluster these two variables. If we, for example, take one minus the correlation coefficients, we can create the following distance matrix.

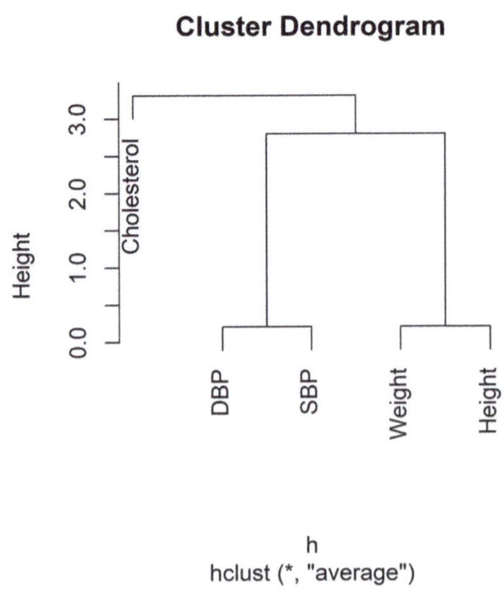

Fig. 12.7 A dendrogram showing how the variables cluster based on the standardized data, using Euclidean distance and the average linkage function

```
cor_dist=1-cor(t(df))
h=as.dist(cor_dist)
round(h,2)
             DBP      SBP       Weight     Height
SBP          0.01
Weight       0.91     1.01
Height       0.95     1.05       0.01
Cholesterol  1.04     0.96       1.78          1.82
```

We see that the shortest distances can be found between the two variables Weight and Height, and between the SBP and the DBP. We can now generate a dendrogram based on these distances:

```
# Change to complete linkage to get the same dendrogram as in
the video
hp=hclust(h,method="average")
plot(hp,ylab="1-Pearson's correlation")
```

We see that this dendrogram (Fig. 12.8), which is generated based on the correlation matrix, is quite similar to the dendrogram generated based on the standardized data. This is due to that the calculations of the correlation coefficients involve normalization of the variables.

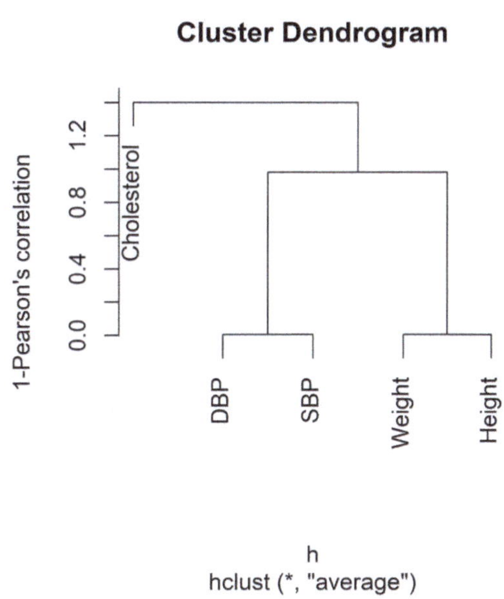

Fig. 12.8 A dendrogram showing how pairs of variables cluster based on one minus the Pearson correlation coefficients in the correlation matrix

12.1.5 Transposing the Data Frame

If we instead would like to analyze the similarities between the individuals A-E (similarities between the columns), we can simply transpose the data frame with the function "t":

```
t_df=t(df) # Transpose data frame
t_df # Print transposed df
   DBP  SBP    Weight    Height    Cholesterol
A  70   130     100       180        190
B  86   147      90       170        215
C  78   137     100       181        192
D  60   121      90       171        215
E  75   134     106       185        200
```

Note that the previous columns are now presented as rows and vice versa. The corresponding profile plot for the transposed data frame can be generated by:

```
library(GGally)
t_df2=data.frame(t_df,ind=colnames(df))
ggparcoord(t_df2, columns=1:5, groupColumn=6,
scale="globalminmax")
```

The green and red lines seem to be close to each other, which suggests that individuals A and C have the most similar health profiles (Fig. 12.9). A dendrogram will help us to identify individuals with similar heath profiles:

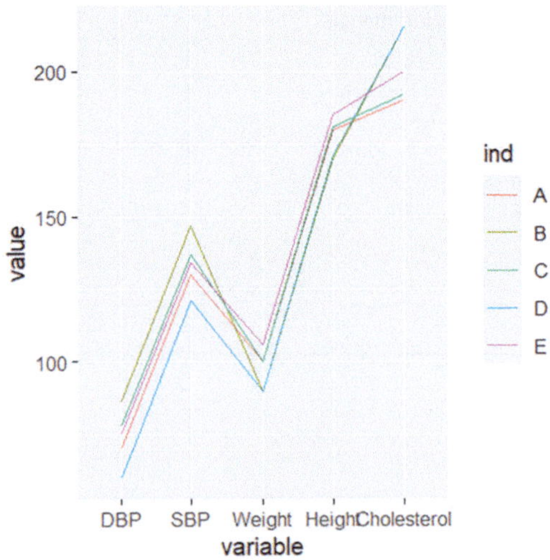

Fig. 12.9 A profile plot showing the values of the five variables for each individual (A-E) in the dataset

```
h=dist(t_df, method = "euclidean")
hp=hclust(h,method="average")
plot(hp,ylab="Euclidean distance")
```

From this dendrogram (Fig. 12.10), we can see that individuals A and C have the most similar health profiles and that individual E has a similar profile to these two individuals. However, one problem with this analysis is that variables with large values will have more impact on the clustering compared to variables with small values. It might therefore be a good idea to first standardize the variables before we cluster, such as:

```
s_t_df=scale(t_df)
h=dist(s_t_df, method = "euclidean")
hp=hclust(h,method="average")
plot(hp,ylab="Euclidean distance")
```

Using standardized variables did, in this case, not change the clusters (Fig. 12.11).

12.1.6 Robustness of Clusters and Evaluation of Linkage Functions

If we would repeat the whole study again with five new individuals, we would probably not identify the exact same clusters of the variables since five new individuals would not show the exact same correlations between the measured variables.

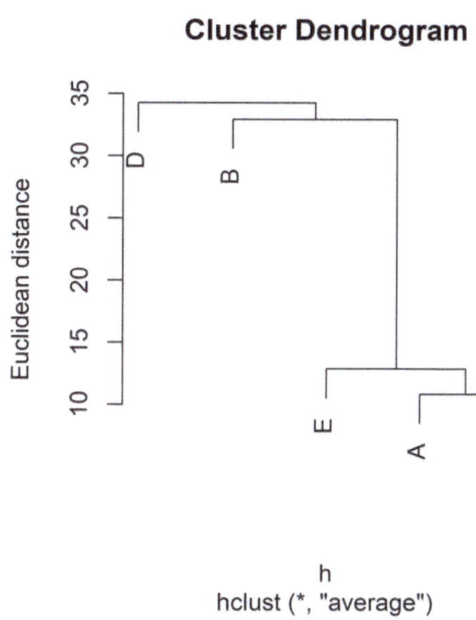

Fig. 12.10 A dendrogram showing how the individuals cluster based on the Euclidean distance and the average linkage function

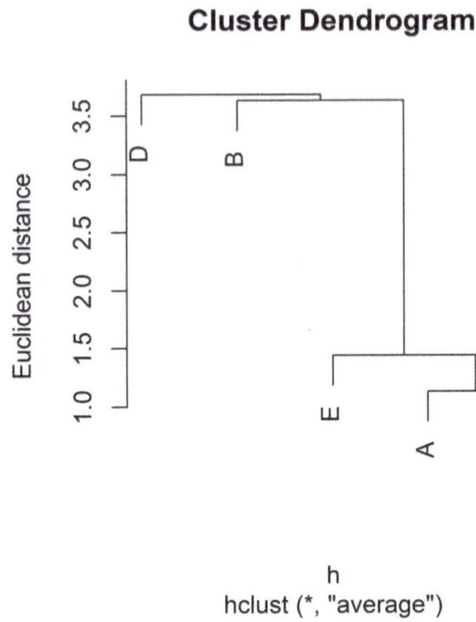

Fig. 12.11 A dendrogram showing how the individuals cluster based on the standardized variables, using the Euclidean distance and the average linkage function

However, variables with a very similar profile that cluster in the first experiment are likely to also cluster in the second experiment, whereas variables with a weak similarity of the profiles are likely to cluster differently between the experiments. Hence, clusters with a very strong association should be robust to variation, meaning that we expect to identify the same clusters even if we repeat the experiment with five new individuals. One method to measure the robustness of our clusters is to build many dendrograms by taking a bootstrap of the original data. If a cluster is identified many times from these bootstraps, then the cluster can be considered as being robust. Bootstrap is a resampling method where numbers are repeatedly drawn, with replacement, from a single original data. For example, suppose that we have a variable with the numbers 1–10:

```
v=1:10
```

We now randomly select ten of these numbers with replacements, which means that the same number can be selected many times:

```
sample(v,replace=TRUE)
2   9   1   1  10   5   2   7   8   8
```

Note that the numbers 3, 4, and 6 were never selected because some numbers were selected more than once. Try to run the above function many times and note that you will get different random numbers every time.

The function "pvclust" in the **pvclust** package can perform bootstrapping and generate a dendrogram based on the original data that shows how often the clusters are identified from the sampled data. Note that this function, in comparison to our previous code, clusters the columns in the data frame instead of the rows. To illustrate how the function works, we will here cluster the four numeric variables in the Iris dataset:

```
df=iris[,1:4] # Extract the continuous variables
library(pvclust)
set.seed(1970) #For reproducibility
fit = pvclust(df, method.hclust="average",
method.dist="euclidean",nboot=100)
plot(fit)
```

Note that we here only run 100 bootstrap replicates to save computation time. It is recommended to run at least 10.000 bootstraps (Suzuki & Hidetoshi, 2006). The values in green (bp = bootstrap probability) show the fraction of times the original cluster is identified in the 100 bootstrap replicates (Fig. 12.12). Hence, the cluster with the variables petal width, sepal width, and petal length forms a cluster about 53% of the time. Try to run the code below many times and note that the dendrogram sometimes forms different clusters:

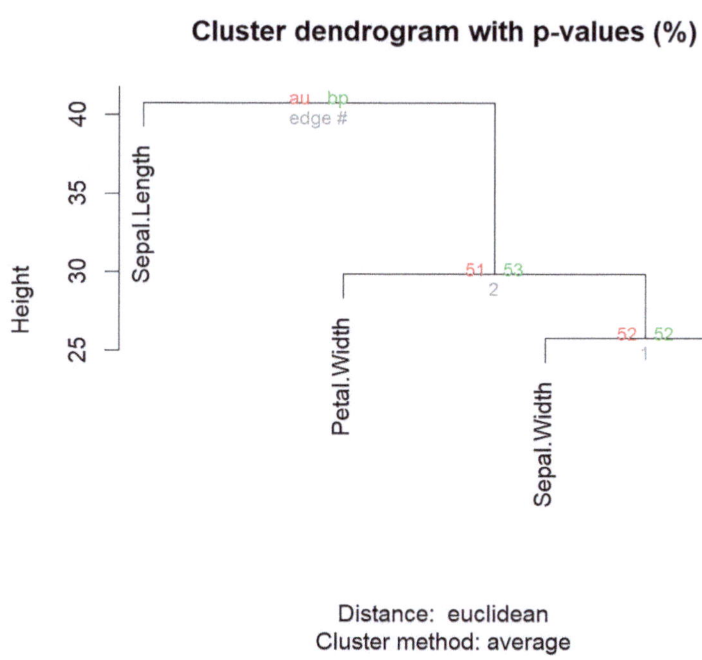

Fig. 12.12 A dendrogram displaying hierarchical clustering of the numeric variables in the Iris dataset. 100 bootstraps were used to compute the approximately unbiased p-values (au, red) and bootstrap probabilities (bp, green)

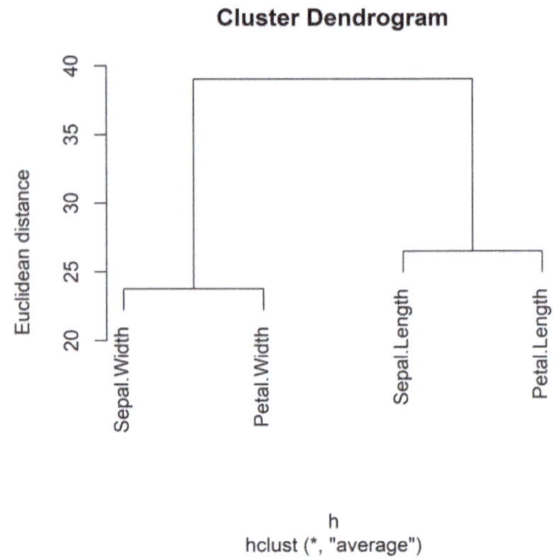

Fig. 12.13 An alternative dendrogram that is generated in some bootstraps due to chance

```
i=sample(1:150,replace=TRUE)
df1=df[i,]
h=dist(t(df1), method = "euclidean")
hp=hclust(h,method="average")
plot(hp,ylab="Euclidean distance")
```

In about half of the time, we will generate the dendrogram as shown in Fig. 12.13. This means that the generated dendrogram is sensitive to which flowers we select in our bootstrap. Thus, the clusters are not robust. Maybe there is another linkage function that generates more robust clusters. One can estimate this by computing the mean bp value for different clusters. Let's compute the mean bp value for four different linkage functions:

```
set.seed(1980) #For reproducibility
fit_aver=pvclust(df, method.hclust="average",
method.dist="euclidean",nboot=100)
fit_single=pvclust(df, method.hclust="single",
method.dist="euclidean",nboot=100)
fit_comp=pvclust(df, method.hclust="complete",
method.dist="euclidean",nboot=100)
fit_ward=pvclust(df, method.hclust="ward.D",
method.dist="euclidean",nboot=100)
mean(fit_aver$edges$bp)
0.6853233
mean(fit_single$edges$bp)
0.8328354
mean(fit_comp$edges$bp)
0.6847625
mean(fit_ward$edges$bp)
0.6727002
```

We see that the single linkage function generates the highest mean bp value, which indicates that this linkage function creates the most robust cluster. Try to run the code below many times and note that the dendrogram barely changes between the runs when we use the single linkage function:

```
i=sample(1:150,replace=TRUE)
df1=df[i,]
h=dist(t(df1), method = "euclidean")
hp=hclust(h,method="single")
plot(hp,ylab="Euclidean distance")
```

Thus, using the single linkage clearly generates the most robust cluster out of the four linkage functions that we have tested for this example data.

12.2 Exercises

1. Cluster the 200 crabs based on the numerical variables of the Crab dataset, using average linkage and the Euclidean distance based on standardized data. Show a dendrogram of the clustering.
2. Can you identify a crab that is far away from the other crabs?
3. Cut the tree at 1.3. How many clusters do you then obtain? In which cluster can you find crab number 122?
4. Transpose the dataset so that you instead cluster the standardized numerical variables. Which variables have the most similar profiles across the crabs according to the dendrogram?
5. Cluster the standardized numerical variables in the Crab dataset. Check which of the linkage functions: average, single, and complete that generates the most robust clusters. Use the Euclidean distance and 1000 bootstraps.

12.3 Cluster Heatmaps

A heatmap is a graphical illustration of a data matrix, where numbers in each cell are illustrated by a square of color. A heatmap can be combined with clustering where rows and columns are rearranged based on the order of the dendrogram. Watch the video to understand how to create and interpret a heatmap and how different normalizations affect the appearance of the heatmap.

12.3.1 Video

https://youtu.be/gEJSdHrboVo
www.tilestats.com/ml/

To illustrate how to generate a heatmap, we will here use the same dataset as we used in the previous section about hierarchical clustering:

```
rm(list=ls()) # Clear environment
A=c(70,130  ,100 ,180, 190 )
B=c(86,147  ,90 ,170,215)
C=c(78, 137 ,100, 181, 192)
D=c(60, 121 ,90 ,171 ,215)
E=c(75,134  ,106 , 185, 200  )
df=data.frame(A,B,C,D,E)
rownames(df)=c("DBP","SBP","Weight","Height","Cholesterol")
```

As discussed in the video, it usually makes sense to first standardize the variables, which can be done by:

```
s_df=t(scale(t(df)))
```

To create a heatmap of the standardized data, we can use the function "heatmap". To be consistent with our earlier clustering, we will here use the average linkage function for the two dendrograms that determine the order of the rows and columns. Also, since we have already standardized the data, we set the argument "scale" to none:

```
heatmap(as.matrix(s_df),scale="none",
hclustfun=function(d) hclust(d, method="average"))
```

This heatmap shows high numbers with dark red color and low numbers with white color (Fig. 12.14). The dendrograms correspond to the ones we previously generated with hierarchical clustering on the standardized data. From this heatmap, we can see that persons D and B have the highest cholesterol levels out of the five individuals and that these two persons have a relatively low weight and height. The individuals with the most similar health profiles are persons A and C. Thus, by analyzing the heatmap, we can now get an understanding of why certain individuals form a cluster.

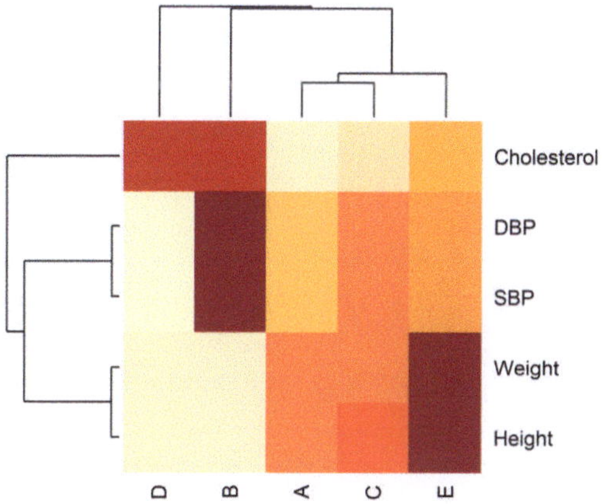

Fig. 12.14 A heatmap based on standardized data showing the variables on the rows and the individuals on the columns. Rows and columns are ordered based on hierarchical clustering, using Euclidean distances and the average linkage function

12.3.2 The Package Pheatmap

We have so far used the function “heatmap”, which is a function that we can use without any package. However, using the package **pheatmap** allows us to customize the heatmap a lot more. To generate the same heatmap as in Fig. 12.14, we can use the function “pheatmap”:

```
library(pheatmap)
pheatmap(as.matrix(s_df),scale="none",
clustering_method="average")
```

This will result in the same heatmap but note that individual E has been placed on the left-hand side of cluster A-C (Fig. 12.15). The placement of variables on either side of a dendrogram is arbitrary, as long as the clustering structure is preserved. When we interpret a dendrogram or a heatmap, we should therefore focus on the clustering patterns rather than the exact layout. For example, variables grouped together are more similar to each other than to variables in other clusters, regardless of their visual placement.

To see the power of the **pheatmap** package, let's compute a heatmap of the Iris dataset where we will add an annotation to indicate the species of each flower (each row) in the heatmap. We first standardize the numeric variables in the Iris dataset and make sure that the data is stored as a matrix since the input must be a matrix in the “pheatmap” function:

```
rm(list=ls())
# Create a matrix of the standardized numeric variables
df_scale=as.matrix(scale(iris[,-5]))
```

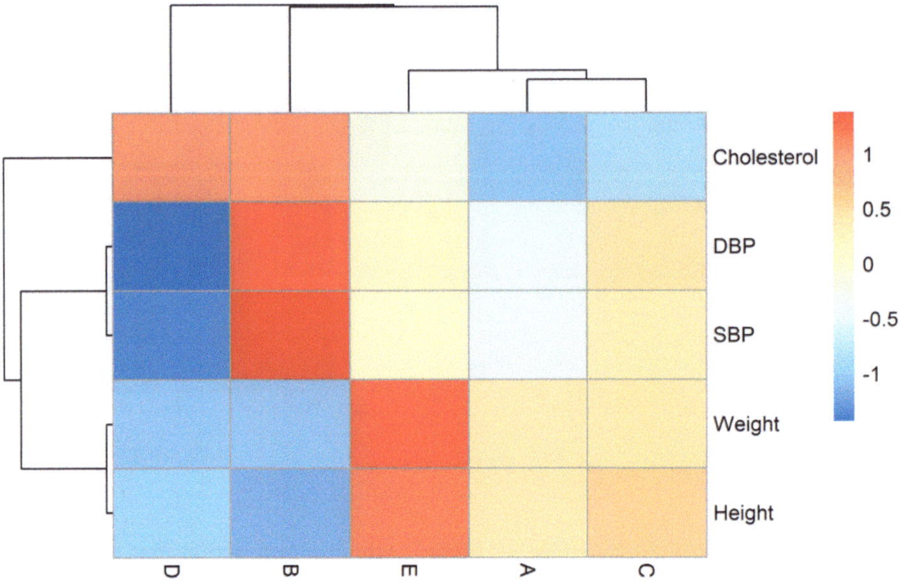

Fig. 12.15 A heatmap based on standardized data showing the variables on the rows and the individuals on the columns. Rows and columns are ordered based on hierarchical clustering, using Euclidean distances and the average linkage function. The heatmap was generated by the **pheatmap** package

Then we need to restore the original row names because we will display these in the heatmap:

```
rownames(df_scale)=rownames(iris)
```

We now plug in this matrix in the "pheatmap" function and use, for example, the complete linkage function for creating the dendrograms. To use an appropriate size of the row names (flowers 1–150), we set a smaller font size by the argument "fontsize_row". To annotate the rows so that we can identify the species of the flowers, we set the argument "annotation_row" equal to the column Species in the Iris dataset, which must be in the form of a data frame:

```
library(pheatmap)
pheatmap(df_scale,scale="none",clustering_method="complete",
fontsize_row = 2,annotation_row = data.frame
(Species=iris$Species))
```

From this heatmap (Fig. 12.16), we can learn a lot. The Setosa flowers form one distinct cluster at the bottom of the heatmap. What deviates the flowers in this cluster is that they have a relatively large sepal width but small sepal length, petal length, and petal width. However, there is one Setosa flower, flower number 42, in the

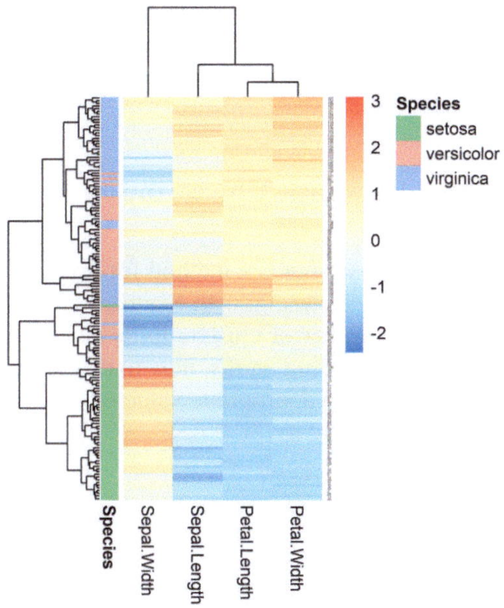

Fig. 12.16 A heatmap based on standardized variables in the Iris dataset. The rows show the individual flowers, whereas the columns show the numeric variables. Rows and columns are ordered based on hierarchical clustering, using Euclidean distances and the complete linkage function. The heatmap was generated with the **pheatmap** package

middle of the heatmap that deviates from the other Setosa flowers because this flower has a relatively small sepal width. Another interesting cluster is the cluster with Virginicas in the middle. In comparison to the other Virginicas, the flowers in this cluster have a relatively large sepal length. However, note that the cluster in the middle could have arbitrarily been placed on the first rows of the heatmap. This would then have put the Virginicas closer to each other. In summary, by using a heatmap, we can explain why certain flowers form a cluster, which would be impossible if we only study a dendrogram.

12.4 Exercises

1. Create a heatmap of the standardized numerical variables in the Crab dataset, using the **pheatmap** package. Use complete linkage and the Euclidean distance for the dendrograms. Annotate the rows so that one can see if a crab is a female or male. Tip: export the figure to PDF for a better resolution and set a smaller font size so that you can see the row numbers clearly (fontsize_row = 1.5).
2. Based on the heatmap, can you explain why crab number 200 deviates from the other crabs in the dendrogram?
3. Based on the dendrogram of the crabs, do you think that male and female crabs are well separated?
4. There is a distinct cluster of crabs in the middle of the heatmap. What characterizes this cluster?

5. Create a similar heatmap as before but use annotations also for the species of the crabs so that one can identify both the sex and the species. Which type of crabs have the longest rear width (RW) according to the heatmap?

12.5 K-Means Clustering

K-means clustering is a method for dividing the data into *k* clusters. Hence, unlike hierarchical clustering, with K-means clustering we can already from the beginning select the number of clusters to be generated. Watch the video to understand how K-means clustering works, how to calculate the within-cluster sum of squares, and how to select an appropriate value of *k* based on the elbow method.

12.5.1 Video

https://youtu.be/V9RqMFR1_Ys
www.tilestats.com/ml/

Let's run k-means clustering on the same data as shown in the video:

```
rm(list=ls()) # Clear environment
x=c(1,2,4,5,7,8,10,11,9,12)
y=c(9,7,3,3,2,4,11,9,10,8)
df=data.frame(x,y)
plot(x,y,cex=2,xlim=c(0,13),ylim=c(0,13),las=1)
text(x,y,1:10,cex=0.8)
```

To run K-means clustering on this data (Fig. 12.17) where we like to, for example, identify three clusters, we can use the function "kmeans". The argument "nstart"

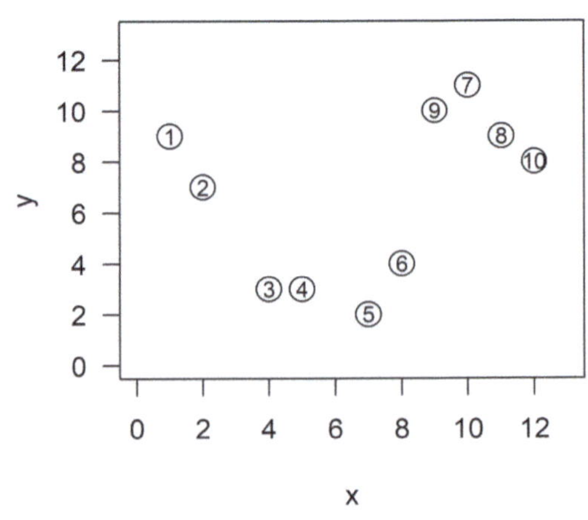

Fig. 12.17 A scatter plot of the example data for k-means clustering

determines how many initial random positions of the three centroids that should be evaluated:

```
set.seed(1990) #For reproducibility
# generate 3 cluster and try 100 different initial random positions
k_clust = kmeans(df, 3,nstart=100)
k_clust
K-means clustering with 3 clusters of sizes 2, 4, 4

Cluster means:
     x    y
1   1.5  8.0
2  10.5  9.5
3   6.0  3.0

Clustering vector:
 [1] 1 1 3 3 3 3 2 2 2 2

Within cluster sum of squares by cluster:
[1]  2.5   10.0   12.0
 (between_SS / total_SS =  89.2 %)
```

We can see that the first two data points belong to cluster 1, data points 3–6 belong to cluster 3, whereas the last four data points belong to cluster 2. The within-cluster sum of squares (WCSS) for the three clusters are 2.5, 10, and 12. The sum of the WCSS can be extracted by:

```
k_clust$tot.withinss
24.5
```

Let's put some colors in the figure so that we can identify the clusters in the plot (Fig. 12.18):

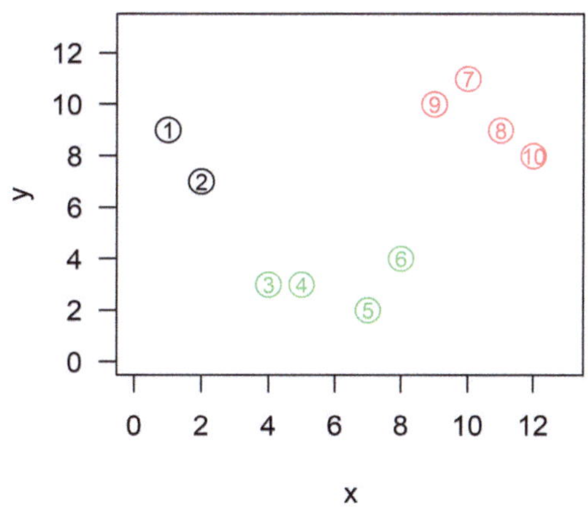

Fig. 12.18 A scatter plot that shows which data points that belong to cluster 1 (black), cluster 2 (red), and cluster 3 (green)

```
plot(x,y,cex=2,xlim=c(0,13),ylim=c(0,13),las=1,
col=k_clust$cluster)
text(x,y,1:10,cex=0.8,col=k_clust$cluster)
```

12.5.2 Elbow Plot

To compute an elbow plot as the one shown in the video, we need to compute the sum of the WCSS for a range of different values of k. The code below computes the sum of the WCSS where k goes from 1 to 8. The sum of the WCSS is then plotted against the different values of k:

```
Ks=1:8
WCSS=NULL
for (i in Ks) {
  WCSS[i]=kmeans(df, i, nstart = 25 )$tot.withinss
}
plot(Ks, WCSS,type="b", pch = 19, frame=FALSE,
xlab="Number of clusters (k)",
ylab="Total within cluster sum of squares")
```

The optimal value of k is the value at the "elbow" of the curve, which seems to be equal to three in this example (Fig. 12.19). Finding the optimal value of k this way is called the elbow method.

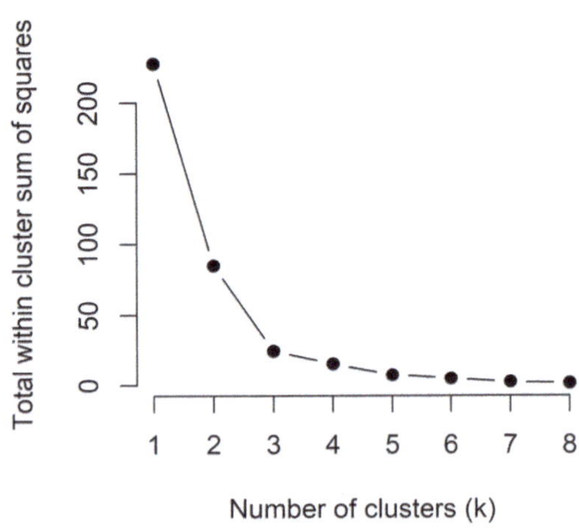

Fig. 12.19 An elbow plot that shows how the total within-cluster sum of squares changes with different numbers of clusters (k)

12.5.3 K-Means Clustering with the Iris Dataset

Let's apply K-means clustering to cluster the flowers in the Iris dataset. It is recommended that we first standardize the data before computing the clustering so that all variables contribute equally. To identify an appropriate number of clusters to use, we can first generate an elbow plot:

```
Ks=1:12
WCSS=NULL
for (i in Ks) {
  WCSS[i]=kmeans(scale(iris[,1:4]), i,
  nstart = 100 )$tot.withinss
}
plot(Ks, WCSS,type="b", pch = 19, frame=FALSE,
xlab="Number of clusters (k)",
     ylab="Total within cluster sum of squares")
```

From Fig. 12.20, it seems like the elbow is visible at two or three clusters. We will here set *k* to three and compute K-means clustering by using 100 initial random positions of the three centroids:

```
set.seed(1) #For reproducibility
clust=kmeans(scale(iris[,1:4]), 3, nstart = 100)
Cluster=as.factor(clust$cluster)
table(Cluster)
Cluster
 1     2    3
53    47   50
```

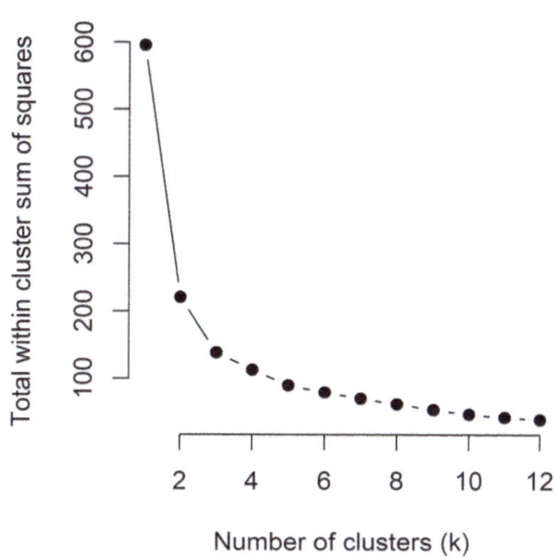

Fig. 12.20 An elbow plot that shows how the total within-cluster sum of squares changes with different numbers of clusters (*k*) based on the standardized numeric variables in the Iris dataset

For example, we see that the first cluster includes 53 flowers.

One way to visualize the three clusters is to combine the variables with PCA so that we can plot the data in a two-dimensional scatter plot (Fig. 12.21):

```
pca=prcomp(iris[,-5],scale=TRUE) # Compute PCA
dataset = data.frame(pca$x,Species=iris$Species)
library(ggplot2)
ggplot(dataset) +
  geom_point(aes(PC1, PC2, colour = Cluster), size = 3)
```

Let's view the corresponding PCA plot (Fig. 12.22) where we instead label the known species:

```
ggplot(dataset) +
  geom_point(aes(PC1, PC2, colour = Species), size = 3)
```

By comparing these plots, we can see that cluster 3 (Fig. 12.21) includes all Setosa flowers (Fig. 12.22) and that clusters 1 and 2 almost resemble Versicolor and Virginica, respectively. Thus, in comparison to supervised ML models that train on labeled data, K-means clustering, which has no information about the species, identifies the species quite well.

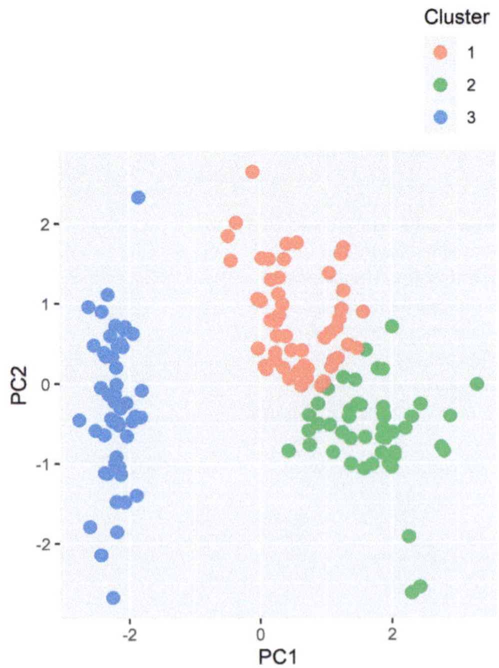

Fig. 12.21 A PCA plot, generated based on the "prcomp" function and the **ggplot2** package, showing the distribution of the 150 Iris flowers along the first two principal components (PC1 and PC2). The colors have been set according to which cluster the flowers belong to by using K-means clustering

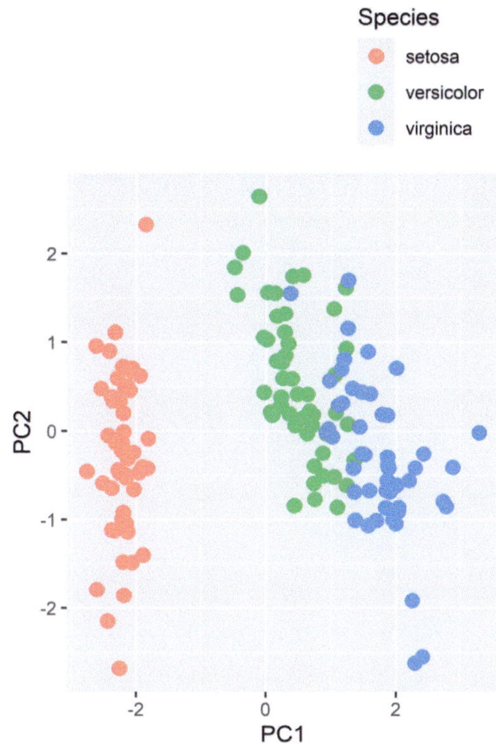

Fig. 12.22 A PCA plot, generated based on the "prcomp" function and the **ggplot2** package, showing the distribution of the 150 Iris flowers along the first two principal components (PC1 and PC2). The colors have been set according to known species type

12.6 Exercises

1. Compute K-means clustering on the standardized numerical variables in the Crab dataset. Use the elbow method to determine the optimal value of *k*. Use 25 random initial positions of the centroids.
2. Use K-means clustering to generate four clusters. How many crabs are included in the first cluster (note that the computation involves random processes, which means that you might get different results each time you run your code)?

Reference

Suzuki, R., & Hidetoshi, S. (2006). Pvclust: An R package for assessing the uncertainty in hierarchical clustering. *Bioinformatics, 22*, 1540–1542.

Chapter 13
PCR, PLS, and Lasso Regression

One of the major problems with multiple linear regression analysis is multicollinearity, which occurs when the predictor variables are highly correlated with one another. Multicollinearity may cause unreliable coefficient estimates and inflated standard errors. This is especially problematic with high-dimensional datasets, where at least some predictors are likely to strongly correlate. To overcome these problems, principal component regression and partial least squares regression combine highly correlated predictors. These combined variables are then used in the regression model. In this chapter, we will cover these two methods and see how to calculate a confidence interval based on bootstrapping. We will also discuss Lasso regression, which is a regularization method that can shrink parameter values down to zero. If multiple features are highly correlated, Lasso regression may randomly select one and discard the others.

13.1 Principal Component Regression

Principal component regression (PCR) is a regression technique that is based on PCA. PCR is often used as an alternative to multiple linear regression when strong correlations are observed between the predictor (explanatory or independent) variables. Thus, PCR can deal with multicollinearity in multiple linear regression by reducing the number of predictors with minimal loss of important information. Watch the video to understand how PCR works.

13.1.1 Video

https://youtu.be/Za4mOh_jc8M
www.tilestats.com/ml/

A. Tilevik, *Multivariate Statistics and Machine Learning in R For Beginners*,
https://doi.org/10.1007/978-3-032-01851-9_13

PCR generally involves the following steps:

1. Rotate/combine the predictor variables by PCA.
2. Decide the number of principal components to use.
3. Use multiple linear regression on the extracted principal components.

As a simple example, let's consider the same dataset as in the video where we like to predict the systolic blood pressure (SBP) based on age and cholesterol level:

$$\text{SBP} = \text{intercept} + \text{Chol} + \text{Age}$$

```
rm(list=ls()) # Clear environment
SBP=c(120,125,130,121,135,140)
Chol=c(126,128,128,130,130,132)
Age=c(38,40,42,42,44,46)
df=data.frame(SBP,Chol,Age)
```

Let's first check the correlation between the predictor variables Cholesterol and Age:

```
cor(Chol,Age)
0.9438798
```

Since there is a very strong correlation between the two predictor variables, a linear model will therefore suffer from collinearity, which means that the interpretation of the model coefficients will not be reliable due to inflation in the standard errors. Let's see what happens if we use linear regression:

```
fit=lm(SBP~Chol+Age)
confint(fit)
                    2.5 %        97.5 %
(Intercept)   -292.92874334   1086.928743
Chol           -10.64019837      3.140198
Age              0.01509213     10.234908
```

We see that the confidence intervals are very wide, which means that we cannot trust the estimated parameters of the model. If we use the **car** package to calculate the variance inflation factor (VIF), which quantifies the severity of the multicollinearity,

```
library(car)
vif(fit)
    Chol        Age
9.166667   9.166667
```

we see that the VIF is much greater than 5, which is a lower rule-of-thumb threshold for problems with multicollinearity.

We will now use PCR to combine the two predictor variables with PCA. We combine the two variables Cholesterol and Age by:

```
pca=prcomp(cbind(Chol,Age))
a1=pca$rotation[1,1] # Extract the first weight
a1
0.5890632
a2=pca$rotation[2,1] # Extract the second weight
a2
0.808087
PC1=a1*Chol+a2*Age
```

The linear combination of the two variables can be described by the following equation:

$$\text{PC1} = 0.589 \cdot \text{Chol} + 0.808 \cdot \text{Age}$$

We can now perform linear regression of the combination of the two variables (PC1):

```
fit = lm(SBP ~ PC1, data=df)
fit
Coefficients:
(Intercept)          PC1
  -83.933            1.932
```

Our linear model is:

$$\text{SBP} = -83.933 + 1.932 \cdot \text{PC1}$$

We can plot the fitted regression line by (Fig. 13.1):

```
plot(PC1,SBP)
abline(fit)
```

If we substitute PC1 in our model:

$$\text{SBP} = -83.933 + 1.932 \cdot \text{PC1}$$

by

$$\text{PC1} = 0.589 \cdot \text{Chol} + 0.808 \cdot \text{Age}$$

we get:

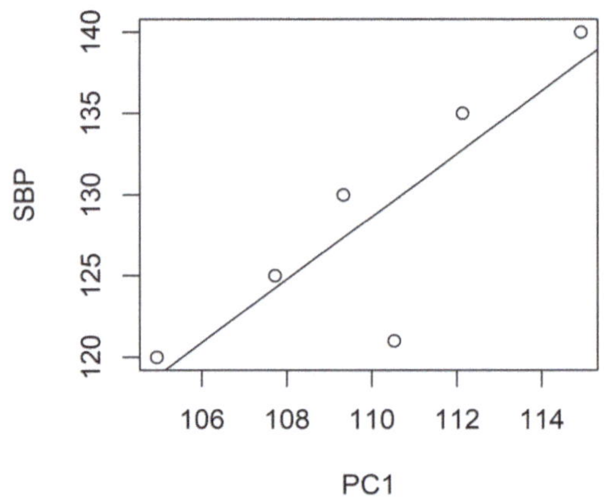

Fig. 13.1 A scatter plot that shows the systolic blood pressure (SBP) on the y-axis and the scores of the first principal component (PC1) on the x-axis. The line represents the fitted line from simple linear regression

$$\text{SBP} = -83.933 + 1.932 \cdot (0.589 \cdot \text{Chol} + 0.808 \cdot \text{Age})$$

If we multiply the weights (0.589 and 0.808) with the slope (1.932), then we get the following equation:

$$\text{SBP} = -83.933 + 1.14 \cdot \text{Chol} + 1.56 \cdot \text{Age}$$

13.1.2 *Using the pls Package*

In the **pls** package, there is a function called "pcr", which will produce the same calculations as above. We simply include the equation and the data frame in the function and say that we like to extract the first component:

```
library(pls)
pcr_fit=pcr(SBP~ Chol + Age,data=df,ncomp=1)
coef(pcr_fit,intercept = TRUE)
(Intercept)          -83.932901
Chol                   1.138340
Age                    1.561595
```

Note that these estimated parameters correspond exactly to the ones in our final equation that we previously calculated by hand.

13.1.3 Calculate Bootstrap Confidence Intervals

Standard errors and confidence intervals for a PCR model are usually obtained by some sort of iterative method. For example, one can compute a non-parametric 95% confidence interval based on many bootstrap samples. Watch the video below to learn how to generate a 95% bootstrap confidence interval.

13.1.4 Video

https://youtu.be/KlqOyGf5I6A
www.tilestats.com/ml/

There are different methods for computing non-parametric confidence intervals, but we will here only focus on the percentile method. The code below uses the **boot** package to draw 1000 bootstraps of the original data:

```
library(boot)
set.seed(10) #For reproducibility
bs=function(formula, data, indices){
  # Allows the function boot to select a sample
  bootstrap=data[indices,]
  fit = pcr(formula, data=bootstrap,ncomp=1)
  return(coef(fit,intercept = TRUE))
}
results = boot(data=df, statistic=bs, R=1000,
formula=SBP ~Chol+Age)
```

If we run the above code, we will get 1000 different estimated values of the parameters. For example, we can plot the 1000 different estimated parameters associated with the variable Age (the third parameter) by:

```
hist(results$t[,3],breaks=30)
```

A simple 95% confidence interval can now be defined by the 2.5% and 97.5% percentile. The values that define the interval that covers 95% of the middle values in Fig. 13.2 can be used as our 95% confidence interval based on the bootstraps. Such interval can be computed by:

```
boot.ci(results, type="perc", index=3)# Age
Level      Percentile
95%     ( 0.125,   2.622 )
```

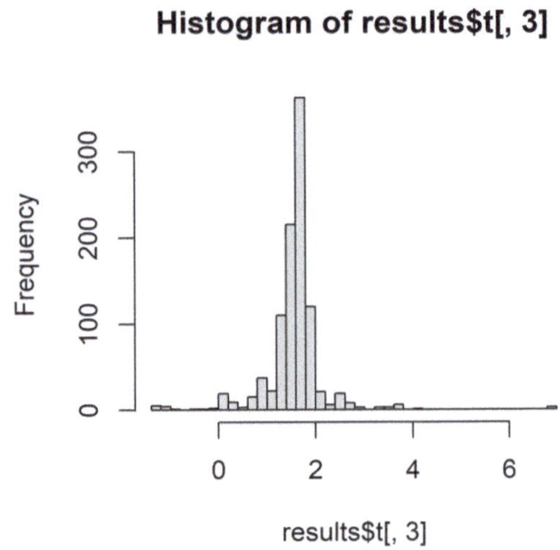

Fig. 13.2 A histogram of the parameter associated with the variable Age based on 1000 bootstraps

We see that the interval for the third parameter (the one associated with Age) spans between 0.125 and 2.622. The intervals for the intercept and the parameter associated with the variable Cholesterol can be computed by:

```
# get 95% confidence intervals
boot.ci(results, type="perc", index=1)# Intercept
Level        Percentile
95%      (-209.61,   102.58 )
boot.ci(results, type="perc", index=2)# Chol
Level       Percentile
95%      ( 0.038,   1.782 )
```

The estimated parameter associated with the variable Cholesterol spans between 0.038 and 1.782. What is interesting is that the intervals associated with the two predictor variables are much narrower compared to the ones from the multiple linear regression model. None of these two intervals includes the value zero, which means that both parameters associated with the predictor variables are significantly different from zero. This is the main advantage of using principal component regression because we have solved the problem with collinearity which is problematic in linear regression.

13.1.5 Predict

Let's use the model that we created earlier to predict the SBP based on an age of 40 and a cholesterol level of 125:

```
new=data.frame(Chol=125, Age=40)
predict(pcr_fit,new)
120.8234
```

The predicted systolic blood pressure is about 121.

13.1.6 Standardize the Predictors

As we discussed in the chapter about PCA, it is often recommended to standardize the variables before we compute PCA. In the case of PCR, the predictors are therefore usually first standardized. This is especially important if the predictors are on different scales or have a large difference in variances. Standardizing ensures that all predictors contribute equally to the analysis, regardless of their original units or spread. To standardize the predictors, we can set the argument "scale" to TRUE:

```
library(pls)
pcr_fit=pcr(SBP~ Chol + Age,data=df,ncomp=1, scale=TRUE)
```

If we would use this model to predict:

```
new=data.frame(Chol=125, Age=40)
predict(pcr_fit,new)
119.835
```

we see that we get approximately the same predicted value as when we did not standardize the predictors.

13.1.7 Choosing the Number of Components Based on Cross-Validation

We will here use a bit larger dataset, which is the same as the one in the video, so that we can practice how to extract an appropriate number of components for our model. In addition to SBP and cholesterol, we here also have data on weight and height:

```
rm(list=ls()) # Clear environment
library(pls)
SBP=c(120,125,130,121,135,140)
Chol=c(126,128,128,130,130,132)
Age=c(38,40,42,42,44,46)
```

```
Weight=c(60,80,70,85,90,87)
Height=c(165,180,170,185,190,187)
df=data.frame(SBP,Chol,Age,Weight,Height)
```

By, for example, using the leave-one-out cross-validation (LOOCV), we can calculate the root mean squared error of the prediction (RMSEP). By setting the validation argument to "LOO", we run a LOOCV:

```
pcr_fit.cv=pcr(SBP~ Chol + Age + Weight + Height,data=df,
validation="LOO")
summary(pcr_fit.cv)
VALIDATION: RMSEP
Cross-validated using 6 leave-one-out segments.
        (Intercept)  1 comps   2 comps   3 comps    4 comps
CV          8.729      8.069     5.205     6.196      2.198e+16
adjCV       8.729      7.884     5.031     6.062      2.176e+16
```

The output shows two cross-validation estimates where CV is the ordinary cross-validation estimate, whereas adjCV is the adjusted cross-validation estimate. For LOOCV, there is virtually no difference between these estimates (Mevik & Wehrens, 2007). We can see that a model based on two principal components results in the lowest root mean squared error of prediction. We should aim to use as few components as possible that result in a relatively small error, which means that we should extract only the first two components in this example by:

```
pcr_fit=pcr(SBP~ Chol + Age + Weight + Height, data=df,
ncomp=2)
summary(pcr_fit)
...
TRAINING: % variance explained
        1 comps   2 comps
X         97.99     99.58
SBP       33.85     77.52
coef(pcr_fit,intercept=TRUE)
                      SBP
(Intercept)       -63.91887431
Chol                1.22263244
Age                 2.35643309
Weight              0.08920853
Height             -0.39715119
```

The coefficients correspond exactly to the ones as shown in the video. We see that the variance in the SBP, the response (or the dependent) variable, is explained by 77.52% of the model when using two principal components. The value 99.58 in the output corresponds to the percentage of variance in the predictor variables

(Cholesterol, Age, Weight, and Height) that is explained by the first two principal components in the model.

13.2 Partial Least Squares Regression

Partial least square regression (PLSR) works very similarly to PCR. The difference between PCR and PLSR is that PCR maximizes the variance of the combined predictor variables, whereas PLSR maximizes the covariance between the scores from the combined predictor variables and the response variable. Thus, PLSR, in contrast to PCR, involves the response variable when the data is rotated. PLSR therefore often needs fewer components than PCR to generate the same prediction error (Mevik & Wehrens, 2007). Watch the video to understand the difference between PCR and PLSR.

13.2.1 Video

https://youtu.be/CzSvCuVm_l0
www.tilestats.com/ml/

Let's try to use PLSR on our previous data. To run PLSR, we use the function "plsr":

```
plsr_fit=plsr(SBP~ Chol + Age + Weight + Height,data=df,
ncomp=2)
summary(plsr_fit)
TRAINING: % variance explained
       1 comps     2 comps
X       97.95       99.58
SBP     35.29       78.78
coef(plsr_fit,intercept=TRUE)
, 2 comps
                        SBP
(Intercept)       -46.75607767
Chol                0.96439911
Age                 2.54643647
Weight              0.03340407
Height             -0.32718399
```

We see that the first two principal components explain 78.78% of the variation in the SPB, which is higher compared to when we used PCR (77.52%). Since PLSR components are optimized for predicting the response variable (SBP), they capture more of the relevant variability for the response variable compared to PCR components.

13.3 Lasso Regression

Lasso (Least Absolute Shrinkage and Selection Operator) regression is a technique used in machine learning and regression analysis. It extends ordinary least squares (OLS) regression by incorporating regularization, which shrinks the coefficients in the model. Such shrinking can remove the effect of redundant explanatory variables (predictors). In comparison to PCR and PLS, which combine variables to reduce the dimensions, Lasso regression can reduce the number of explanatory variables in the regression model. Thus, Lasso regression can be used for feature/variable selection, which generates a simpler model to prevent overfitting. Have a look at the following video, which explains how Lasso regression works and how to find an appropriate value of lambda based on cross-validation.

13.3.1 Video

https://youtu.be/7FjVjbhRkB8
www.tilestats.com/ml/

We will first begin to reproduce some of the results shown in the video by using the same dataset. The example data includes the systolic blood pressure (BP), Age, and Score on a math test of seven individuals.

```
rm(list=ls())
BP=c(120,115, 127, 130, 122, 132, 137)
Age=c(22,  33, 35,  44,  52,  62, 65)
Score=c(65,34, 35, 43, 54,60, 22)
df=data.frame(BP,Age,Score)
```

Let's first use linear regression (ordinary least squares) to compute the coefficients and the R-squared values of three different models to predict the BP as shown in the video:

```
# Predict blood pressure with Age
fit1=lm(BP~Age)
coef(fit1)
(Intercept)        Age
109.8631380   0.3640832
summary(fit1)$r.squared
0.5776147
```

```
# Predict blood pressure with Score on a math test
fit2=lm(BP~Score)
coef(fit2)
(Intercept)       Score
132.7519577   -0.1478074
summary(fit2)$r.squared
0.09192303

# Predict blood pressure with both Age and Score
fit3=lm(BP~Age+Score)
coef(fit3)
(Intercept)         Age            Score
113.17385534    0.34956742    -0.05952585
summary(fit3)$r.squared
0.5916053
```

The output tells us that a model including the explanatory variable Age explains 57.76% of the variance in the BP because the R-squared value is equal to 0.5776. Thus, age is an important predictor of the BP. In contrast, the explanatory variable Score seems to be useless in predicting the BP because the R-squared value of such a model is only 0.092. However, a model including both Age and Score has the highest R-squared value (0.592). As explained in the video, a model with more explanatory variables generally fits better to the data and has a higher R-squared value although some explanatory variables are useless to predict the outcome. It is therefore desirable to remove useless explanatory variables from the model to avoid overfitting and to only keep variables that are useful for predictions. Let's try to use Lasso regression on the model including both age and math score as explanatory variables. We first need to store the explanatory variables (Age and Score) in a matrix (X), and then we store the response variable (BP) in y:

```
# Store the explanatory variables in matrix X
X = as.matrix(df[,-1])
y = df$BP # Store the response variable in Y
```

We will here first use the **ncvreg** package and later see how to use the **glmnet** package.

```
library(ncvreg)
```

The first thing that we should do is to find an appropriate value of lambda, which can be done with the function "cv.ncreg", which computes cross-validation of the model:

```
cv_model = cv.ncvreg(X, y, family="gaussian",
penalty="lasso")
plot(cv_model)
```

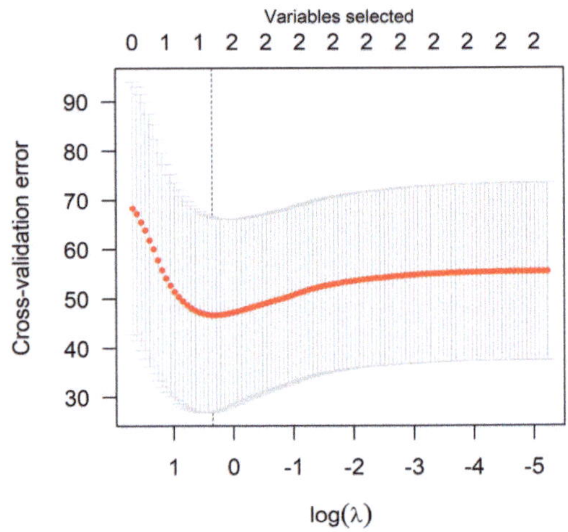

Fig. 13.3 A plot showing how the cross-validation error changes over different values of lambda (λ). The red squares represent the mean cross-validation error, whereas the error bars display the standard deviation. The dashed vertical line represents the lambda value that generates the smallest error. The values at the top of the plot show the number of variables that are used in the model for different values of lambda

Figure 13.3 shows the result of the cross-validation. A lambda value of about 1.42 (log(1.42) = 0.35) seems to be the optimal value since it results in the lowest cross-validation error. This value can be extracted by:

```
cv_model$lambda.min
 1.42098
```

We will now fit a Lasso model to the data:

```
lasso_model = ncvreg(X, y, family="gaussian",
penalty="lasso")
lasso_model # Print output
```

However, note that the function "ncvreg" fits a range of models with different values of lambda. To extract the coefficients of the model where lambda is equal to 1.42, we need to set lambda to 1.42 (cv_model$lambda.min) in the "coef" function:

```
coef(lasso_model, lambda=cv_model$lambda.min)
 (Intercept)          Age           Score
114.1871743        0.2673795      0.0000000
```

These coefficients are the same as shown in the video. Note that the coefficient associated with the math score has been reduced to zero, which means that we can remove this variable from the model. Let's fit a Lasso regression model again but without the variable math score:

```
# Use only Age as the explanatory variable
X=as.matrix(data.frame(Age))
```

```
lasso_model_red = ncvreg(X, y, family="gaussian",
penalty="lasso")
coef(lasso_model_red, lambda=cv_model$lambda.min)
(Intercept)          Age
114.1871743      0.2673795
```

We see that we get the same coefficients for the intercept and the age with the model where the variable math score has been deleted.

13.3.2 Predict

We can now use the reduced model for prediction. Suppose that we like to predict the systolic blood pressure of a person with an age of 50, then we type:

```
Xnew=as.matrix(data.frame(Age=50))
predict(lasso_model_red,Xnew,lambda=cv_model$lambda.min)
1.4210
127.5561
```

We see that a person with an age of 50 is predicted to have a systolic blood pressure of 127.55. The value 1.4210 corresponds to the lambda that is used in the Lasso model.

13.3.3 The glmnet Package

We will now repeat the same analysis on the same data but instead use the **glmnet** package. To find an appropriate value of lambda, we first use the function "cv.glmnet" where we set the parameter alpha to 1 in order to use Lasso regression. If alpha is set to 0, the function will instead perform Ridge regression, and if the value is somewhere between 0 and 1, Elastic Net will be used.

```
library(glmnet)
# Store the explanatory variables in matrix X
X = as.matrix(df[,-1])
y = df$BP    # Store the response variable in Y
cv.lasso=cv.glmnet(X, y,family = c("gaussian"),alpha=1)
plot(cv.lasso)
```

We see in Fig. 13.4 that we get approximately the same plot as we got from using the **ncvreg** package. We can extract the lambda value that results in the lowest error by:

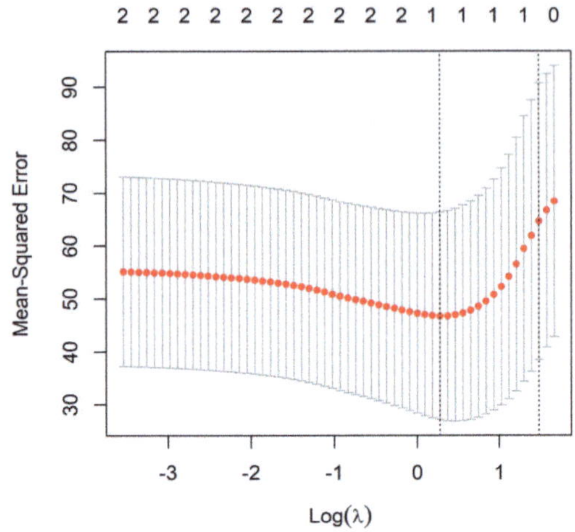

Fig. 13.4 A plot showing how the cross-validation error changes over different values of lambda (λ). The red squares represent the mean cross-validation error, whereas the error bars display the standard deviation. The left dotted vertical line represents the lambda value that generates the smallest error, whereas the right dotted line represents the largest lambda value within one standard error of the lambda that results in the smallest error. The values at the top of the plot show the number of variables that are used in the model for different values of lambda

```
cv.lasso$lambda.min
1.32521
```

The **glmnet** package results in a slightly different value of lambda compared to the **ncvreg** package. This is due to that the two packages are based on different numerical methods. We can also extract the lambda value that corresponds to the right dotted line in Fig. 13.4 by:

```
cv.lasso$lambda.1se
4.441578
```

This value corresponds to the largest lambda value within one standard error of lambda.min. By instead using this value, we will generally get a simpler model since more coefficients will be reduced to zero for larger values of lambda.

We can now fit a Lasso model with the optimal value of lambda, here defined as the value that results in the lowest cross-validation error, and extract the coefficients of the model by:

```
lasso.fit=glmnet(X, y,family=c("gaussian"),alpha=1,
intercept=TRUE, lambda=cv.lasso$lambda.min)
coef(lasso.fit)
...
(Intercept)  113.895749
Age            0.273897
Score          .
```

Note that the coefficients are a bit different from the **ncvreg** package and that the "glmnet" function displays a dot (.) for a coefficient that has been reduced to zero by the regularization process.

13.3.4 Logistic Regression with Lasso Regularization

Lasso regression can also be used in association with logistic regression. To illustrate this, we will here use the Crab dataset, which is stored in the package **MASS**:

```
rm(list=ls())          # Clear environment
library(MASS)          # To access the Crab dataset
```

We will here try to use logistic regression with Lasso regularization to create a model that can predict the sex of a crab based on the numeric variables in the Crab dataset:

```
# Feature matrix
X = as.matrix(crabs[, c("FL", "RW", "CL", "CW", "BD")])
y = crabs$sex  # Response variable Male (M) or Female (F)
```

We first find an optimal value of lambda by performing cross-validation. Note that we here set "family" to "binomial" because our predictor variable is now on a binary scale:

```
set.seed(1) # For reproducibility
cv_model = cv.glmnet(X, y, family="binomial", alpha=1)
cv_model$lambda.min # Print optimal value of lambda
```

Then we fit a model based on the optimal lambda value and print its coefficients:

```
lasso_model=glmnet(X, y, family="binomial", alpha=1,
intercept=TRUE, lambda=cv_model$lambda.min)
coef(lasso_model)
(Intercept)       11.7053385
FL               -1.4026422
RW               -9.8455076
CL                4.0569227
CW                .
BD                0.4944496
```

Note that the regularization has shrunk the coefficient associated with the variable CW down to zero, which suggests that this variable is unnecessary for predicting the sex of the crabs. To compute the accuracy of this model, we can use the "predict" function to compute the predicted sex of the crabs and then calculate the accuracy by comparing it with the true sex of the crabs (y):

```
pred = predict(lasso_model, newx=X, type="class")
sum(pred == y) / length(y)
0.975
```

We see that we get an accuracy of 97.5%. Note that we have here used the same data for both training and validation. To get a better estimate of the true performance of the model, we can use the same validation methods as explained in Chap. 11.

13.3.5 Multinomial Logistic Regression with Lasso Regularization

The previous example code only works when we have a binary outcome (two categories to predict). By instead using a multinomial logistic regression, we can create a model that can predict more than two categories. Let's use the Iris dataset to create a model that can predict the three species:

```
rm(list=ls())   # Clear environment
X = as.matrix(iris[,-5])  # Feature matrix
# Response variable: Species (Setosa, Versicolor and Virginica)
y = iris$Species
set.seed(1) # For reproducibility
# Find optimal value of lambda
cv_model = cv.glmnet(X, y, family="multinomial", alpha=1)
cv_model$lambda.min # Print optimal value of lambda
lasso_model = glmnet(X, y, family="multinomial", alpha=1,
lambda=cv_model$lambda.min)
coef(lasso_model)
                  $setosa
5 x 1 sparse Matrix of class "dgCMatrix"
                    s0
                 11.705197
Sepal.Length  .
Sepal.Width   3.497447
Petal.Length -2.749511
Petal.Width  -1.742940

$versicolor
5 x 1 sparse Matrix of class "dgCMatrix"
```

```
                s0
             5.899985
Sepal.Length 1.428125
Sepal.Width  .
Petal.Length .
Petal.Width  .

$virginica
5 x 1 sparse Matrix of class "dgCMatrix"
                   s0
              -17.605182
Sepal.Length    .
Sepal.Width   -3.334131
Petal.Length   5.117537
Petal.Width   10.105956
```

This output shows the results from three dependent binary logistic regression models that have been trained together with a shared penalty. For example, the first part of the output shows a logistic regression model where Setosa is predicted. This part of the model therefore only predicts if the flower is a Setosa or not. Since the coefficient associated with the variable sepal width is positive (3.497447), it means that a flower with a large sepal width increases the probability that the flower will be predicted to be of class Setosa. In comparison, a larger petal length or petal width reduces the probability of predicting the flower as a Setosa since the associated coefficients are negative. The coefficient of the sepal length has been shrunk to zero, which suggests that this variable is not important to predict if the flower is a Setosa. We can now compare the predicted classes of the model with the true classes to compute the accuracy:

```
pred = predict(lasso_model, X, type="class")
sum(pred == y) / length(y)
0.98
```

We see that we get an accuracy of 98%. Note that you can validate this model, just as we did in Chap. 11, by the hold-out method or cross-validation. For example, we can use the **caret** package to perform hyperparameter tuning based on a ten-fold cross-validation. Let's first see which parameters we can tune:

```
library(caret)
modelLookup("glmnet")
  model    parameter label for                Reg    forClass  probModel
1 glmnet   alpha     Mixing Percentage        TRUE   TRUE      TRUE
2 glmnet   lambda    Regularization Parameter TRUE   TRUE      TRUE
```

We can tune the parameters lambda and alpha. If we tune the parameter alpha between zero and one, we will use Elastic Net, which might improve the performance of the model. However, to be consistent with our previous examples, we will here fix alpha to 1 so that we only use Lasso regression:

```
cv_control = trainControl(method = "cv", number = 10)
lambda_grid=expand.grid(alpha = 1, lambda = 10^seq(-10, 2,
length = 100))
set.seed(123)  # For reproducibility
model = train(Species ~ ., data = iris, method = "glmnet",
trControl = cv_control,
  family = "multinomial", tuneGrid = lambda_grid)
print(model)
  ...
  2.009233e-04  0.9800000  0.97
  2.656088e-04  0.9800000  0.97
  3.511192e-04  0.9733333  0.96
  ...

  Tuning parameter 'alpha' was held constant at a value of 1
  Accuracy was used to select the optimal model using the
largest value.
  The final values used for the model were alpha = 1 and lambda
= 0.0002656088.
```

We see that the Lasso model, with lambda set to 0.0002656, results in an accuracy of 0.98 based on a ten-fold cross-validation.

13.4 Exercises

1. Use a multiple linear regression model to predict the frontal lobe size (FL) based on the variables RW, CL, CW, and BD from the Crab dataset:

$$FL \sim RW + CL + CW + BD$$

   Once you have generated the model, check if your model involves multicollinearity.
2. Use instead the **pls** package to compute PCR where you extract only the first principal component. Show the equation with the estimated parameters for this model.
3. Compute 95% confidence intervals for the parameters in the PCR model based on 1000 bootstrap samples.

4. Use your PCR model to predict the FL size of a crab with the following measurements: RW = 6.7, CL = 16.1, CW = 19.0, BD = 7.0.
5. Use Lasso regression to predict the frontal lobe size (FL) based on the variables RW, CL, CW, and BD in the Crab dataset:

$$\text{FL} \sim \text{RW} + \text{CL} + \text{CW} + \text{BD}$$

   Which variable is suggested by the Lasso model to be unnecessary to predict FL?
6. Use Lasso regression to predict the sex of the crabs based on the variables sp, FL, RW, CL, CW, and BD in the Crab dataset:

$$\text{sex} \sim \text{sp} + \text{FL} + \text{RW} + \text{CL} + \text{CW} + \text{BD}$$

   Which variable is suggested by the Lasso model to be unnecessary to predict sex? Note that you need to convert the variable species (sp) to ones and zeros so that the feature matrix only includes numeric data.

Reference

Mevik, B., & Wehrens, R. (2007). The pls package: Principal component and partial least squares regression in R. *Journal of Statistical Software, 18*, 1–24.

Chapter 14
Case Studies

In this final chapter, we will reproduce the results from two different scientific papers. The aim is to see how some of the multivariate statistical methods we have covered so far can be applied to reproduce the results in these papers. The two papers that we will try to reproduce are:

- Wallner, F. K., Hopkins, M. H., Lindvall, T., Olofsson, P., & Tilevik, A. (2017). Cytokine correlation analysis based on drug perturbation. *Cytokine*, *90*, 73–79.
- Lin, W. C., Chen, C. W., Chao, L., Chao, J., & Lin, Y. S. (2017). Plasma Kallistatin in critically ill patients with severe sepsis and septic shock. *PloS one*, *12*(5), e0178387.

The first paper (paper 1) by Wallner et al. (2017) analyzes the correlation between cytokines that are produced by the immune system in the presence of different drugs. In the second paper by Lin et al. (2017), a range of different biomarkers have been analyzed from 86 patients with severe sepsis or septic shock for 60-day mortality prediction.

14.1 Paper 1

Cytokines are proteins that are mainly produced by immune cells that are used for cell communication. Usually, these cytokines bind to a receptor on the cell surface of an immune cell, which provides a signal to the cell to, for example, become activated. In this study, the authors stimulated immune cells in vitro for 44 hours with ConA. The supernatant was then harvested to analyze the production of cytokines. To analyze how drugs affect cytokine production by the immune cells, a range of different drugs were added to the cell cultures in which the immune cells were stimulated. Thus, cell cultures without any drug were used as controls that could then be compared to cell cultures with a certain drug to analyze the effect of the

A. Tilevik, *Multivariate Statistics and Machine Learning in R For Beginners*, https://doi.org/10.1007/978-3-032-01851-9_14

```
Treatment;IL1a;IL1b;IL2;IL5;IL6;IL7;IL10;IL1
actarit1;285,1;957,31;11520,6;99,18;175;67,3
astaxanthin1;1417,59;4119,02;10186,39;101,09
bardoxolone methyl1;102,96;885,59;9417,59;54
bortezomib1;128,04;1007,6;967,32;48,62;21,4;
bucillamine1;279,12;836,25;7865,97;89,27;146
cinchophen1;247,88;946,71;7663,34;93,54;188,
diacerein1;214,78;874,94;10178,52;82,62;185,
doramapimod1;417,47;646,39;22478,17;85,14;64
```

Fig. 14.1 A screenshot that illustrates how the data is arranged

drug on the cytokine production by the immune cells. By analyzing the correlation of the perturbated cytokine production by the drugs, one can identify cytokines that are likely to be co-regulated in the presence of these drugs.

You can download the dataset as a CSV file from:

https://www.tilestats.com/ml/

To illustrate how the data is arranged in this file, you can open the file in a text editor, such as Notepad or TextEdit. In Fig. 14.1, I have opened the file in Notepad.

We see that the first row includes the names of the columns and that the columns are separated with a semi-colon (Fig. 14.1). We also see that the decimals of the numerical values are separated with a comma.

The easiest way to read in the file into R is to run:

```
df=read.csv(file.choose(),header=TRUE,sep=";",dec=",")
```

If you run the above line in R, a window should pop up in R that allows you to select the CSV file that you have downloaded. In the code above, we set the argument header to TRUE because our file has names for the columns. We also set sep to ";" and dec to "," because the columns in this file are separated by semi-colons, whereas the decimals of the numerical values are separated by commas.

The code above is convenient to use for beginners because no path to the file is required. However, it is tedious to locate the file every time you run the code. If you read in the same data file many times, it is convenient to instead use the path to the file. For example, if you have stored the file in the folder C:/data, you can instead read in the file by:

```
df=read.csv("C:/data/Cytokines.csv",header=TRUE,sep=";",
dec=",")
```

You should change "C:/data" to the path to the folder where you have saved the data file "Cytokines.csv". To print the path of your current working directory in R, you can type:

```
getwd()
```

which might help you to understand how to set a correct path.

It is also possible to read in the CSV file directly from the website:

```
df=read.csv(
"https://www.tilestats.com/wp-content/uploads/2024/12/Cytokines.csv",
header=TRUE,sep=";",dec=",")
```

Once you have read in the file, you should print the data frame to make sure it looks fine. Since it is a large dataset, we print only the first four rows and columns by:

```
df[1:4,1:4]
        Treatment              IL1a        IL1b       IL2
1       actarit1             285.10      957.31  11520.60
2    astaxanthin1           1417.59     4119.02  10186.39
3 bardoxolone methyl1        102.96      885.59   9417.59
4     bortezomib1            128.04     1007.60    967.32
```

We see that the first column includes the type of treatment (drug) the immune cells have been exposed to. Note that the same drug was used twice in two different biological replicates. Thus, if the drug was used in the first biological replicate, its name ends with a 1, whereas if it was used in the second biological replicate, it ends with a 2.

To check the dimension of the data frame, we can run:

```
dim(df)
126  18
```

which tells us that the data frame has 126 rows and 18 columns. The first column includes the type of treatment, whereas the other 17 columns include the concentrations of the 17 different cytokines after 44 hours of stimulation in the presence or absence of a certain drug.

In RStudio, we can get a full view of the data by:

```
View(df)
```

Note that the last rows of the dataset, rows 111–126, represent two different controls. If the row includes the name ConA, it means that the immune cells were stimulated with ConA but in the absence of drugs. Since some drugs were diluted in DMSO, the corresponding control for these drugs was stimulated with ConA in the presence of DMSO but in the absence of drugs (ConA_DMSO).

To simplify the analysis, we will here separate the data frame into three new data frames. The first data frame will include only the cytokine concentrations in the presence of the drugs. We therefore exclude the controls from this data frame:

```
library(dplyr)
library(tibble)
Drugs = df %>%
  filter(!Treatment %in% c("ConA_DMSO", "ConA")) %>%
  column_to_rownames(var = "Treatment")
```

Note that we here also set the drug names in the column "Treatment" as row names of the new data frame with the function "column_to_rownames".

We then define the other two data frames to include the controls (ConA only and ConA with DMSO):

```
ConA = df %>% filter(Treatment %in% c("ConA"))
ConA_DMSO = df %>% filter(Treatment %in% c("ConA_DMSO"))
```

To check if our three data frames include any missing data (NAs), we can run the following code:

```
any(is.na(Drugs))
FALSE
any(is.na(ConA))
FALSE
any(is.na(ConA_DMSO))
TRUE
```

We see that the data frame ConA_DMSO includes at least one missing data that we later need to deal with.

14.1.1 Table 1: Descriptive Statistics

We are now ready to reproduce some of the descriptive statistics that are shown in Table 1 in the paper:

```
MEDIAN=apply(Drugs,2,median)
IQR=apply(Drugs,2,IQR)
MEAN=apply(Drugs,2,mean)
SD=apply(Drugs,2,sd)
CV=SD/MEAN
round(data.frame(MEDIAN,IQR,MEAN,SD,CV), 1)
        MEDIAN     IQR      MEAN      SD      CV
IL1a     227.9    94.2     243.6    184.8     0.8
IL1b     925.3   381.0     981.5    581.7     0.6
IL2     8729.7  7154.0   11201.5  11362.6     1.0
IL5       78.9    31.3      73.1     20.7     0.3
IL6      109.8    68.0     118.6     81.2     0.7
...
```

This table shows the median, interquartile range (IQR), mean, standard deviation (SD), and coefficient of variation (CV) of the cytokine concentrations from all the cell cultures in the presence of the drugs. A larger value of the CV means that the cytokine has a large spread relative to its mean value.

14.1.2 Figure 1: Descriptive Statistics

We will now calculate the log2 fold change (FC), which represents how much the drugs affect the cytokine production relative to the controls. We therefore first calculate the mean of the biological replicates of the two different controls:

```
mean_ConA_DMSO=colMeans(ConA_DMSO[,-1],na.rm = TRUE)
mean_ConA=colMeans(ConA[,-1])
```

Note that we here specify that we want to remove any missing data (na.rm. = TRUE) before we compute the means of the data frame ConA_DMSO because this data frame included missing values. Also, to compute the means of each column, we exclude the first column ([,-1]) because this column does not include any numeric values. Print the above vectors and note that the mean of each cytokine has been calculated for the two controls.

The drugs that were not diluted with DMSO are the ones located on rows 98–103 and 105–110 in the data frame Drugs. Let's store these row numbers in a vector:

```
conA_ind=c(98:103,105:110) # Rows of drugs without DMSO
```

We will now calculate the FC, where drugs stored in DMSO will be divided by the mean cytokine concentration in controls with DMSO, whereas the drugs stored without DMSO will be divided by the mean cytokine concentration in the controls with no DMSO:

```
FC=Drugs # Create a new data frame to store FC in
for (i in 1:ncol(Drugs)){ # Loop over all cytokines
  # DMSO
  FC[-conA_ind,i] = Drugs[-conA_ind,i] /
  mean_ConA_DMSO[i]
  # No DMSO
  FC[ conA_ind,i] = Drugs[ conA_ind,i] / mean_ConA[i]
}
```

Next, we compute the log2 FC and show these as boxplots, which will reproduce figure 1 in the paper:

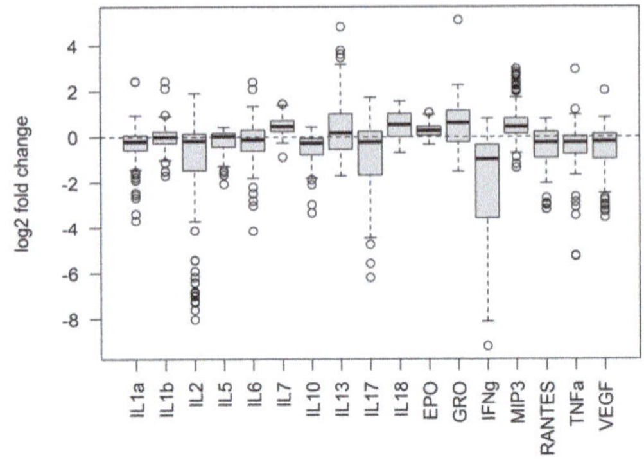

Fig. 14.2 A boxplot that reproduces figure 1 in paper 1. The log2 fold change is shown for each cytokine. Circles define outliers

```
log2_FC=log2(FC)
boxplot(log2_FC,las=2,ylab="log2 fold change")
abline(h=0,col="black",lty=2)
```

From this plot (Fig. 14.2), one can see that most of the drugs downregulate the cytokines IL-2, IL-17, and IFN-γ because most of the log2 FC values are negative. A large spread in the FC values indicates that the drugs have a large effect on the cytokine production where some drugs may have an inhibitory effect, whereas other drugs may have a stimulatory effect.

14.1.3 Table 2 Correlation Matrix

In this study, any value above the detection limit of the standard curve was set to the maximum value of the standard curve. One problem with this method is that the spread of the data might be constrained within a certain range, which will affect the calculations of the correlation coefficients. To avoid such constraints, one can instead compute correlations directly on the fluorescence intensity values, which was done in the follow-up study (Wallner et al., 2018). To compute the correlation matrix shown in table 2 in paper 1, the values were first log10 transformed because the variables were highly skewed:

```
log10.Drugs=log10(Drugs)
```

The Pearson correlation coefficients were then computed based on the log10 values. The reason for selecting the Person correlation, instead of the Spearman correlation, was to focus on drugs that actually affected the cytokine production. The matrix which is printed at the last line of this code generates the correlation matrix as shown in the paper:

```
library(Hmisc)
pears=rcorr(as.matrix(log10.Drugs), type="pearson")
pearsr=pears$r # Save the correlation coefficients
diag(pearsr) = NA # Set the main diagonal to NA
# Set the upper triangle to NA
pearsr[upper.tri (pearsr)] = NA
print(round(pearsr,2)) # Print the correlation matrix
```

The corresponding *p*-values were calculated by:

```
pearsP=pears$P # Save the p-value
diag(pearsP) = NA
pearsP[upper.tri (pearsP)] = NA
print(round(pearsP,3))
```

To create a table where we can easily sort the pairs of cytokines based on the correlation coefficients, and to adjust the *p*-values by the Bonferroni method, we can reshape the two matrices into vectors:

```
library(reshape)
correlations=na.omit(melt(pearsr))
pval=na.omit(melt(pearsP))[,3]
padjust=p.adjust(pval,method="bonferroni")
```

We can now create a data frame of these vectors and sort the data frame based on the correlation coefficients:

```
correlations=data.frame(correlations,pval,padjust)
sort_correlations=correlations[order(correlations$value,
decreasing = TRUE),]
```

Finally, we can print the numeric values in this data frame with four decimal places where we easily can identify correlations with an adjusted *p*-value <0.01, which was the significance level used in this paper:

```
sort_correlations %>%
  mutate(across(where(is.numeric), ~ round(., 4)))
          X1       X2       value     pval      padjust
47        IFNg     IL2      0.8662    0.0000    0.0000
164       EPO      IL18     0.8358    0.0000    0.0000
43        IL17     IL2      0.7942    0.0000    0.0000
96        EPO      IL7      0.7746    0.0000    0.0000
149       IFNg     IL17     0.7405    0.0000    0.0000
...
```

From the output, we can, for example, see that the strongest positive correlation ($r = 0.8662$) can be found between IFN-γ and IL-2.

14.1.4 *Figure 2: Cluster Analysis*

To identify groups that consist of cytokines that have a strong correlation to each other, hierarchical clustering with distances based on one minus the Pearson correlation coefficients was computed with the average linkage method. To assess the robustness of the generated dendrogram, bootstrapping was performed using the **Pvclust** package. To save simulation time, we will here run just 1000 bootstraps:

```
library(pvclust)
set.seed(2) #For reproducibility
fit = pvclust(log10(Drugs), method.hclust="average",
method.dist="cor",use.cor="pairwise.complete.obs",nboot=1000)
plot(fit)
mean(fit$edges$bp) # To compute the mean of the bp value
```

From this dendrogram (Fig. 14.3), we can, for example, see that there is one robust cluster, including the cytokines IL-17, IL-2, and IFN-γ. To better understand why these cytokines form a cluster, we can create a heatmap where we cluster the columns (the cytokines) based on one minus the Pearson correlation coefficients to be consistent with the generated dendrogram in Fig. 14.3.

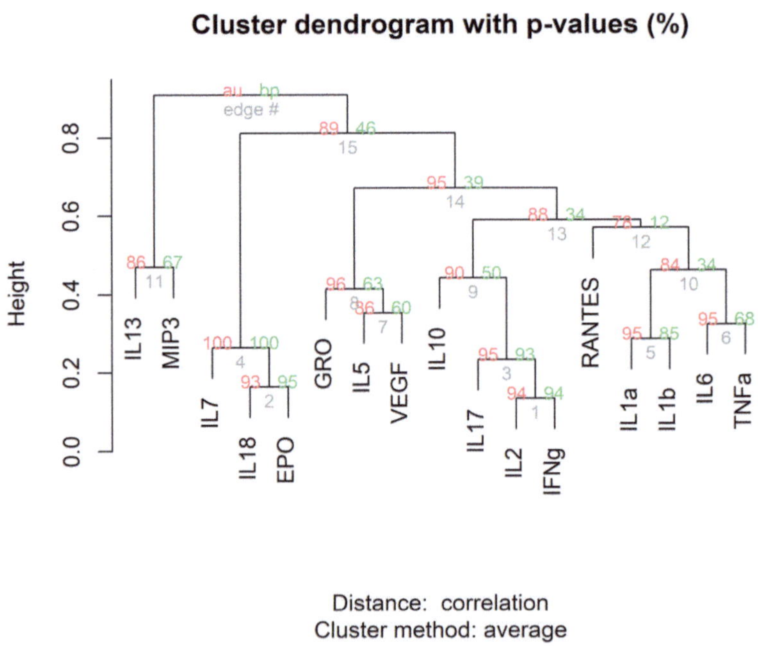

Fig. 14.3 A dendrogram that reproduces figure 2 in paper 1. The dendrogram was computed based on one minus the Pearson correlation distances and the average linkage function. One thousand bootstraps were used to compute the approximately unbiased *p*-values (au, red) and bootstrap probabilities (bp, green)

```
library(pheatmap)
pheatmap(as.matrix(log10.Drugs),scale="column",
        clustering_distance_cols="correlation",
        clustering_method = "average",
        fontsize_row=4)
```

From this heatmap (Fig. 14.4), we can see that the production of the cytokines IL-17, IL-2, and IFN-γ is similarly affected by the drugs. For example, they are inhibited in the presence of, for example, the calcineurin inhibitors cyclosporine A and tacrolimus. In comparison, the production of the cytokines IL-13 and MIP-3 is instead increased in the presence of the same drugs.

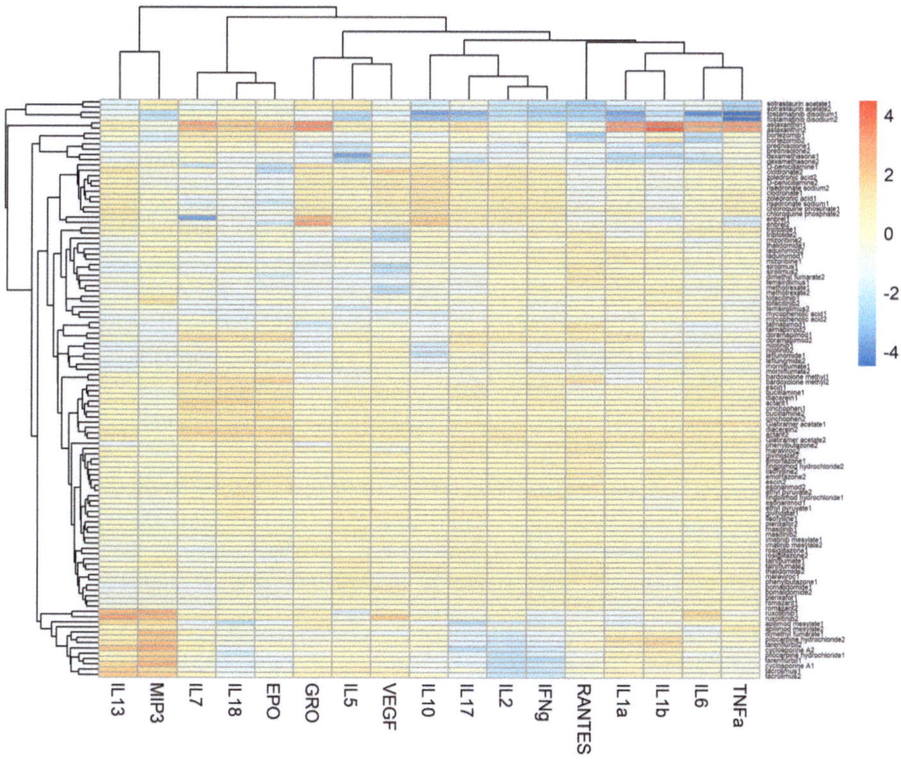

Fig. 14.4 A heatmap that shows the drugs on the rows and the cytokines on the columns. The dendrogram for the columns was computed based on one minus the Pearson correlation distances and the average linkage function, whereas the rows were clustered based on the Euclidean distance (default setting)

14.1.5 *Table 3: Principal Component Analysis (PCA)*

A PCA was also conducted to identify groups of cytokines that correlated. We will here compute a PCA of the log10 data and calculate the variance of each component to know how many components to extract:

```
pca=prcomp(log10(Drugs),scale=TRUE)
pca$sdev^2
6.34119579 2.61114345 2.43181018 1.84016908 0.89897544
0.66962321 ...
```

The Kaiser's criterion was used to determine the number of components to extract. Since the PCA is here based on the standardized data, we extract the first four components because these have an eigenvalue, or variance, larger than one. Next, we compute the Varimax rotation of the first four components:

```
library(psych)
principal(log10(Drugs), nfactors = 4, rotate = "varimax")
Standardized loadings (pattern matrix) based upon
correlation matrix
             RC1   RC4    RC2    RC3    h2    u2    com
IL1a         0.78  0.27   0.14  -0.08  0.72  0.285  1.3
IL1b         0.67  0.07   0.43  -0.38  0.78  0.215  2.4
IL2          0.52  0.32  -0.04   0.69  0.84  0.161  2.3
IL5          0.32  0.70   0.13   0.14  0.62  0.377  1.6
IL6          0.61  0.52   0.18   0.05  0.68  0.318  2.2
IL7          0.16  0.04   0.88  -0.12  0.81  0.186  1.1
IL10         0.52  0.55  -0.26   0.14  0.66  0.337  2.6
IL13         0.15  0.64   0.08  -0.52  0.71  0.292  2.1
IL17         0.40  0.57   0.12   0.62  0.89  0.115  2.8
IL18         0.04  0.18   0.86   0.34  0.89  0.107  1.4
EPO          0.15  0.04   0.93   0.08  0.90  0.100  1.1
GRO          0.07  0.87  -0.06  -0.08  0.78  0.224  1.0
IFNg         0.65  0.20  -0.02   0.67  0.91  0.089  2.2
MIP3         0.20  0.18  -0.22  -0.84  0.82  0.176  1.4
RANTES       0.80 -0.19   0.07   0.16  0.71  0.288  1.2
TNFa         0.76  0.32   0.15   0.07  0.71  0.292  1.4
VEGF        -0.02  0.85   0.21   0.12  0.79  0.214  1.2
```

For example, one distinct group of cytokines with IL-7, IL-18, and EPO loaded on the same factor because the absolute loading values are relatively large compared to the other cytokines. A cutoff value of 0.6 was used in the study because this value can separate cytokines to load on just one factor in most cases. Thus, a cytokine with an absolute loading value larger than 0.6 was considered to load on one of the four factors. For example, the cytokines IL-17, MIP3, IL-2, and IFN-γ all load on the same factor (RC3) although IFN-γ also loads on the first factor.

14.2 Paper 2

We will now have a look at the paper published by Lin et al. (2017). In this study, they measured several clinical variables on 86 patients with severe sepsis or septic shock. Sepsis is a life-threatening condition that arises when the body responds to an infection that causes widespread inflammation. For example, a pathogen that enters the bloodstream may trigger a too strong immune reaction. Common symptoms include fever, rapid heart rate, confusion, and difficulty in breathing. The SOFA score (Sequential Organ Failure Assessment) is usually used to measure the severity of sepsis by evaluating a number of critical organ systems. In addition to the SOFA score, inflammatory biomarkers in blood such as CRP and IL-6 are also used in the assessment. Out of the 86 patients who were enrolled, 33 patients were diagnosed with severe sepsis and 53 with septic shock where septic shock is the most severe type of sepsis. Blood samples were collected from the patients at days 1, 3, and 5 from entering the intensive care unit (ICU). The blood plasma concentrations of Kallistatin, Kallikrein, TNF-α, IL-1β, IL-6, and IL-8 were then measured. Patients were followed for 60 days after they had entered the ICU in order to record the survival time. One aim of the study was to investigate if plasma Kallistatin could predict the survival of patients with severe sepsis or septic shock. In addition, they also analyzed how the Kallistatin level correlated with the other biomarkers that were measured in the blood samples.

Note that they have used SPSS and GraphPad Prism for the analysis in this paper. Thus, there might therefore be some differences in the output and plots of the paper since we here use R.

To download the dataset used in this paper, use the link below or search for the paper:

https://doi.org/10.1371/journal.pone.0178387

Once you have found the paper at PLOS One, navigate to the supporting information and download the Excel file under **S1 Data: The dataset of all enrolled patients**. If you open this Excel file, the first rows and columns should look similar to (Table 14.1).

Note that missing data in the file has been coded as "#NULL!".

I will now show two different ways you can import this dataset into R.

If you use RStudio, you can import this dataset by selecting the tab "Environment" and then click:

Import Dataset → from Excel…

A window with the title "Import Excel Data" should now pop up. In this window, click "Browse…" and navigate to where you have saved the Excel file.

Fill in #NULL! in the box "NA:" so that R knows how missing values have been coded. Then click "Import". When you click import, RStudio will read in the data

Table 14.1 First rows and columns of data from paper 2

Case no	Age	Sex	Appropriate antibiotics	Days (ICU)	Days (hospital)
1	90	2	1	67	67
2	85	2	0	22	65
3	73	1	1	12	13
4	55	1	1	6	9
5	89	1	1	2	9
6	61	1	1	4	46
7	82	2	0	32	37
8	84	1	0	8	23
9	72	2	1	2	16
10	55	1	1	5	36
11	66	1	1	9	9

and run the function "View", which then shows the data viewer window that can be used to view the imported data. Close this tab and view the code in the Console:

```
library(readxl)
pone_0178387_s001 <- read_excel("C:/data/pone.0178387.
s001.xlsx")
View(pone_0178387_s001)
```

We can see that when we click import, RStudio runs the above code. The dataset will be stored as a tibble with the same name as the data file (pone_0178387_s001). The second option to read in the file is to instead use a similar code as the one above. Note that you need to change the path "C:/data/" to the folder where you have saved the Excel file:

```
library(readxl)
pone_0178387_s001 <- read_excel(
"C:/data/pone.0178387.s001.xlsx", na = "#NULL!")
```

Our tibble (similar to a data frame) has currently the name "pone_0178387_s001". To use a shorter name, we can run the following code where we create a new tibble with the name "df":

```
df=pone_0178387_s001
```

Our tibble "df" should have 86 rows (86 patients) and 46 columns (46 variables).

```
dim(df)
86 46
```

If you print df, note that some of the columns have spaces and parentheses in their names. To, for example, extract the first column we can run:

```
df$`Case No`
```

However, to use simpler column names without spaces and backticks, we can use the function "make.names", which replaces, for example, spaces with dots.

```
colnames(df) = make.names(colnames(df))
```

If you now print the tibble, note that the column names have changed a bit and that we now can extract the first column by:

```
df$Case.No
```

If you run:

```
str(df)
```

you will see that all variables are defined as numeric variables. We therefore first need to convert some of the variables into factors so that R interprets these variables as categorical variables:

```
df$Sex=factor(df$Sex) # 1 = men, 2 = women
df$Appropriate.antibiotics=factor(df$Appropriate.antibiotics)
# 0 = survival, 1 = death
df$Hospital.death=factor(df$Hospital.death)
# 0 = survival, 1 = death
df$X60.day.death=factor(df$X60.day.death)
df$DM=factor(df$DM)
df$Lung.Dz=factor(df$Lung.Dz)
df$Cardiac.Dz=factor(df$Cardiac.Dz)
df$Liver.Dz=factor(df$Liver.Dz)
df$Kidney.Dz=factor(df$Kidney.Dz)
df$Malignancy=factor(df$Malignancy)
df$Pneumonia.Extrapulmonary=factor(
df$Pneumonia.Extrapulmonary)
# 0 = negative, 1 = positive
df$Blood.Culture=factor(df$Blood.Culture)
df$Mechanical.ventilation=factor(df$Mechanical.ventilation)
# 0 = severe sepsis, 1 = Septic chock
df$Shock=factor(df$Shock)
df$ARDS=factor(df$ARDS)
```

14.2.1 Table 1: Demographic Data and Clinical Variables

We are now ready to reproduce some of the results in the paper. In table 1, they report survivors (n = 57) and non-survivors (n = 29), which can be found in the column "Hospital.death":

```
table(df$Hospital.death)
 0    1
 57   29
```

Survivors are coded as zeros, and non-survivors as ones. Thus, 57 patients survived during the 60 days the patients were followed.

To reproduce the statistics on the first row of table 1 in paper 2, which is the mean age of the survivors and non-survivors, we can, for example, use the following code:

```
tapply(df$Age,df$Hospital.death,mean) # Compute mean
   0           1
69.57895    74.37931
# Compute standard deviation
tapply(df$Age,df$Hospital.death,sd)
   0           1
16.405517   9.567108
t.test(df$Age~df$Hospital.death,var.equal=FALSE)

          Welch Two Sample t-test


data:  df$Age by df$Hospital.death
t = -1.7103, df = 82.322, p-value = 0.09098
….
```

Based on the results from the t-test, we can draw the conclusion that there is no significant difference in age between survivors and non-survivors because the p-value is larger than the significance level 0.05.

Continuous variables were compared with a t-test, if they were considered to have a normal distribution according to the Shapiro-Wilk test or the corresponding non-parametric Mann-Whitney U test. For example, to check if the variable Age is normally distributed in the two groups, we can run the Shapiro-Wilks test in R by:

```
# Shapiro-Wilk test on the survivors
shapiro.test(df$Age[df$Hospital.death == 0])
  Shapiro-Wilk normality test
data:  df$Age[df$Hospital.death == 0]
W = 0.96357, p-value = 0.08374
# Shapiro-Wilk test on the non-survivors
shapiro.test(df$Age[df$Hospital.death == 1])
  Shapiro-Wilk normality test
data:  df$Age[df$Hospital.death == 1]
W = 0.97357, p-value = 0.6598
```

Since both *p*-values from these tests are greater than the significance level of 0.05, the variable age of the two groups can be assumed to be normally distributed. To know if we should run the Welch two-sample t-test (var.equal = FALSE) or the classical t-test, which assumes equal variance (var.equal = FALSE), one can run the Levene's test:

```
library(car)
leveneTest(df$Age ~ df$Hospital.death)
Levene's Test for Homogeneity of Variance (center = median)
        Df    F value   Pr(>F)
group   1     5.9743    0.01661 *
        84
```

Since the *p*-value from this test is less than the significance level, we reject the null hypothesis that the two groups have equal variance, which explains why the Welch two-sample t-test (var.equal = FALSE) was performed on the variable Age in this study.

For variables on a numeric scale that were not considered as normally distributed according to the Shapiro-Wilk test, or variables on an ordinal scale, they report the median and the interquartile range (quartile 1 and quartile 3) and a *p*-value from the Mann-Whitney U test. For example, the statistics based on the qSOFA score can be calculated by:

```
# Compute median
tapply(df$qSOFA,df$Hospital.death,median,na.rm=TRUE)
0   1
2   3
# Compute IQR
tapply(df$qSOFA,df$Hospital.death,quantile,na.rm=TRUE)
$`0`
  0%  25%  50%  75% 100%
  1   2    2    3    3

$`1`
```

```
  0%   25%   50%   75% 100%
  2     2     3     3    3
# Compute the Mann-Whitney U test
wilcox.test(df$qSOFA~df$Hospital.death)
Wilcoxon rank sum test with continuity correction
data:  df$qSOFA by df$Hospital.death
W = 583, p-value = 0.01305
```

From these results, we can conclude that survivors had a significantly lower qSOFA score compared to the non-survivors.

For variables on a nominal scale, frequency and proportions were reported. The corresponding *p*-values were computed by a chi-squared test or a Fisher's exact test if the assumptions of a chi-squared test were not fulfilled. For example, the statistics for the variable sex can be calculated by:

```
# 1 = men, 2 = women,  0 = survival, 1 = non-survival
tab=table(df$Sex,df$Hospital.death)
tab
       0    1
  1   40   17
  2   17   12
# Calculate proportions based on the columns
round(prop.table(tab,2),2)
      0       1
  1 0.70   0.59
  2 0.30   0.41
chisq.test(tab)
   Pearson's Chi-squared test with Yates' continuity
   correction
data:  tab
X-squared = 0.68941, df = 1, p-value = 0.4064
```

Since the *p*-value from the chi-squared test is larger than the significance level of 0.05, they concluded that there was no significant difference in survival between men and women.

14.2.2 Table 3: Comparisons of Plasma Biomarkers Between Survivors and Non-survivors

In Table 3, they analyzed if there was a significant difference in the concentrations of the plasma biomarkers between survivors and non-survivors. For example, let's reproduce the statistics of day 1 Kallistatin:

```
tapply(df$Kallistatin.D1., df$Hospital.death,median ,
na.rm=TRUE) # Median
  0     1
3.68   2.76
tapply(df$Kallistatin.D1., df$Hospital.death,quantile ,
na.rm=TRUE) # IQR
# Mann-Whitney U test
wilcox.test(df$Kallistatin.D1.~ df$Hospital.death)
    Wilcoxon rank sum test with continuity correction
data:  df$Kallistatin.D1. by df$Hospital.death
W = 1062, p-value = 0.03182
```

We can see that the Kallistatin level at day 1 is significantly higher in patients who survived (coded as zero) compared to the non-survivors (coded as ones). The median blood concentration of the survivors was 3.68 μg/mL, whereas the median concentration of the non-survivors was 2.76 μg/mL.

14.2.3 Figure 2A: Kallistatin Levels at Day 1, 3, and 5 in Patients with Severe Sepsis and Septic Shock

Kallistatin was measured in blood samples of patients taken on the day they entered the ICU (day 1) and on days 3 and 5. To see if there was a difference in the Kallistatin concentration between patients with severe sepsis and patients with septic shock, they created a boxplot and computed the *p*-values with the Mann-Whitney U test.

Mann-Whitney U tests:

```
wilcox.test(df$Kallistatin.D1.~df$Shock)
wilcox.test(df$Kallistatin.D3.~df$Shock)
wilcox.test(df$Kallistatin.D5.~df$Shock)
```

To reproduce the boxplot in figure 2A in paper 2, we can first extract the variables that we want to plot:

```
library(dplyr)
df_subset <- df %>%
  select(Kallistatin.D1.,Kallistatin.D3., Kallistatin.D5.,
  Shock)
```

Note, if you have previously loaded the package **MASS**, that package also uses a function called "select". Thus, if you get an error when you run the "select" function, it might be due to that you are using the "select" function from the package MASS and not from the **dplyr** package. To prevent this issue, you can either unload the package MASS or instead use "dplyr::select" in the code above.

Then we create a long format where we put all numeric variables (Kallistatin day 1, 3, and 5) in one column that we name "value":

```
library(tidyr)
df_long <- df_subset %>%
  pivot_longer(
  cols = 1:3,                    # Columns to stack
  # Name of the column with labels: Kallistatin day 1, 3 and 5
  names_to = "variable",
  # Name of the column with all the values
  values_to = "value"
)
```

Next, we compute the log2 of the Kallistatin values and save these in a new column with the name "log2value".

```
df_long$log2value=log2(df_long$value)
```

Finally, we make a boxplot of the log2 values that will give us a similar plot as in the paper.

```
library(ggplot2)
ggplot(df_long, aes(x = variable, y = log2value, fill =
Shock)) +
  # Dodge to separate the boxes
  geom_boxplot(position = position_dodge(width = 0.8)) +
  labs(y = "Kallistatin (log2 µg/ml)", x = "", fill =
  "Sepsis") + # Manual labels
  # Manual labels on the x-axis
  scale_x_discrete(labels = c("Day 1", "Day 3","Day 5")) +
  scale_fill_manual(
    # Custom colors
    values = c("0" = "skyblue", "1" = "orange"),
    # Custom legend text
    labels = c("Severe sepsis", "Septic shock")
  ) +
  ylim(-1, 9) + # Change the height of the y-axis
  annotate("text",x = 1, y = 7, label = "p=0.004",
  size = 4) + # Add p-value at coordinate (1,7)
  annotate("text",x = 2, y = 9, label = "p=0.010",
  size = 4) + # Add p-value in the plot
  annotate("text",x = 3, y = 7.5, label = "p=0.555",
  size = 4) + # Add p-value in the plot
  theme_minimal() # Use white background
```

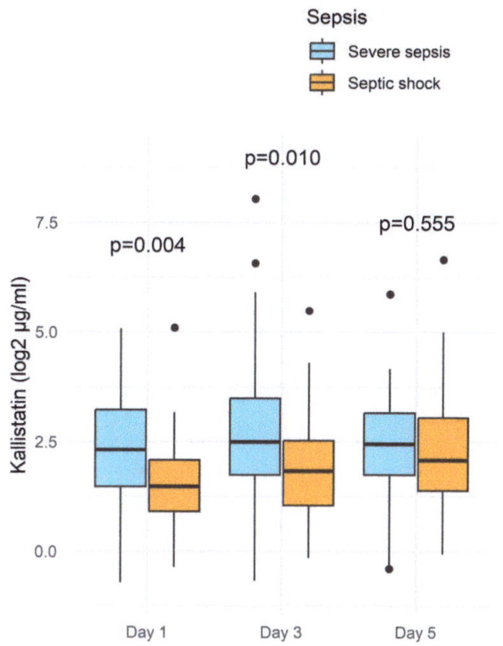

Fig. 14.5 A boxplot of the log2 values of Kallistation at day 1, 3, and 5 from blood samples of patients with severe sepsis and septic shock. This figure corresponds to figure 2A in paper 2

Note that the outliers (Fig. 14.5) do not correspond to the ones in the paper, which is likely due to that they have used another statistical software tool. There are several different ways to calculate quartiles and define outliers and different software tools may use different methods. From this plot, it seems like the ones with septic shock have lower levels of Kallistatin at the given time points.

14.2.4 Relationship between Kallistatin and Other Biomarkers at Day 1

To investigate the relationship between Kallistatin and other biomarkers, they used the Spearman correlation method. For example, the Spearman's rank correlation coefficient between Kallistatin and IL-6 on day 1 can be calculated by:

```
cor.test(df$Kallistatin.D1.,df$IL.6.D1.,method="spearman")
    Spearman's rank correlation rho
data:  df$Kallistatin.D1. and df$IL.6.D1.
S = 139919, p-value = 0.002664
alternative hypothesis: true rho is not equal to 0
sample estimates:
       rho
-0.3200529
```

We see that the Spearman's rank correlation coefficient is −0.32, which is significant because the corresponding p-value is 0.0027. If you compute the correlation between Kallistatin and the other plasma biomarkers, you will see that Kallistatin is negatively correlated to all other biomarkers. Note that different software tools may handle ties with different methods, which might explain differences in R compared to the values in the paper.

In summary, a high level of Kallistatin seems to be associated with the severity of sepsis. Patients with more severe sepsis (septic shock) have lower levels of Kallistatin. A higher level of Kallistatin is found in the survivors compared to the non-survivors. Also, Kallistatin is negatively correlated with other biomarkers that are often high in patients with more severe sepsis. Thus, in comparison with the other biomarkers, a high level is a good sign when it comes to Kallistatin.

14.2.5 Figure 3A: ROC Curve of Kallistatin at Day 1 of 60-Day Mortality

To find the best cutoff value of Kallistatin on day 1 that could separate the patients that survived 60 days and the ones that did not survive longer than 60 days, they created an ROC curve and used the Youden Index. Let's compute an ROC curve and save metrics like the AUC, best cutoff value, and sensitivity and specificity:

```
library(pROC)
roc1=roc(df$X60.day.death, df$Kallistatin.D1.,smooth=FALSE)
AUC=roc1$auc # Extract AUC
# Compute the p-value
pval=wilcox.test(df$Kallistatin.D1.~df$X60.day.death)$p.val
# Find best cutoff
cord=coords(roc1,"best", best.method="youden")
```

Then we make a plot similar to fig 3A in the paper:

```
plot(roc1)
text(0.85,0.95,paste("AUC=",round(AUC,2)))
text(0.80,0.85,paste("p-value=",round(pval,3)))
text(0.35,0.25,paste("Cutoff value=",round(cord$threshold,2),
"µg/ml"))
text(0.35,0.15,paste("Sensitivity=",
round(cord$sensitivity,2)))
text(0.35,0.05,paste("Specificity=",round(cord$specificity,2)))
```

From the ROC curve (Fig. 14.6), we can conclude that the best cutoff value to use for Kallistatin to predict 60 days survival, according to the Youden Index, is a

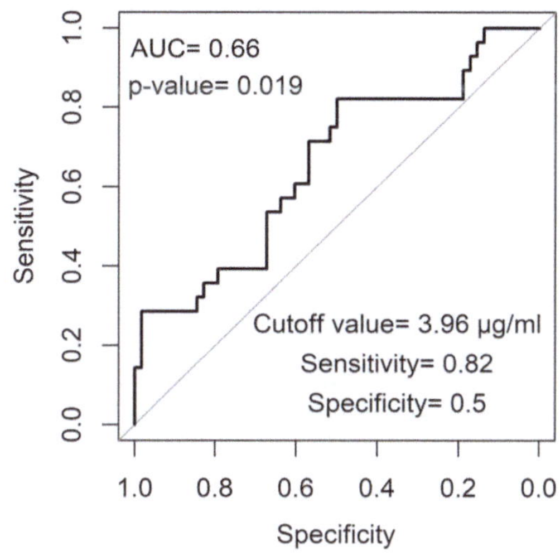

Fig. 14.6 An ROC curve that illustrates the performance of Kallistation at day 1 to discriminate between survivors and non-survivors. The figure corresponds to figure 3A in paper 2

value of 3.96 µg/mL or rounded to 4.0 as in the paper. By using this cutoff value, the sensitivity is 82%, whereas the specificity is 50%. Using Kallistatin as a biomarker for survival results in an AUC value of 0.66, which is significantly larger than 0.5 (*p*-value = 0.019).

14.3 Table 4: Combine Biomarkers with Logistic Regression

To evaluate if Kallistatin could be combined with other biomarkers to increase the accuracy, they used logistic regression as an ML model. We will here have a look at a model that combines Kallistatin with IL-8. One could simply set up a logistic regression model with the two biomarkers like this:

```
fit = glm(X60.day.death~Kallistatin.D1.+ IL.8.D1.,
data = df,family=binomial)
```

However, in this study, they converted the numeric variables into binary variables based on the best cutoff values from the ROC curves: 4.0 for the Kallistatin and 42.3 for IL-8. We can categorize the numerical variables and save them in a data frame like this:

```
Kallistatin=factor(ifelse(df$Kallistatin.D1.<4.0,"low",
"high"))
IL8=factor(ifelse(df$IL.8.D1.<42.3,"low","high"))
Death=factor(ifelse(df$X60.day.death==0,"Survival",
"Nonsurvival"))
data=data.frame(Kallistatin,IL8,Death)
```

Then we can use logistic regression on these new categorical variables, which will result in an AUC of about 0.78 which corresponds to the value in the paper.

```
fit = glm(Death~Kallistatin+IL8, data = data,family=binomial)
pred.prob=predict(fit,type="response")
ROC=roc(Death, pred.prob)
plot(ROC)
ROC$auc
Area under the curve: 0.7774
```

Thus, by combining Kallistatin with IL-8, using optimal cutoff values, the AUC increases from 0.66 to 0.78. However, the authors did not perform any validation of the models to prevent possible overfitting.

14.3.1 Figure 3B: Kaplan–Meier Analysis

In figure 3B, they have created a Kaplan–Meier curve that shows the survival of patients that had a Kallistatin level that was higher or lower than a cutoff value of 4.0 μg/mL, as they previously determined based on the ROC curve. By using a Kaplan–Meier curve, one can show the proportion of patients that have survived up to a certain time point. To compare the survival rate between two or more groups, one can use a log-rank test. If you like to learn about Kaplan–Meier analysis, have a look at these two videos.

14.3.2 Video

https://youtu.be/irhFmq5Rz04
https://youtu.be/rAVGd8hgNv8
www.tilestats.com/ml/

To create the Kaplan–Meier curve and to compute a log-rank test, we will here use the package **survival**:

```
library(survival)
```

We first separate the patients into two groups, where the ones with a Kallistatin level lower than 4.0 are coded as zeros, whereas the ones with a Kallistatin level greater than 4.0 are coded as ones. The survival times of the patients can be found in the column "Days.60.day.death". Since the patients were followed for 60 days, day 60 is the endpoint of the study. Patients that survived longer than 60 days are therefore defined as censored observations. The column "X60.day.death" defines the censored observations (coded as 0) and events/deaths (coded as 1) during the 60 days. However, using this column does not generate the same Kaplan–Meier curve and *p*-value as shown in the paper. Instead, they seem to have used the column "Hospital.death". The only difference between these two columns is the data recorded for the first person. Anyway, to be consistent with the results in the paper, we will here use the column "Hospital.death". Note that we previously defined "Hospital.death" as a factor and that we here need to convert it back to a numeric scale:

```
# Kallistatin groups
Group=factor(ifelse(df$Kallistatin.D1.<4,0,1))
ST=df$Days.60.day.death. # Survival times
# 0= Censor, 1 = Event
State=as.numeric(as.character(df$Hospital.death))
df_surv=data.frame(Group,State,ST)
```

We can now create a survival object with the function "Surv":

```
survobj=Surv(ST,State)
```

By using this object in the "survfit" function, we can plot the survival curve:

```
fit=survfit(survobj~Group, data=df_surv,conf.type="plain")
summary(fit)
plot(fit,ylab="Percent survival (%)",xlab="Days",las=1,
col=c("gray","black"),lwd=2)
legend("bottomleft",c("Kallistatin<4.0 µg/ml",
"Kallistatin>4.0 µg/ml"), col=c("gray","black"),
lty=1, lwd=2)
```

Next, we compute the log-rank test with the function "survdiff" and used the chi-squared test statistic from this function to compute the *p*-value with three decimal places:

```
m=survdiff(survobj ~ Group, data=df_surv) # Log-rank test
p_value = 1 - pchisq(m$chisq, df = 1)
text(50,0.4,paste("p-value = ",round(p_value,3)),cex=0.8)
```

Our final figure should look like the one shown in Fig. 14.7.

From this plot (Fig. 14.7), we can see that the patients with a Kallistatin level greater than 4.0 have a significantly longer survival time compared to the ones with a level lower than 4.0.

We can create a bit nicer plot (Fig. 14.8) if we use the **survminer** package that can be used to draw survival curves based on the **ggplot2** package:

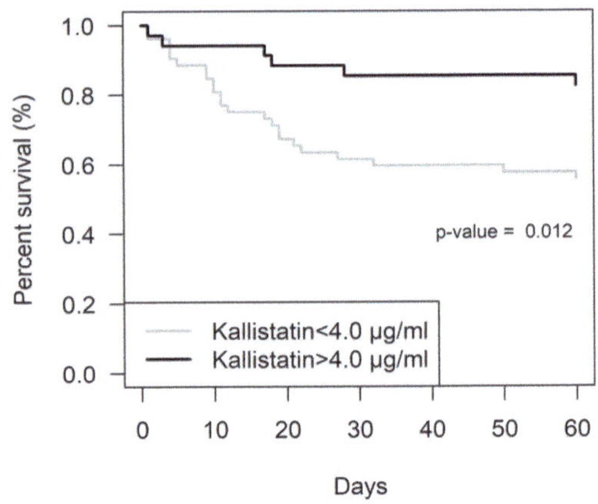

Fig. 14.7 A Kaplan–Meier curve that illustrates the survival of the patients with a high or low level of Kallistatin at day 1. The figure corresponds to figure 3B in paper 2

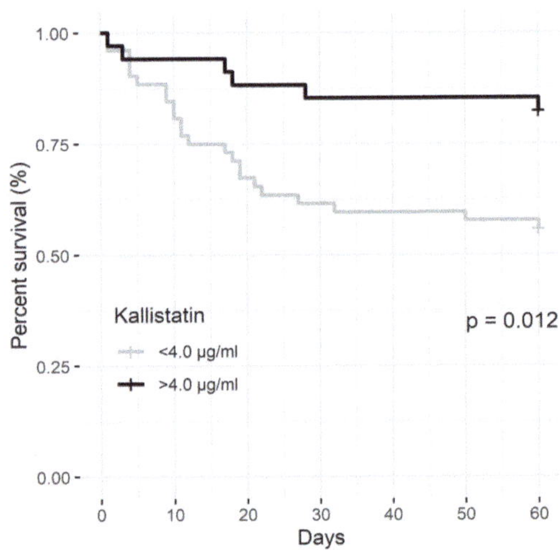

Fig. 14.8 A Kaplan–Meier curve, generated with the **survminor** package, which illustrates the survival of the patients with a high or low level of Kallistatin at day 1. The figure corresponds to figure 3B in paper 2

```
library(survminer)
ggsurvplot(
  fit,
  conf.int = FALSE, # Disable confidence intervals
  pval = TRUE,  # Add p-value to the plot
  pval.coord = c(50, 0.35),  # Coordinate of the p-value
  pval.size = 4,  # Text size of the p-value
  legend.title = "Kallistatin",  # Legend title
  # Legend labels
  legend.labs = c("<4.0 μg/ml", ">4.0 μg/ml"),
  palette = c("gray", "black"),  # Line colors
  xlab = "Days",  # X-axis label
  ylab = "Percent survival (%)",  # Y-axis label
  ggtheme = theme_minimal(),  # Minimal theme
  legend = c(0.2, 0.3)   # Position of legend
)
```

14.3.3 *Figure 3C: Difference in SOFA Score between Individuals with Low and High Kallistatin Levels*

In figure 3C, they plot the mean SOFA score determined on days 1, 3, and 5 separately for the patients with a Kallistatin level greater than 4.0 μg/mL and for the patients with a Kallistatin level lower than this cutoff value. The error bars were based on ± one standard deviation. To create such a plot, we can first extract the relevant variables: the SOFA scores at day 1, 3, and 5 and the patient number:

```
library(dplyr)
df_subset <- df %>%
  select(SOFA.D1.,SOFA.D3.,SOFA.D5.,Case.No)
```

Then, we create a categorical variable that tells if the patient has a Kallistatin level lower or higher than 4.0 μg/mL at day 1 and add this to the data frame:

```
df_subset$Kallistatin.group=
factor(ifelse(df$Kallistatin.D1.<4,0,1))
```

Next, we create a long format where we put all SOFA scores (day 1, 3, and 5) in one column that we name "value":

```
library(tidyr)
df_long <- df_subset %>%
  pivot_longer(
  cols = 1:3,                    # Columns to stack
  # Name of the column with labels: SOFA day 1, 3 and 5
  names_to = "variable",
  # Name of the column with all the SOFA scores
  values_to = "value"
)
```

Finally, we add the time points (day 1, 3, and 5) for which the SOFA score was measured of the 86 patients:

```
df_long$time=rep(c(1,3,5),86)
```

We can now calculate the mean and standard deviation of the two groups for the three time points by using, for example, the "summarySE" function in the **Rmisc** package:

```
library(Rmisc)
stats = summarySE(df_long, measurevar="value",
groupvars=c("Kallistatin.group","time"), na.rm = TRUE)
```

Then we add a column to this data frame that holds appropriate labels for the plot:

```
stats$group=ifelse(stats$Kallistatin.group==0,
"Kalli <4.0","Kalli>4.0")
```

We will now make a plot of the means and the standard deviations. To avoid that the means and error bars overlap in the plot for the two groups, we use dodging:

```
library(ggplot2)
# Dodge to prevent plotting on the same x-coordinate
dodge=0.7
ggplot(stats, aes(x=factor(time), y=value, color = group,
group=group)) +
  geom_point(position = position_dodge(width = dodge),
  size = 3) +
  geom_errorbar(aes(ymin=value-sd, ymax=value+sd), width=.2,
  position =   position_dodge(width =   dodge)) +
  geom_line(position = position_dodge(width = dodge))   +
  # Custom x-axis labels
  scale_x_discrete(breaks = c(1, 3, 5), labels = c("Day 1",
  "Day 3", "Day 5")) +
  theme_bw() + # White background with a box
  labs(y = "SOFA score", x = "")
```

We see that the mean SOFA score is lower over the 3 days for the ones with a high Kallistatin level (Fig. 14.9).

14.3.4 Linear Mixed-Effects Model

A linear mixed-effects model is a type of regression model that includes both fixed effects and random effects. These types of regression models are commonly used in situations where observations are not independent. Since the SOFA scores of the same patients are measured at three time points, the observations in Fig. 14.9 are not independent. To learn more about linear mixed-effects models, have a look at the following two videos:

https://youtu.be/IY3NF33W6RA
https://youtu.be/X0cXH_iECoc
www.tilestats.com/ml/

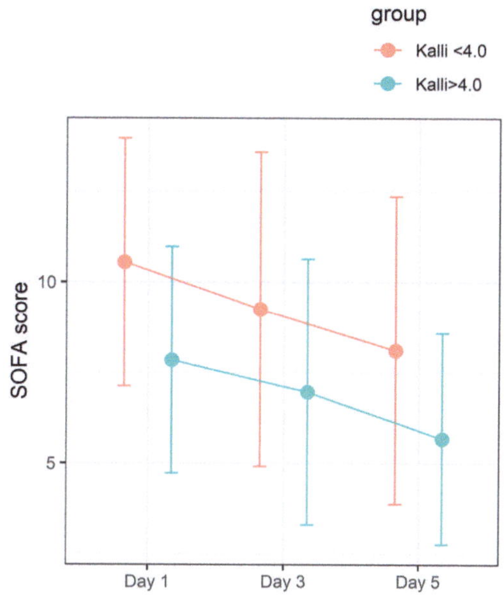

Fig. 14.9 A line chart that illustrates the SOFA scores on day 1, 3, and 5 for two groups: patients with Kallistatin levels <4.0 (red) and those with Kallistatin levels >4.0 (blue). Mean SOFA scores are shown with error bars representing ± one standard deviation

To compute a linear mixed-effects model, we will here use the "lme" function in the **nlme** package. However, you may also use the "lmer" function in the **lmerTest** package. To predict the SOFA score with a random intercept model, we will here use the variables time (day 1, 3, and 5) and the Kallistatin group as the fixed effects in the model and the patients (subjects) as the random effect. The "~1" in the code below defines that we like to use a random intercept model, which I assume is the model they have used in the study:

```
library(nlme)
fit = lme(value ~ time + Kallistatin.group,
random =~ 1 | Case.No,data = df_long,na.action =  na.omit)
summary(fit)
Fixed effects: Sofa ~ time + Kallistatin.group
                        Value     Std.Error  DF    t-value    p-value
(Intercept)          11.076223 0.5259523  163   21.059366   0.0000
time                 -0.566689 0.0801566  163   -7.069769   0.0000
Kallistatin.group1 -2.539388  0.7490100   84   -3.390326   0.0011
```

From this output, we can see that the ones with a Kallistatin level greater than 4.0 µg/mL have an overall intercept that is 2.53 lower than the ones with a Kallistatin level lower than 4.0 µg/mL who have an intercept of 11.07. The corresponding p-value for the difference in the intercepts is equal to 0.0011. Based on this result, the authors concluded that a higher level of Kallistatin is associated with a lower SOFA score over the first 5 days at the ICU.

14.3.5 S2 Table: Cox Univariate and Multivariable Analysis

In the supporting information, one can find the S2 table where they have performed Cox regression modeling. The Cox proportional hazards model can be used as a regression technique in survival analysis, which, in comparison to the Kaplan–Meier analysis, can adjust for possible cofounders. To learn about the Cox proportional hazards model, have a look at the following video:

14.3.6 Video

https://youtu.be/JfZr9kmntTM
www.tilestats.com/ml/

In Table S2, they have performed both univariate and multivariable analyses for the 60-day survival of the patients. The code below is very similar to the code we used for the Kaplan–Meier analysis but where we here use the "coxph" function to perform Cox regression. Also, to define censoring observations and events, we here use the column "X60.day.death" instead of the column "Hospital.death" because that generates the same results as in the paper. The example below shows how to compute the hazard ratio (HR) and its 95% confidence interval of the variable Sex:

```
library(survival)
ST=df$Days.60.day.death. # Survival times
# 0= Censor, 1 = Event
State=as.numeric(as.character(df$ X60.day.death))
# 1 = men, 2 = women
res.cox = coxph(Surv(ST, State) ~ df$Sex)
summary(res.cox)
...
           coef     exp(coef)     se(coef)      z          Pr(>|z|)
df$Sex2  0.2918     1.3389         0.3871    0.754         0.451

             exp(coef)   exp(-coef)    lower .95       upper .95
df$Sex2       1.339        0.7469        0.627           2.859
```

Note that the HR is shown for the women, whereas in the paper, they show the HR for the men. To be consistent with the paper, we should set the women (the twos) as the baseline by:

```
# Set the women (2) as the baseline
sex = factor(df$Sex, levels = c(2, 1))
```

Also, the function "coxph" uses, per default, the Efron approximation to deal with ties, whereas the statistical software SPSS uses the Breslow method. To be consistent with the paper, we will therefore use the Breslow method:

```
res.cox = coxph(Surv(ST, State) ~ sex, ties = "breslow")
summary(res.cox)
...
         coef      exp(coef)    se(coef)      z        Pr(>|z|)
sex1    -0.2929     0.7461       0.3871    -0.757     0.449

       exp(coef)     exp(-coef)      lower .95     upper .95
sex1    0.7461          1.34          0.3494         1.593
...
```

We see that we now get the exact same p-value (0.449) and HR (0.75) as well as the same 95% confidence interval (0.35–1.59) as in the S2 table. Since the 95% confidence interval includes the value one, men and women do not have a significantly different hazard.

To adjust for confounders in order to evaluate the HR for Kallistatin, they adjusted for the variables with a p-value less than 0.05 in the univariate analysis: age, sex, septic shock, ARDS, SOFA score, and APACHE II score.

```
Kallistatin=factor(ifelse(df$Kallistatin.D1.<4.0,"low",
"high"),levels=c("low","high"))
res.cox = coxph(Surv(ST, State) ~ df$Shock+df$ARDS+
Kallistatin+df$IL.1β.D1.+
df$IL.6.D1.+df$IL.8.D1.+df$CRP+df$SOFA.D1.+df$APACHE.II,
ties = "breslow")
summary(res.cox)
...
n= 86, number of events= 28

                       coef     exp(coef)    se(coef)       z      Pr(>|z|)
df$Shock1        -3.496e-02   9.656e-01   5.588e-01  -0.063   0.9501
df$ARDS1         -1.156e-01   8.908e-01   5.226e-01  -0.221   0.8250
Kallistatinhigh  -3.310e-01   7.182e-01   5.648e-01  -0.586   0.5579
df$IL.1ß.D1       1.016e-01   1.107e+00   5.344e-02   1.901   0.0573.
df$IL.6.D1.       1.253e-05   1.000e+00   2.320e-05   0.540   0.5890
df$IL.8.D1.      -3.510e-05   1.000e+00   3.057e-05  -1.148   0.2509
df$CRP            4.171e-03   1.004e+00   2.143e-03   1.946   0.0516.
df$SOFA.D1.       2.180e-01   1.244e+00   9.623e-02   2.266   0.0235*
df$APACHE.II      3.586e-02   1.037e+00   4.615e-02   0.777   0.4372
---
```

```
Signif. codes:  0 '***' 0.001 '**' 0.01 '*' 0.05 '.' 0.1 ' ' 1

                exp(coef)  exp(-coef)  lower .95  upper .95
df$Shock1          0.9656      1.0356     0.3230      2.887
df$ARDS1           0.8908      1.1225     0.3199      2.481
Kallistatinhigh    0.7182      1.3923     0.2374      2.173
df$IL.1ß.D1.       1.1069      0.9034     0.9968      1.229
df$IL.6.D1.        1.0000      1.0000     1.0000      1.000
df$IL.8.D1.        1.0000      1.0000     0.9999      1.000
df$CRP             1.0042      0.9958     1.0000      1.008
df$SOFA.D1.        1.2436      0.8041     1.0298      1.502
df$APACHE.II       1.0365      0.9648     0.9469      1.135

   Concordance= 0.783  (se = 0.047 )
   Likelihood ratio test= 35.55  on 9 df,   p=5e-05
   Wald test            = 30.47  on 9 df,   p=4e-04
   Score (logrank) test = 45.78  on 9 df,   p=7e-07
```

In this multivariable analysis, Kallistatin is no longer significant because its 95% confidence interval of the HR includes the value one and the *p*-value is larger than 0.05.

14.3.7 S3 Table: Univariate and Multivariable Logistic Regression

In the supplementary table (S3), they performed logistic regression to test if there was an association between, for example, patients with severe sepsis or septic shock and some of the variables that were measured in this study. Let's, for example, reproduce the odds ratio (OR) and *p*-value of CRP as the independent variable and septic shock as the dependent variable:

```
fit = glm(df$Shock~df$CRP,family=binomial)
summary(fit)
....
Coefficients:
               Estimate   Std. Error   z value    Pr(>|z|)
(Intercept)   -0.279668   0.378229     -0.739     0.4597
df$CRP         0.006074   0.002597      2.339     0.0194*
```

We see that we get the exact same *p*-value as in the paper. To reproduce the OR and its 95% confidence interval, we can run:

```
exp(cbind(coef(fit),confint.default(fit)))
                              2.5 %      97.5 %
(Intercept)    0.7560345    0.3602405    1.586685
df$CRP         1.0060920    1.0009837    1.011226
```

The OR is 1.006 (rounded to 1.01 in the paper) and the 95% confidence interval of the OR is 1.00–1.01. Thus, CRP is significantly associated with the degree of sepsis since the confidence interval does not include the value one.

They also created a multivariable logistic regression with Kallistatin and variables that were significant (i.e., $p < 0.05$) in the univariate analysis. For example, using the septic shock variable as the dependent variable in a model with Kallistatin and CRP as the independent variables they applied backward elimination of this model, which resulted in that only Kallistatin was included in the final model:

```
Kallistatin=factor(ifelse(df$Kallistatin.D1.<4.0,"low",
"high"),levels=c("low","high"))
fit = glm(df$Shock~Kallistatin+df$CRP,family=binomial)
fit.back=step(fit,method="backward") # Backward elimination
summary(fit.back)
Coefficients:
                 Estimate   Std. Error   z value    Pr(>|z|)
(Intercept)       0.9985      0.3126       3.194    0.00140 **
Kallistatinhigh  -1.2349      0.4659      -2.651    0.00803 **
exp(cbind(coef(fit.back),confint.default(fit.back)))
                                2.5 %        97.5 %
(Intercept)      2.7142857    1.4707380    5.0092857
Kallistatinhigh  0.2908587    0.1167148    0.7248336
```

The OR of the model including Kallistatin was 0.29 with a 95% confidence interval of 0.12–0.73.

References

Lin, W. C., Chen, C. W., Chao, L., Chao, J., & Lin, Y. S. (2017). Plasma Kallistatin in critically ill patients with severe sepsis and septic shock. *PLoS One, 12*(5), e0178387.

Wallner, F. K., Hopkins, M. H., Lindvall, T., Olofsson, P., & Tilevik, A. (2017). Cytokine correlation analysis based on drug perturbation. *Cytokine, 90*, 73–79.

Wallner, F. K., Hopkins, M. H., Woodworth, N., Bark, T. L., Olofsson, P., & Tilevik, A. (2018). Correlation and cluster analysis of immunomodulatory drugs based on cytokine profiles. *Pharmacological Research, 128*, 244–251.

Answers to the Exercises

Answers to the Exercises in Chapter 2

Exercises 2.2

1. Create the following matrix in R and print only its second column.

$$A = \begin{bmatrix} 4 & 1 \\ 1 & 5 \\ 0 & 9 \end{bmatrix}$$

```
A=matrix(c(4,1,0,1,5,9),3,2)
A[,2]
1  5  9
```

2. Create the following matrix in R. Once you have created this matrix, extract only the last two columns and the last row (the values 3 and 1) and save these in a vector with the name V.

$$A = \begin{bmatrix} 5 & 2 & 4 \\ 6 & 3 & 1 \end{bmatrix}$$

```
A=matrix(c(5,6,2,3,4,1),2,3)
V=A[2,2:3]
V
3  1
```

This also works:

```
V=A[2,-1] # Extract the second row and exclude the first column
V
3  1
```


A. Tilevik, *Multivariate Statistics and Machine Learning in R For Beginners*,
https://doi.org/10.1007/978-3-032-01851-9

3. Create a four-by-four identity matrix and print its transpose.

```
I=diag(4)
t(I)
```

4. Check if matrix A is a symmetric matrix.

$$A = \begin{bmatrix} 3 & 2 & 4 \\ 2 & 1 & 3 \\ 4 & 3 & 2 \end{bmatrix}$$

```
A=matrix(c(3,2,4,2,1,3,4,3,2),3,3)
A==t(A)
isSymmetric(A)
TRUE
```

5. Compute $A - B$.

$$A = \begin{bmatrix} 3 & 2 \\ 1 & 2 \end{bmatrix}$$

$$B = \begin{bmatrix} 4 & 3 \\ 2 & 2 \end{bmatrix}$$

```
A=matrix(c(3,1,2,2),2,2)
B=matrix(c(4,2,3,2),2,2)
A-B
      [,1]  [,2]
[1,]    -1    -1
[2,]    -1     0
```

6. Compute $A \times v$.

$$A = \begin{bmatrix} 3 & 2 & 4 \\ 2 & 1 & 3 \\ 4 & 3 & 2 \end{bmatrix}$$

$$v = \begin{bmatrix} 2 \\ 1 \\ 3 \end{bmatrix}$$

```
A=matrix(c(3,2,4,2,1,3,4,3,2),3,3)
v=matrix(c(2,1,3),3,1)
A%*%v
```

```
        [,1]
[1,]     20
[2,]     14
[3,]     17
```

7. Is it possible to compute $v \times A$? Explain why, or why not.

No, because the first matrix (v) does not have the same number of columns as the number of rows of the second matrix (A).

8. Multiply matrix A with an identity matrix of appropriate size.

$$A = \begin{bmatrix} 2 & 3 \\ 2 & 3 \\ 1 & 3 \end{bmatrix}$$

```
A=matrix(c(2,2,1,3,3,3),3,2)
I=diag(2)
A%*%I
        [,1]    [,2]
[1,]     2        3
[2,]     2        3
[3,]     1        3
# This also works
I=diag(3)
I%*%A
```

Exercises 2.4

1. Compute the inverse and the determinant of the following matrix.

$$A = \begin{bmatrix} 5 & 2 & 3 \\ 5 & 5 & 5 \\ 3 & 2 & 3 \end{bmatrix}$$

```
A=matrix(c(5,5,3,2,5,2,3,5,3),3,3)
det(A)
10
solve(A)
# The inverse will look a bit nicer if we round the numbers:
round(solve(A),1)
      [,1]  [,2]   [,3]
[1,]  0.5   0.0   -0.5
[2,]  0.0   0.6   -1.0
[3,] -0.5  -0.4    1.5
```

2. Explain why it is not possible to compute the inverse of the following matrix.

$$A = \begin{bmatrix} 4 & 2 \\ 8 & 4 \end{bmatrix}$$

```
A=matrix(c(4,8,2,4),2,2)
solve(A)
Error in solve.default(A):
  Lapack routine dgesv: system is exactly singular:
  U[2,2] = 0
```

It is not possible because the determinant is equal to zero:

```
det(A)
0
```

3. Solve the following system of equations.

$$\begin{aligned} 2x + 3y - 2z &= 10 \\ 3x - 2y + 2z &= 20 \\ 4x + 4y + 3z &= 30 \end{aligned}$$

```
A=matrix(c(2,3,4,3,-2,4,-2,2,3),3,3)
B= matrix(c(10,20,30),3,1)
solve(A,B)
          [,1]
[1,] 5.9154930
[2,] 0.4225352
[3,] 1.5492958
c=solve(A,B)
A%*%c # check if A*c is equal to B
      [,1]
[1,]    10
[2,]    20
[3,]    30
```

Exercises 2.6

1. Draw the following vector in a plot and compute its length.

$$v = \begin{bmatrix} 4 \\ 3 \end{bmatrix}$$

```
v=c(4,3)
origin=c(0,0)
plot(NULL,NULL,xlim=c(0,5),ylim=c(0,5),las=1,xlab="x",
ylab="y")
grid()
arrows(origin[1],origin[2],v[1],v[2],length = 0.15)
# Length
sqrt(sum(v^2))
5
```

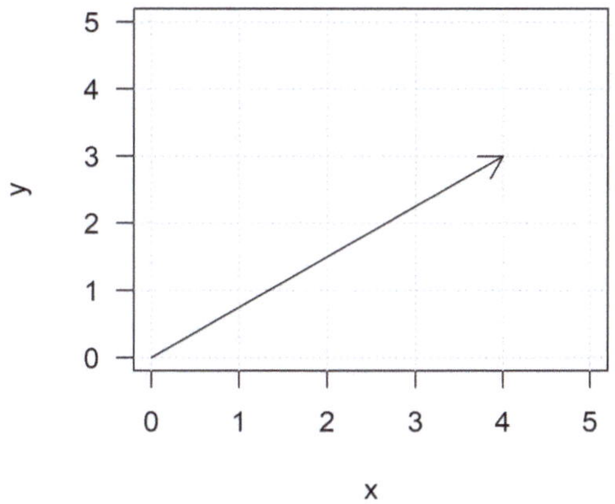

2. Check if the above vector is an eigenvector of the following matrix.

$$A = \begin{bmatrix} 1 & 2 \\ 1 & 0 \end{bmatrix}$$

Use a plot to illustrate if vector v is an eigenvector of matrix A.

```
v=c(4,3) # Vector to be drawn
origin=c(0,0)
plot(NULL,NULL,xlim=c(0,10),ylim=c(0,10),las=1,xlab="x",
ylab="y")
grid() # Add grid
arrows(origin[1],origin[2],v[1],v[2],length = 0.15)
A=matrix(c(1,1,2,0),2,2)
Av=A%*%v
arrows(origin[1],origin[2],Av[1],Av[2],length = 0.15,
col="red")
```

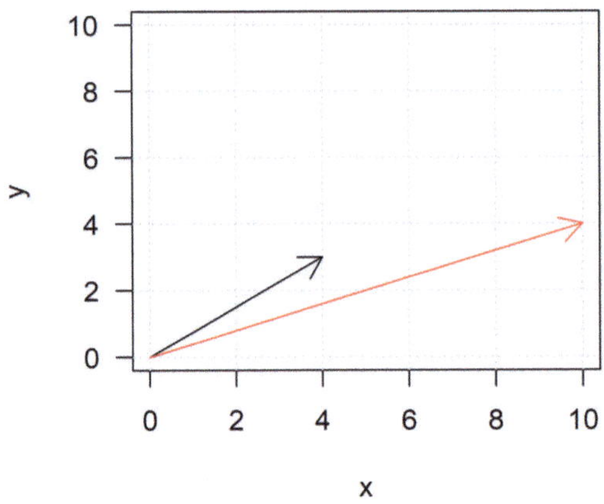

Since the two arrows have different directions, vector v is not an eigenvector of matrix A.

3. Use the function "eigen" in R to compute the eigenvectors, and eigenvalues, of the following matrix:

$$A = \begin{bmatrix} 5 & 2 & 3 \\ 5 & 5 & 5 \\ 3 & 2 & 3 \end{bmatrix}$$

Print the first eigenvector and eigenvalue on the screen after you have extracted them from the output.

```
A=matrix(c(5,5,3,2,5,2,3,5,3),3,3)
Eig=eigen(A)
# Print first Eigenvector
Eig$vectors[,1]
-0.4859332  -0.7798238  -0.3946439
# Print first Eigenvalue
Eig$values[1]
10.646
```

Answers to the Exercises in Chapter 3

Exercises 3.5

1. Use the "str" function on the data frame "crabs" and tell which variables are on a categorical or a numerical scale.

```
library(MASS) # To access the crab dataset
 str(crabs)
'data.frame':   200 obs. of  8 variables:
```

```
$ sp   : Factor w/ 2 levels "B","O": 1 1 1 1 1 1 1 1 1 1 ...
$ sex  : Factor w/ 2 levels "F","M": 2 2 2 2 2 2 2 2 2 2 ...
$ index: int  1 2 3 4 5 6 7 8 9 10 ...
$ FL   : num  8.1 8.8 9.2 9.6 9.8 10.8 11.1 11.6 11.8 11.8 ...
$ RW   : num  6.7 7.7 7.8 7.9 8 9 9.9 9.1 9.6 10.5 ...
$ CL   : num  16.1 18.1 19 20.1 20.3 23 23.8 24.5 24.2 25.2 ...
$ CW   : num  19 20.8 22.4 23.1 23 26.5 27.1 28.4 27.8 29.3 ...
$ BD   : num  7 7.4 7.7 8.2 8.2 9.8 9.8 10.4 9.7 10.3 ...
```

The variables sex and species (sp) are on a categorical scale, whereas FL, RW, CL, CW, and BD are on a continuous/numerical scale. The variable “index” is just an index showing the crab number. This variable should not be included in any statistical analysis.

2. Save the data frame “crabs” as a tibble with the name crab_tibble. Print this tibble and note that the output essentially gives the same information as using the function “str”.

```
library(tibble)
crab_tibble=as_tibble(crabs)
crab_tibble
# A tibble: 200 x 8
      sp    sex   index   FL     RW      CL     CW     BD
   <fct>  <fct>  <int>  <dbl>  <dbl>  <dbl>  <dbl>  <dbl>
 1   B      M      1     8.1    6.7    16.1   19      7
 2   B      M      2     8.8    7.7    18.1   20.8    7.4
 3   B      M      3     9.2    7.8    19     22.4    7.7
….
```

3. Calculate the mean value for all numerical variables in the Crab dataset, separated by sex.

```
aggregate(cbind(FL,RW,CL,CW,BD)~sex,crabs,mean)
     sex    FL       RW       CL       CW        BD
1     F   15.432   13.487   31.360   35.830    13.724
2     M   15.734   11.990   32.851   36.999    14.337
```

or use tapply on each variable, for example:

```
tapply(crabs$FL,crabs$sex,mean)
    F           M
15.432      15.734
```

4. Extract only the Setosa flowers in the Iris dataset.
There are a number of different ways to extract the Setosa flowers. I here show four different ways:

```
Setosa=iris[iris$Species=="setosa",]
Setosa=subset(iris,Species=="setosa")
```

```
library(dplyr)
Setosa=filter(iris, Species=="setosa")
# Use a pipe
Setosa=iris %>% filter(Species=="setosa")
```

5. Extract only Versicolors and Virginicas from the Iris dataset, which have a sepal length larger than 6.8. Tip: use the OR operator "|" to select both Versicolors and Virginicas and the AND operator "&" to select only flowers that have a sepal length larger than 6.8.
   To extract both Versicolors and Virginicas, we can use the logical OR operator "|" where we say that we like to extract all rows where the species are equal to "versicolor" or "virginica". To extract only Versicolors and Virginicas that have a sepal length larger than 6.8, we use the logical AND operator "&":

```
filtered_iris = iris[(iris$Species == "versicolor" |
iris$Species == "virginica") & iris$Sepal.Length > 6.8, ]
# This also works
filtered_iris = subset(iris, (Species == "versicolor" |
Species == "virginica") & Sepal.Length > 6.8)
# This also works
library(dplyr)
filtered_iris = filter(iris, (Species == "versicolor" |
Species == "virginica") & Sepal.Length > 6.8)
# Use a pipe
filtered_iris = iris %>% filter((Species == "versicolor" |
Species == "virginica") & Sepal.Length > 6.8)
```

Answers to the Exercises in Chapter 4

Exercises 4.7

1. Create a scatter plot of the CW and CL in the Crab dataset and label the variable sex with different colors.

```
library(MASS) # To access the crab data
plot(crabs$CW,crabs$CL,col=crabs$sex,pch=16,
xlab="Carapace width (mm)",ylab="Carapace length (mm)")
legend("topleft", legend=c("Female","Male"), pch=16, col=1:2)
```

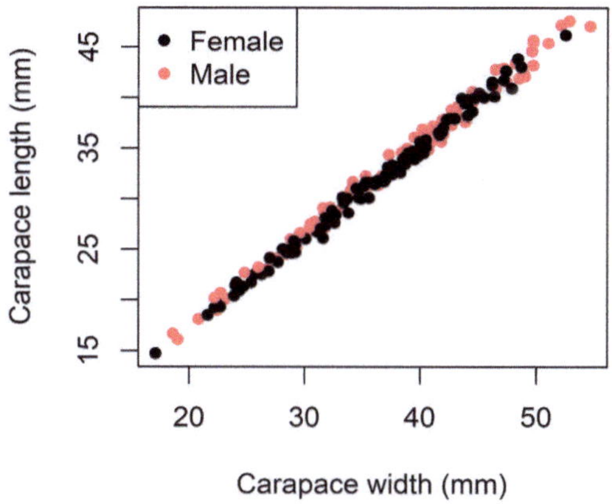

In ggplot:

```
library(ggplot2)
ggplot(data=crabs, aes(x = CW, y = CL, color = sex)) +
  geom_point() +
  labs(x = "Carapace width (mm)", y = "Carapace length (mm)")
```

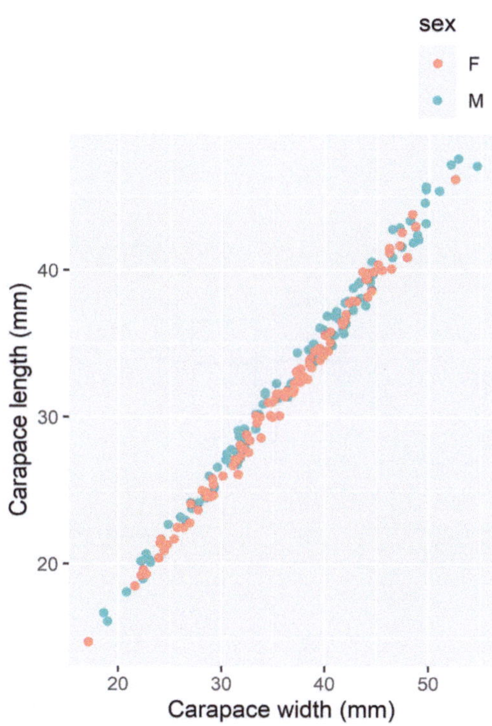

2. Create a boxplot of all the numerical variables in the Crab dataset. Can you identify an outlier in any of the numerical variables?

```
boxplot(crabs[,4:8],ylab="mm")
```

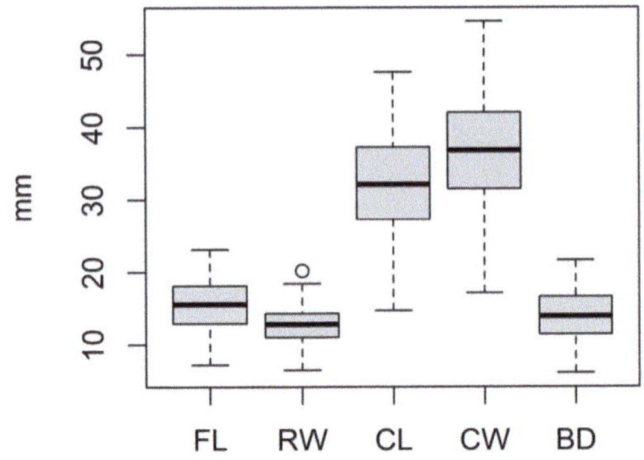

The RW variable includes one outlier (the circle above the box).
In ggplot:

```
library(ggplot2)
library(tidyr)
# Reshape the crab data to long format
crabs_long = crabs %>%
  pivot_longer(cols = 4:8, names_to = "measurement",
  values_to = "value")
# Create the boxplot
ggplot(crabs_long, aes(x = measurement, y = value)) +
  geom_boxplot() +
  labs(y = "Size (mm)")
```

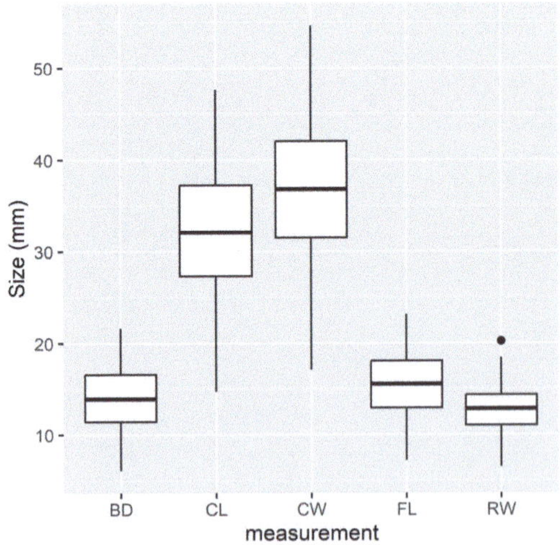

3. Create a boxplot with **ggplot2** of all the numerical variables in the Crab dataset but where you now plot separate boxes for the blue and orange species.

```
ggplot(crabs_long, aes(x = measurement, y = value,
fill = sp)) +
  # Dodge to separate blue from orange
  geom_boxplot(position = position_dodge(width = 0.8))+
```

```
  # Set color for the boxes
  scale_fill_manual(values = c("B" = "blue",
  "O" = "orange"),
    # Labels for the legend
    labels = c("B" = "Blue crab", "O" = "Orange crab")) +
  labs(y = "Size (mm)", x = "Measurement", fill = "Species")
```

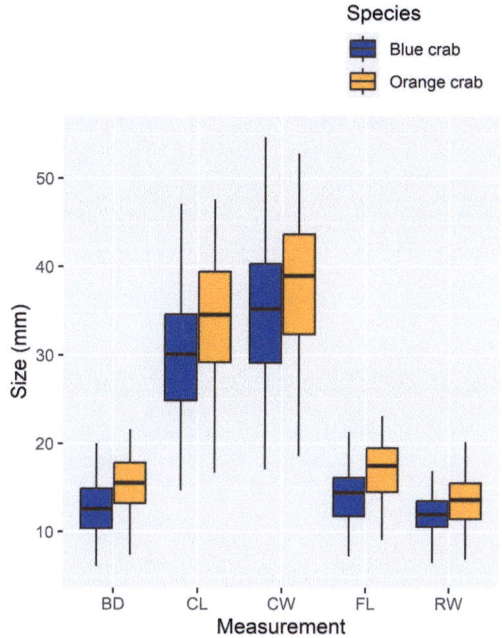

4. Make a one-dimensional scatter plot including all numerical variables in the Crab dataset and set different colors for the variable species.

```
stripchart(crabs[crabs$sp=="B",4:8],vertical = T,
method="jitter",pch=1,cex=0.8, col="blue",ylim=c(0,60),ylab=
"Length (mm)",las=1)
stripchart(crabs[crabs$sp=="O",4:8],vertical = T,
method="jitter", pch=1,cex=0.8, col="orange",add=T)
legend("topleft", legend=c("Blue","Orange"), pch=1,
col=c("Blue","Orange"))
```

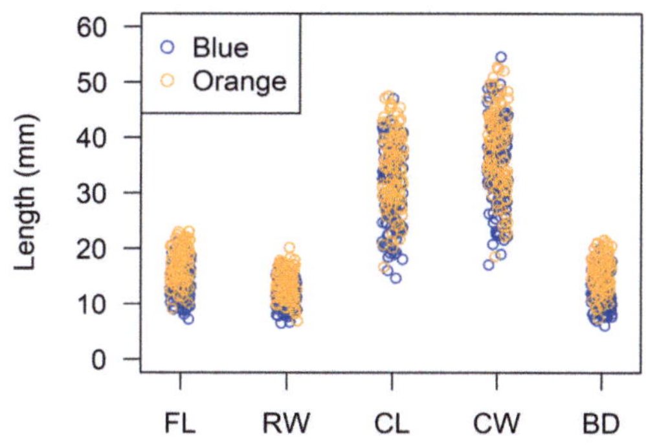

In ggplot:

```
library(ggplot2)
library(tidyr)
library(dplyr)
library(MASS) # To access the crab dataset
# Reshape the crab data to long format and convert labels B
# to Blue and O to Orange
crabs_long <- crabs %>%
  pivot_longer(cols = 4:8, names_to = "measurement",
  values_to = "value") %>%
   # To get nice labels for the legend
   mutate(sp = recode(sp, B = "Blue", O = "Orange"))
ggplot(data=crabs_long, aes(x = measurement, y = value,
color = sp)) +
  geom_jitter(size=2,width=0.1,height=0,alpha = 0.4) +
  scale_color_manual(values = c("Blue" = "blue", "Orange" =
  "orange")) +
  labs(y = "Size (mm)", x = "", color = "Species") +
  theme_minimal()
```

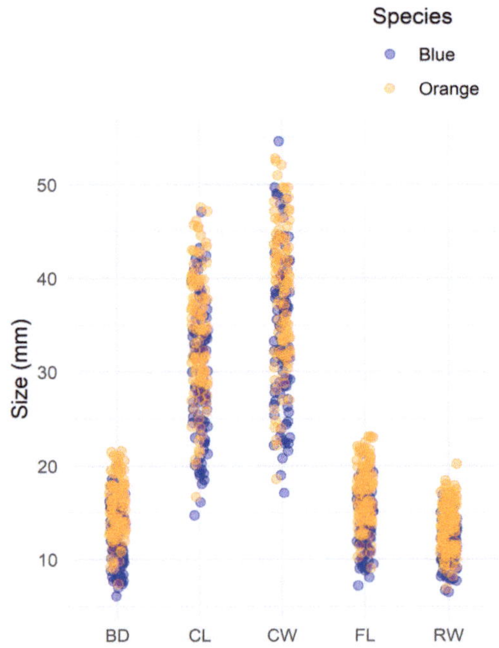

5. Make a scatter plot matrix of all the numerical variables in the Crab dataset and set different colors for the variable sex.

```
pairs(crabs[,4:8], col = crabs$sex ,upper.panel=NULL)
```

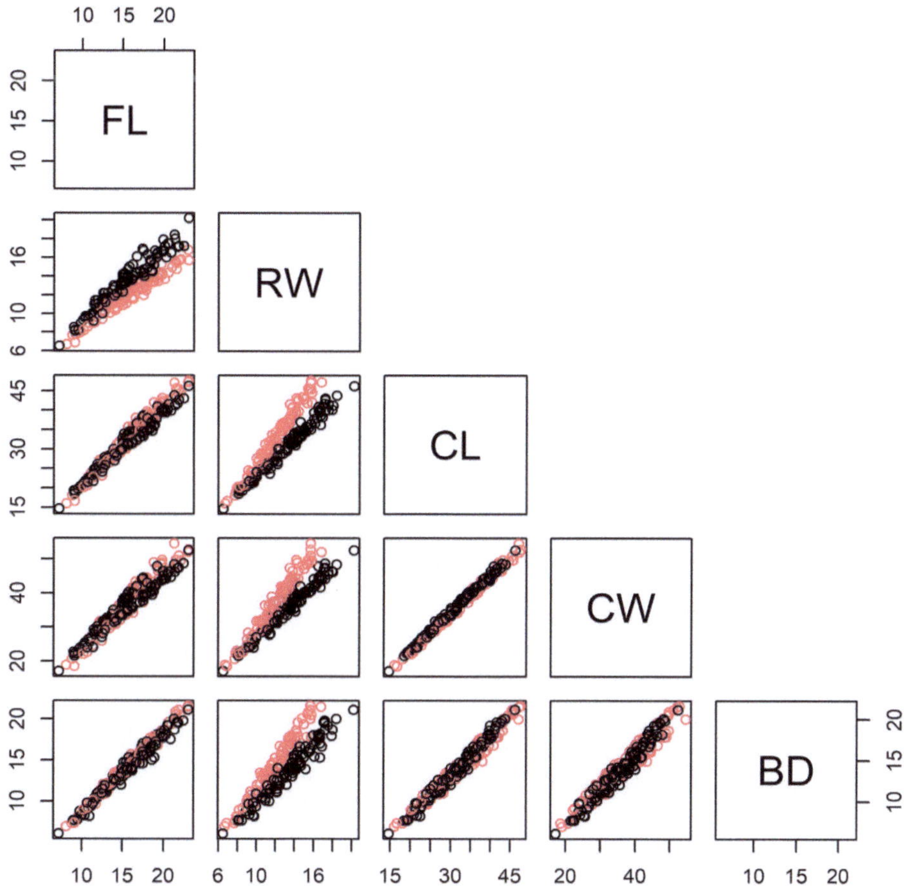

With GGally

```
library(GGally)
ggpairs(crabs, columns = 4:8, aes(color = sex),
upper = list(continuous = "blank"))
```

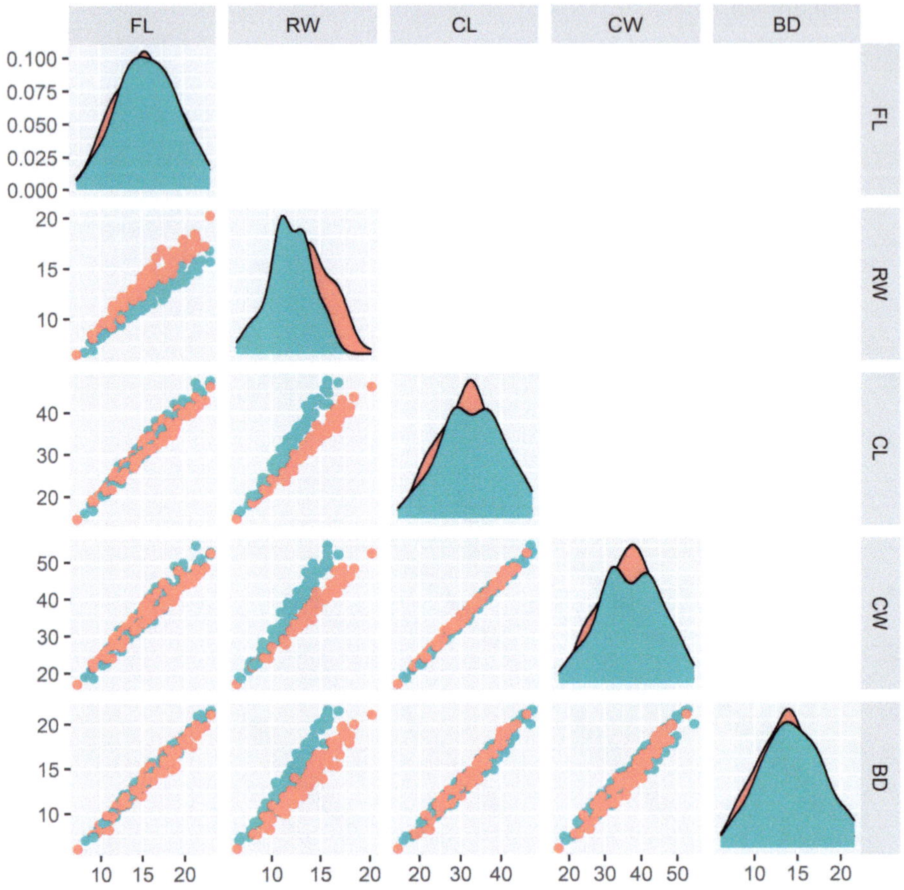

6. Create a profile plot of all the numerical variables in the Crab dataset and set different colors for male and female crabs. Which variables in this plot seem to best separate the sex?

```
library(GGally)
ggparcoord(crabs, columns=4:8, groupColumn = 2,
scale="globalminmax")
```

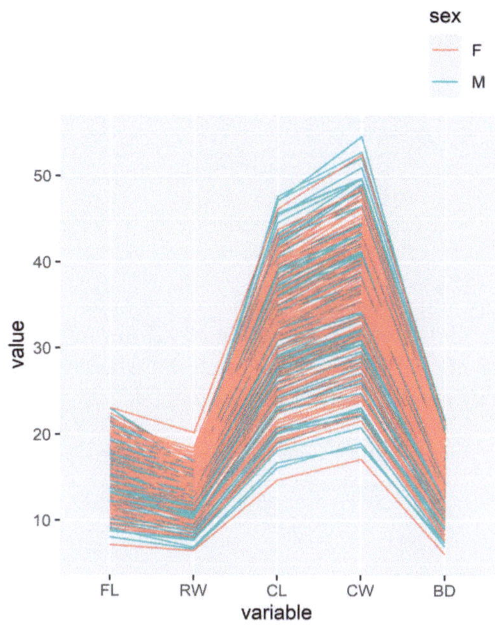

From this plot, it is very hard to tell which variable that shows the best separation between the males and females. However, from the above scatter plot matrix and this profile plot, the variable rear width (RW) seems to best separate the two groups.

Answers to the Exercises in Chapter 5

Exercises 5.4

1. Calculate the correlation matrix of the numerical variables in the Crab dataset and indicate which correlations that are significantly different from zero. Use Bonferroni correction to adjust the p-values.

```
library(Hmisc)
rcorr(as.matrix(crabs[,4:8]), type="pearson")
        FL      RW      CL      CW      BD
FL    1.00    0.91    0.98    0.96    0.99
RW    0.91    1.00    0.89    0.90    0.89
CL    0.98    0.89    1.00    1.00    0.98
CW    0.96    0.90    1.00    1.00    0.97
BD    0.99    0.89    0.98    0.97    1.00
....
```

Bonferroni corrected p-values

```
rcorr(as.matrix(crabs[,4:8]), type="pearson")$P*10
        FL     RW     CL     CW     BD
FL      NA     0      0      0      0
RW      0      NA     0      0      0
CL      0      0      NA     0      0
CW      0      0      0      NA     0
BD      0      0      0      0      NA
```

All 10 p-values are super small and have been rounded to zero, which means that all 10 correlation coefficients are significantly different from zero.

2. Print the correlation coefficients as a sorted list where one easily can see which pair that has the strongest positive correlation.

```
rm(list=ls()) # Clear environment
library(MASS) # To access the crab dataset
cor_mat=cor(crabs[,4:8],method="pearson")
diag(cor_mat) = NA
cor_mat[upper.tri (cor_mat)] = NA
library(reshape)
cor_melt=melt(cor_mat)
cor=na.omit(cor_melt)
cor[order(cor$value,decreasing = TRUE),]
      X1    X2      value
14    CW    CL    0.9950225
5     BD    FL    0.9876272
15    BD    CL    0.9832038
....
```

CW and CL have the strongest correlation.

3. Extract only the female crabs and compute a correlation matrix of the variables FL, RW, and CL.

```
female=crabs[crabs$sex=="F", c("FL","RW","CL")]
# Round correlation coefficients to two decimal places
round(cor(female),2)
       FL      RW      CL
FL    1.00    0.97    0.98
RW    0.97    1.00    0.99
CL    0.98    0.99    1.00
```

Answers to the Exercises in Chapter 6

Exercises 6.2

1. Use PCA to combine the two variables Sepal length and Petal length in the Iris dataset, using both the "manual" way where you compute the eigenvector of the covariance matrix and by using the "prcomp" function. You do not need to standardize or center the data. How much variance is explained by the first PC?

```
rm(list=ls()) # Clear environment
SL=iris$Sepal.Length
PL=iris$Petal.Length
data=cbind(SL, PL)
COV=cov(data) # Calculate covariance
eig=eigen(COV) # Compute eigenvectors and eigenvalues
a11=eig$vectors[1,1]
a12=eig$vectors[2,1]
a21=eig$vectors[1,2]
a22=eig$vectors[2,2]
PC1=a11*SL+a12*PL
PC2=a21*SL+a22*PL
var(PC1)/(var(PC1)+var(PC2))
0.9631579
pca=prcomp(data)
pca$sdev[1]^2/sum(pca$sdev^2)
0.9631579
```

   96% is explained by the first PC.

2. Show the linear equation for the first PC.

```
PC1=a11*SL+a12*PL
```

PC1= 0.39 * SL + 0.92 * PL

3. Compute a PCA based on all numerical variables in the Iris dataset and plot PC1 vs PC2. Standardize the variables before you compute the PCA. Add colors to this plot so that one can identify the three different species and the row numbers so that one can also identify individual flowers.

```
# Simple plot
pca=prcomp(iris[,-5],scale=TRUE)
plot(pca$x[,1],pca$x[,2],col=iris$Species)
text(pca$x[,1],pca$x[,2],1:150,cex=0.3)
```

   In ggplot2

```
library(ggplot2)
pca=prcomp(iris[,-5],scale=TRUE)
prop.pca = (pca$sdev^2/sum(pca$sdev^2)) * 100 # % Variance
dataset = data.frame(species = iris$Species ,pca$x)
ggplot(dataset) +
  geom_point(aes(PC1,PC2,colour =species), size = 3.5) +
  geom_text(aes(PC1, PC2,label=1:length(PC1)),size=2.2) +
  labs( x = paste("PC1 (", round(prop.pca[1]), "%)",
  sep = ""),
        y = paste("PC2 (", round(prop.pca[2]), "%)",
        sep = "")
  )
```

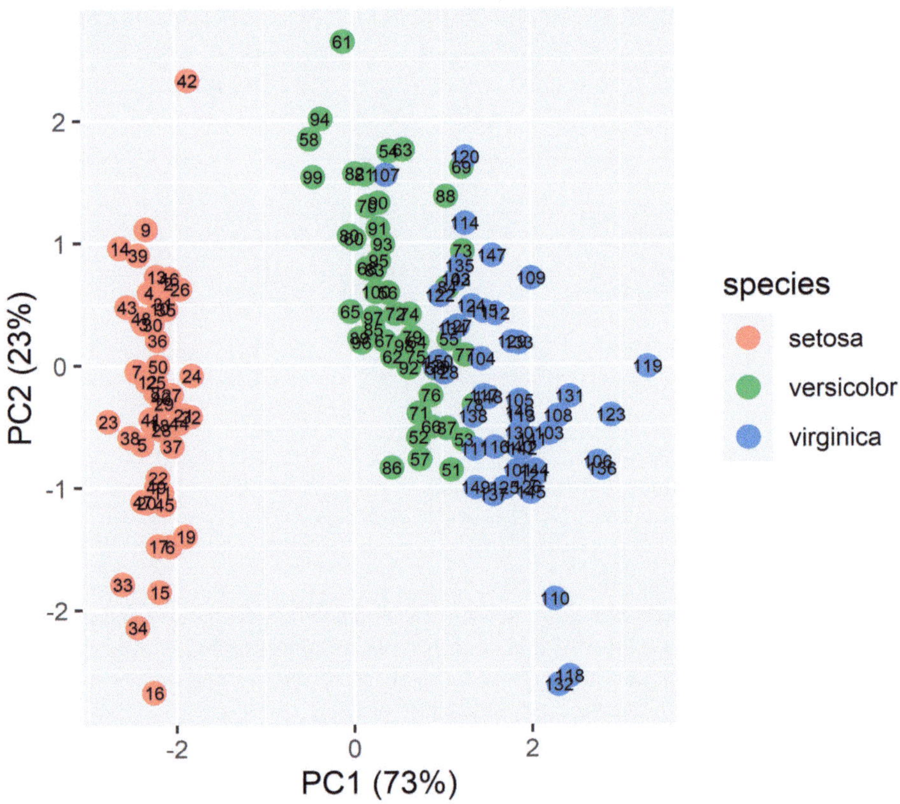

Exercises 6.4

1. Use PCA and the "prcomp" function to combine the four numeric variables in the Iris dataset. Standardize the variables before you compute the PCA. How many PCs should you extract according to the three methods we have discussed in this section?

```
data=scale(iris[,-5])
pca=prcomp(data)
#pca=prcomp(iris[,-5],scale=TRUE) # This also works
summary(pca)
Importance of components:
                          PC1     PC2     PC3      PC4
Standard deviation     1.7084  0.9560  0.38309  0.14393
Proportion of Variance 0.7296  0.2285  0.03669  0.00518
Cumulative Proportion  0.7296  0.9581  0.99482  1.00000
```

We see that the first two PCs explain 96% (73% + 23%) of the total variation. Hence, according to the first method, we would only keep the first two PCs.

```
pca$sdev^2
2.91849782 0.91403047 0.14675688 0.02071484
```

For standardized variables, we keep only components with an eigenvalue greater than 1 (the Kaiser's criterion), which means that we with this method would only extract the first PC.

```
plot(pca,type="l")
```

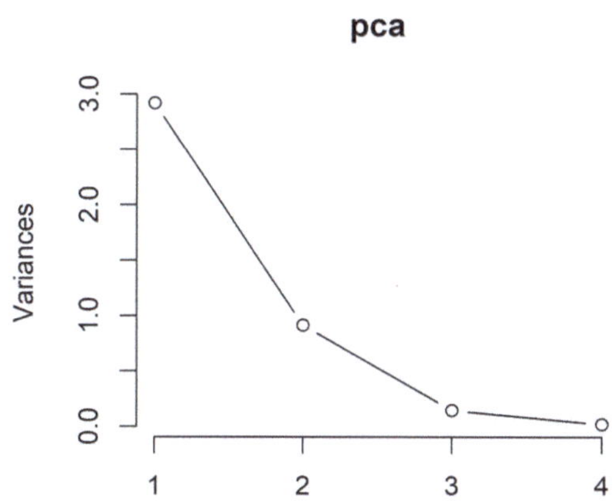

The first two components are involved in the steep part of the curve. Therefore, we extract the first two components with this method.

2. Do the same as in the previous question but use the numeric variables in the Crab dataset.

```
library(MASS) # To access the crab data
# Extract and standardize the numerical variables
data=scale(crabs[,4:8])
pca=prcomp(data)
#pca=prcomp(crabs[,4:8], scale=TRUE) # This also works
summary(pca)   # Proportion of variance
pca$sdev^2       # Variance of each component
plot(pca,type="l") # A scree plot
```

All three methods tell us that we should only extract the first PC.

Exercises 6.6

1. Use a PCA on the standardized numerical variables in the Iris dataset. Extract the two first principal components and print the weights/loadings after Varimax rotation. Which variables load on PC1 and PC2?

```
data=scale(iris[,-5])
pca=prcomp(data)
varmax=varimax(pca$rotation[,1:2])
varmax
Loadings:
                 PC1      PC2
Sepal.Length    0.596   -0.243
Sepal.Width             -0.961
Petal.Length    0.570    0.114
Petal.Width     0.565
....
```

If we use a cutoff value of 0.55, we see that the Sepal width loads on PC2 (because the absolute value of -0.961 is larger than 0.55), whereas the other three variables load on PC1. If we instead use the "principal" function:

```
library(psych)
pr_varmax=principal(data, nfactors = 2, rotate = "varimax")
pr_varmax
Standardized loadings (pattern matrix) based upon
correlation matrix
                 RC1     RC2    h2     u2       com
Sepal.Length    0.96    0.05   0.92   0.0774    1.0
Sepal.Width    -0.14    0.98   0.99   0.0091    1.0
Petal.Length    0.94   -0.30   0.98   0.0163    1.2
Petal.Width     0.93   -0.26   0.94    0.0647   1.2
```

we can use a cutoff value of, for example, 0.9, where we will come to the same conclusion where the Sepal Width loads on PC2, whereas the other three variables load on PC1.

2. Compute a correlation matrix of numerical variables in the Iris dataset and try and understand why your answer in the previous question can be explained by the correlation coefficients.

```
cor(iris[,-5])
               Sepal.Length  Sepal.Width  Petal.Length  Petal.Width
Sepal.Length    1.0000000    -0.1175698    0.8717538     0.8179411
Sepal.Width    -0.1175698     1.0000000   -0.4284401    -0.3661259
Petal.Length    0.8717538    -0.4284401    1.0000000     0.9628654
Petal.Width     0.8179411    -0.3661259    0.9628654     1.0000000
```

The sepal width does not show any strong correlation to the other variables, whereas the other three variables all have a strong correlation to each other.

Exercises 6.8

1. Use a PCoA, based on the Euclidean distances, on the standardized numerical variables of the Iris dataset. Show a PCoA plot where you identify the species with colors and flowers with numbers.

```
sdata = scale(iris[,-5])
D = as.matrix(dist(sdata, upper=T, diag=T))
MDS=cmdscale(D,k=2)
dataset = data.frame(MDS1=MDS[,1],MDS2=MDS[,2],
Species=iris$Species)
ggplot(dataset) +
  geom_point(aes(MDS1,MDS2,color=Species), size = 3.5) +
  geom_text(aes(MDS1,MDS2,label=1:length(MDS1)),size=2.2)
```

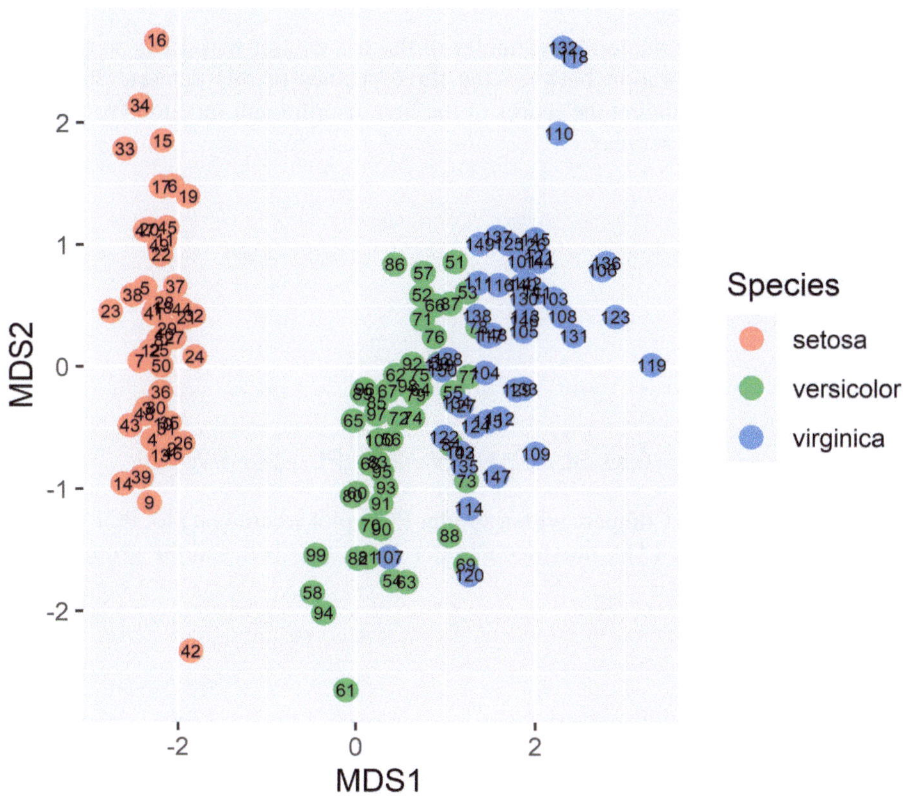

2. Modify the PCoA plot so that it becomes identical to the PCA plot based on the Iris dataset.

```
sdata = scale(iris[,-5])
D = as.matrix(dist(sdata, upper=T, diag=T))
MDS=cmdscale(D,k=2)
dataset = data.frame(MDS1=MDS[,1],MDS2=MDS[,2]*(-1),
Species=iris$Species)
ggplot(dataset) +
  geom_point(aes(MDS1,MDS2,color=Species), size = 3.5) +
  geom_text(aes(MDS1,MDS2,label=1:length(MDS1)),size=2.2)
```

Answers to the Exercises in Chapter 7

Exercises 7.2

1. Combine the four numerical variables of the Iris dataset with LDA so that you optimize the separation between the three species in this dataset. Show the equation for calculating the scores of the first discriminant function (you do not need to center the scores).

```
lda = lda(Species ~ ., iris)
Coefficients of linear discriminants:
                      LD1              LD2
Sepal.Length    0.8293776       0.02410215
Sepal.Width     1.5344731       2.16452123
Petal.Length   -2.2012117      -0.93192121
Petal.Width    -2.8104603       2.83918785
```

$$LD1 = 0.83 \cdot \mathsf{SL} + 1.53 \cdot \mathsf{SW} - 2.20 \cdot \mathsf{PL} - 2.81 \cdot \mathsf{PW}$$

2. Plot LD1 vs LD2. Compare with a similar PCA plot where you plot PC1 vs PC2. Do you think that LDA provides a better separation between the groups compared to PCA?

```
# Simple plot
lda = lda(Species ~ ., iris)
plda = predict(lda)
plot(plda$x[,1],plda$x[,2],col=iris$Species,main="LDA") # LDA
pca=prcomp(iris[,-5],scale=TRUE)
plot(pca$x[,1],pca$x[,2],col=iris$Species,main="PCA") # PCA
```

With **ggplot2**

```
rm(list=ls()) # Clear environment
# PCA
pca = prcomp(iris[,-5],scale. = TRUE)
prop.pca = (pca$sdev^2/sum(pca$sdev^2)) * 100 # % Variance
dataset = data.frame(species = iris$Species, pca$x)
# LDA
lda = lda(Species ~ ., iris)
prop.lda = (lda$svd^2/sum(lda$svd^2)) * 100
plda = predict(lda)
dataset$LD1 = plda$x[,1]
dataset$LD2 = plda$x[,2]
library(ggplot2)
ggplot(dataset) +
  geom_point(aes(LD1,LD2, colour = species), size = 2.5) +
  labs(x = paste("LD1 (", round(prop.lda[1]), "%)", sep=""),
       y = paste("LD2 (", round(prop.lda[2]), "%)", sep=""))
```

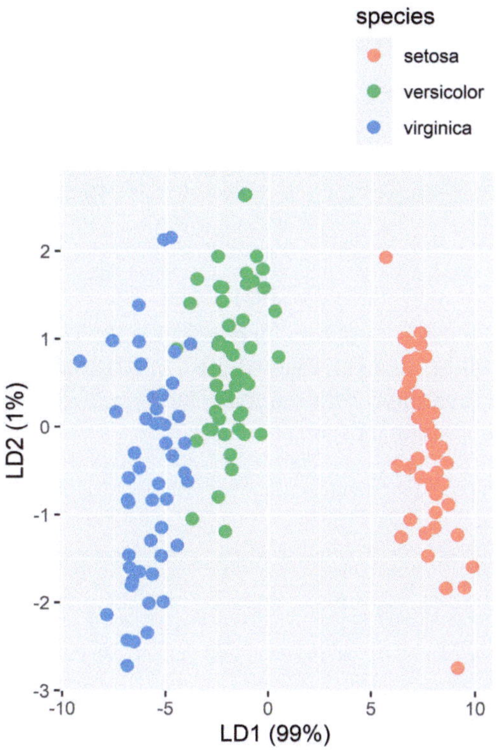

```
ggplot(dataset) +
  geom_point(aes(PC1, PC2, colour = species), size = 2.5) +
  labs(x = paste("PC1 (", round(prop.pca[1]), "%)", sep=""),
       y = paste("PC2 (", round(prop.pca[2]), "%)", sep=""))
```

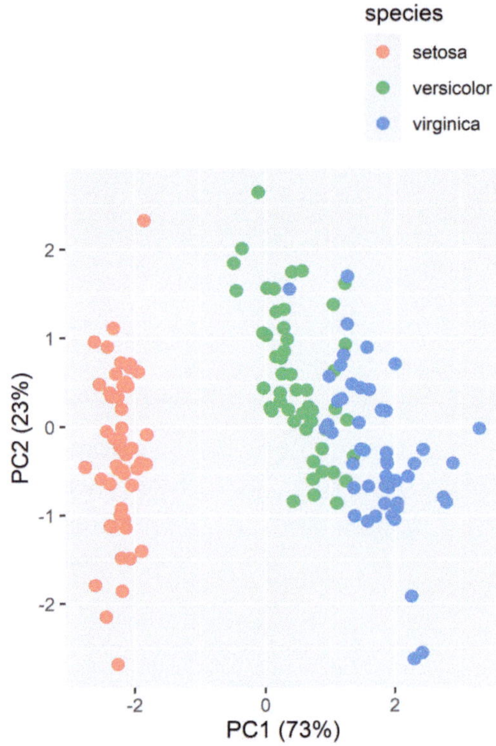

LDA separates the three groups much better than PCA.

3. Combine all the numerical variables of the Crab dataset by using LDA in order to maximize the separation between male and female crabs. Show the equation to calculate the discriminant scores.

```
library(MASS) # To access the crab dataset and the lda function
head(crabs)
fit = lda(sex ~  FL+RW+CL+CW+BD, data=crabs)
fit
              LD1
FL    -0.17509926
RW    -1.61455655
CL     0.90033985
CW    -0.27294518
BD     0.08261892
```

D= -0.17 * FL – 1.61 x RW + 0.90 x CL -0.27 x CW + 0.08 x BD

4. Plot the discriminant scores with a one-dimensional scatter plot where you separate male and female crabs.
   Using the uncentered scores (same as the equation above):

```
D=-0.17*crabs$FL-1.61*crabs$RW+0.90*crabs$CL-0.27*
crabs$CW+0.08*crabs$BD
stripchart(D~crabs$sex,data=crabs,ylab="Discriminant scores",
vertical =TRUE,xlim=c(0.5,2.5))
```

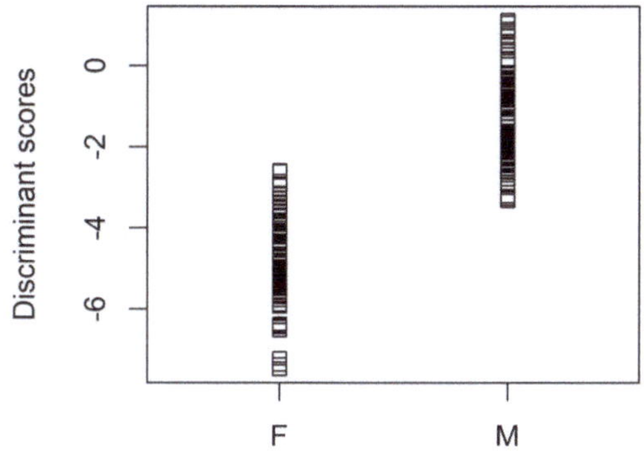

   Using the centered discriminant scores extracted from the object fit by the function "predict":

```
D=predict(fit)$x
stripchart(D~crabs$sex,data=crabs,ylab="Discriminant scores",
vertical =TRUE,xlim=c(0.5,2.5))
```

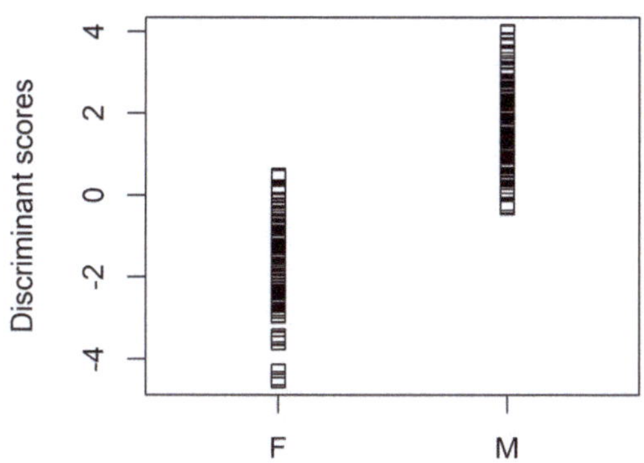

Note that the discriminant scores are now centered around zero!

Answers to the Exercises in Chapter 8

Exercises 8.5

1. Use the Mahalanobis distance in order to identify possible outliers in the numerical variables of the Crab dataset. Use a cutoff value based on the Bonferroni method.

```
df=crabs[,4:8] # Extract the numerical variables
MH2=mahalanobis(df, colMeans(df), cov(df))
p_val=1-pchisq(MH2,df=5)
data3=data.frame(df,MH2,p_val)
# Sort and Print
head(data3[order(data3$MH2,decreasing = TRUE),])
      FL    RW    CL    CW    BD    MH2       p_val
183   18.9  16.7  36.3  41.7  15.3  15.54990  0.008253806
181   18.6  14.5  34.7  39.4  15.0  14.86324  0.010962949
50    21.3  15.7  47.1  54.6  20.0  14.32512  0.013670904
....
```

If we use a cutoff of 0.00025 (0.05/200), no data point is identified as an outlier. It is also possible to adjust the p-values by:

```
p.adjust(p_val,method="bonferroni")
```

which can be compared to a significance level of 0.05. All p-values will in this case be adjusted to 1.

Answers to the Exercises in Chapter 9

Exercises 9.4

1. Use MANOVA on the Crab dataset to test if there is a difference in the means of the numerical variables between male and female crabs. Run t-tests on the individual variables if you reject the null hypothesis.

```
crab_manova = manova(cbind(FL,RW,CL,CW,BD) ~ sex,
data=crabs)
summary(crab_manova)
      Df   Pillai    approx F   num Df den Df     Pr(>F)
sex   1    0.74906    115.82       5     194    < 2.2e-16 ***
```

The p-value is less than 0.05, which means that there is a significant difference in the means of the variables between male and female crabs. Let's continue with post-hoc tests. Since sex has only two categories, we can use unpaired t-tests as post-hoc tests:

```
t.test(FL~sex,data=crabs)
data:  FL by sex
t = -0.60998, df = 197.91, p-value = 0.5426
t.test(RW~sex,data=crabs)
data:  RW by sex
t = 4.2896, df = 187.76, p-value = 2.862e-05
```

Continue with the other variables and adjust the p-values by the Bonferroni method. Only RW is significant between males and females. Female crabs have a significantly bigger rear width (RW).

2. Do you fulfill the assumptions for MANOVA?

```
M=subset(crabs,sex=="M")
F=subset(crabs,sex=="F")
library(mvnormtest)
mshapiro.test(t(M[,4:8]))
data:  Z
W = 0.96947, p-value = 0.02013
mshapiro.test(t(F[,4:8]))
data:  Z
W = 0.95595, p-value = 0.002091
```

Since the Shapiro Wilk's test results in p-values that were less than 0.05 for both groups, we reject the assumption of multivariate normality and conclude that the continuous variables are not normally distributed in the multivariate space. Next, we analyze if there are any outliers in the dataset separately for the variable sex:

```
MD_M=mahalanobis(M[,4:8], colMeans(M[,4:8]), cov(M[,4:8]))
MD_F=mahalanobis(F[,4:8], colMeans(F[,4:8]), cov(F[,4:8]))
sort(1-pchisq(MD_M,df=5))
0.008742058   0.031858787   0.032887593
sort(1-pchisq(MD_F,df=5))
0.005021871   0.010596443   0.037221058
```

Using a cutoff value based on the Bonferroni method, 0.0005 (0.05/100), no data point will be considered as an outlier. Next, we check the assumption of homogeneity of variance-covariance matrices:

```
library(biotools)
boxM(crabs[,4:8], crabs$sex)
data:  crabs[, 4:8]
Chi-Sq (approx.) = 190.7, df = 15, p-value < 2.2e-16
```

Since the p-value is less than 0.05, the null hypothesis of equal population covariance matrices is rejected. Thus, the groups do not have equal population covariance matrices. Finally, we compute the correlation matrix to see if the correlations of our dependent variables are too strong:

```
cor(crabs[,4:8])
          FL          RW          CL          CW          BD
FL   1.0000000   0.9069876   0.9788418   0.9649558   0.9876272
RW   0.9069876   1.0000000   0.8927430   0.9004021   0.8892054
CL   0.9788418   0.8927430   1.0000000   0.9950225   0.9832038
CW   0.9649558   0.9004021   0.9950225   1.0000000   0.9678117
BD   0.9876272   0.8892054   0.9832038   0.9678117   1.0000000
```

Several variables have correlations larger than 0.9 to each other, which is problematic in MANOVA.

In conclusion, the crab data separated by sex does not seem to be appropriate for MANOVA since most assumptions were not fulfilled. One can then try to run the nonparametric alternative called PERMANOVA.

However, the assumption of a linear relationship of the dependent variables seems to be fulfilled, because there is a clear linear relationship between all the variables when we separate the data based on sex:

```
pairs(crabs[,4:8],col = crabs$sex)
```

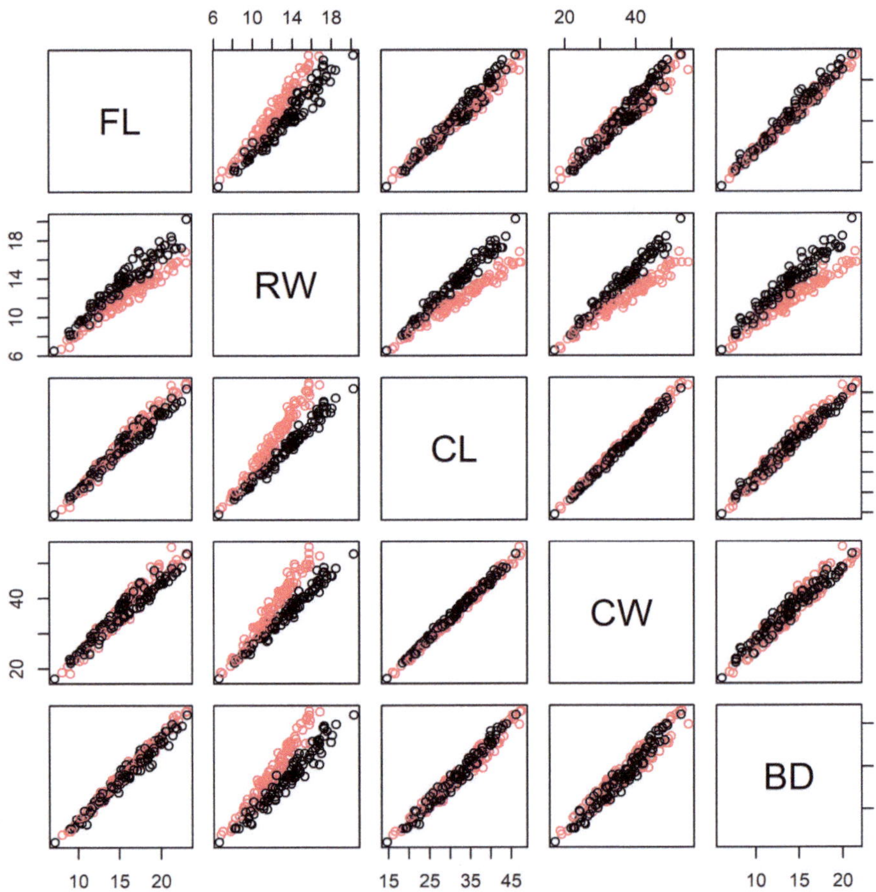

3. Compute a PERMANOVA on the Crab dataset, using the Euclidean distance, to test if there is a difference in the numerical variables between male and female crabs. Standardize the continuous variables before you run the PERMANOVA and run 9999 permutations.

```
library(vegan)
set.seed(1) #For reproducibility
data=data.frame(scale(crabs[,4:8]))
adonis2(data~sex,data=crabs,method = "euclidian",
permutations = 9999)
          Df   SumOfSqs     R2        F      Pr(>F)
sex        1    22.19     0.0223   4.5168   0.035 *
Residual 198   972.81     0.9777
Total    199   995.00     1.0000
```

We see that there is a significant difference in the dependent variables between male and female crabs because the p-value is less than 0.05. However, the p-value is much larger compared to the one from the MANOVA, which is probably due to that we did not fulfill the assumptions of the MANOVA. Note that you might get a different p-value if you have used another seed and/or if you use a different R-version than I used to generate the result (I used version 4.4.2).

4. Run the same PERMANOVA as in the previous question but use both sex and species as independent variables to test if there is a significant interaction between sex and species.

```
library(vegan)
set.seed(1) #For reproducibility
data=data.frame(scale(crabs[,4:8]))
adonis2(data~sex*sp,data=crabs,method ="euclidian",
permutations = 9999,by="terms")
          Df   SumOfSqs     R2        F        Pr(>F)
sex        1    22.19    0.02230   5.2971    0.0230 *
sp         1   119.58    0.12018  28.5440    0.0001 ***
sex:sp     1    32.10    0.03226   7.6626    0.0064 **
Residual 196   821.12    0.82525
Total    199   995.00    1.00000
```

The interaction between sex and species type is significant (p-value = 0.0064). Note that you might get a different p-value if you have used another seed and/or if you use a different R-version than I used to generate the result (I used version 4.4.2). To understand the interaction, let's compute the mean values of the continuous variables separately for sex and species:

```
aggregate(. ~ sex + sp, data = crabs,FUN="mean")
  sex  sp  index    FL      RW      CL      CW      BD
1  F   B   25.5   13.270  12.138  28.102  32.624  11.816
2  M   B   25.5   14.842  11.718  32.014  36.810  13.350
3  F   O   25.5   17.594  14.836  34.618  39.036  15.632
4  M   O   25.5   16.626  12.262  33.688  37.188  15.324
```

We see that male crabs that are blue are generally larger than female crabs, whereas male crabs that are orange are generally smaller than the females. This explains why there is an interaction between sex and species because the overall size difference between blue and orange crabs depends on the sex.

5. In the Iris dataset, we can think of the petal length and petal width as representing the petal size, whereas sepal length and sepal width can be considered as the sepal size of the flowers. Compute the canonical correlation coefficient between petal size and sepal size, using the Iris dataset. Also, compute a p-value by a permutation test.

```
library(CCA)
rm(list=ls()) # Clear environment
X=cbind(iris$Sepal.Length,iris$Sepal.Width)
Y=cbind(iris$Petal.Length ,iris$Petal.Width)
cc(X, Y)
$cor
0.9409690 0.1239369
...
set.seed(1) #For reproducibility
library(CCP)
p.perm.out=p.perm(X, Y, nboot = 1000, type = "Pillai")
plt.perm(p.perm.out)
```

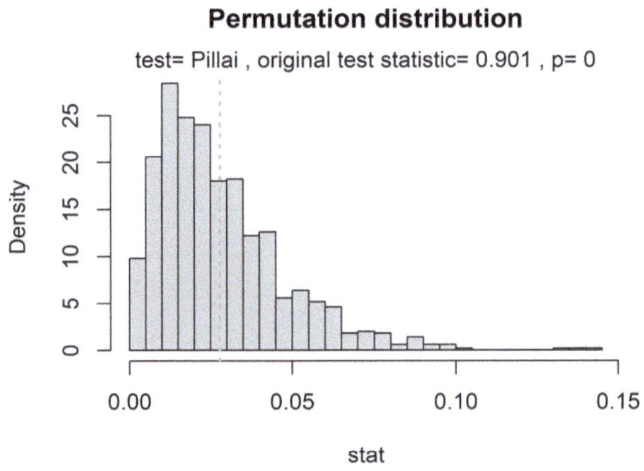

From the results, we see that the canonical correlation coefficient is 0.94 and that the p-value is less than 0.05. Thus, there is a significant linear relationship between the two sets of variables. Note that you might get a different plot if you have used another seed and/or if you use a different R-version than I used to generate the result (I used version 4.4.2).

Answers to the Exercises in Chapter 10

Exercises 10.2

1. Make a one-dimensional scatter plot of the variable body depth (BD) from the Crab data where you separate the two colors (Blue (B) and Orange (O)). Place a cutoff line at 11 and use jittering so that you can see all the data points.

```
library(MASS) # To access the crab dataset
cutoff=11
BD=crabs$BD
Species=crabs$sp
stripchart(BD~Species,method="jitter",ylab=c("body depth (mm)"),
vertical = T,xlim=c(0.7,2.3) ,las=1)
abline(h=cutoff,col="red")
```

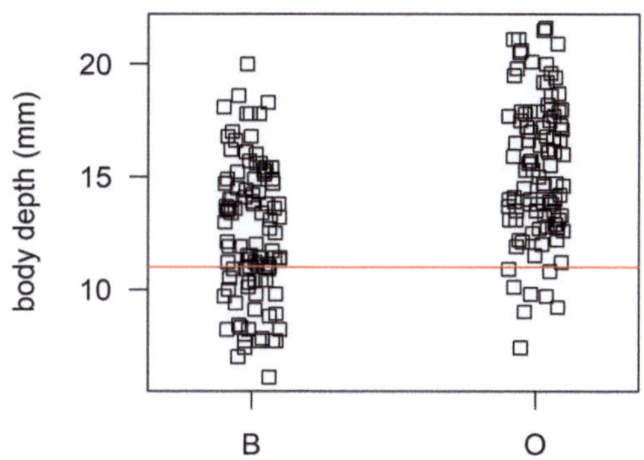

2. Based on the plot you have generated, with the cutoff value of 11, how many false negatives do you have, given that you set the color **blue** as the baseline category (orange is therefore considered as a positive case)?
According to the generated figure, it seems like there are eight orange crabs that are incorrectly predicted to be blue because there are eight data points below the line for the orange group.
3. Based on the same data and the cutoff value as in the previous question, compute sensitivity, specificity, PPV, and NPV.

```
library(caret)
pred=factor(ifelse(BD<cutoff,"B","O"),levels=c("B","O"))
confusionMatrix(data=pred,reference=Species, positive="O")
...
          Sensitivity : 0.9200
          Specificity : 0.3000
       Pos Pred Value : 0.5679
       Neg Pred Value : 0.7895
...
```

Exercises 10.4

1. Use the variable body depth (BD) from the Crab dataset to classify the two-color forms (Blue (B) and Orange (O)). Generate an ROC curve of the data and compute the AUC.

```
library(MASS) # To access the crab dataset
BD=crabs$BD
Group=crabs$sp
library(pROC)
roc1=roc(Group, BD)
data.frame(roc1$thresholds,roc1$sensitivities,
roc1$specificities)
plot(roc1)
roc1$auc
Area under the curve: 0.7364
```

Note the order in Group, where "B" comes before "O". The blue color is therefore our baseline, whereas the orange color is considered as a positive result.

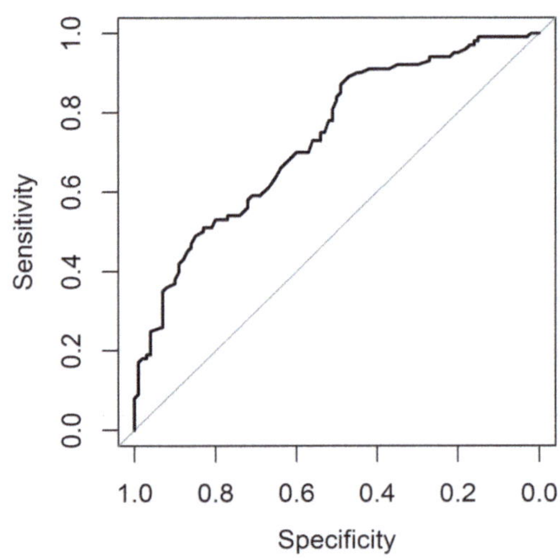

2. Calculate the 95% confidence interval of your AUC value. Is your AUC value significantly greater than 0.5?

```
ci.auc(roc1)
95% CI: 0.6683-0.8045 (DeLong)
```

Yes, because the 95% CI does not include the value 0.5 and the estimated AUC is larger than 0.5.

3. Use the "youden" method to find an appropriate cutoff value. Report the cutoff value and the corresponding sensitivity and specificity based on this cutoff.

```
coords(roc1,"best", best.method="youden")
         threshold       specificity        sensitivity
1          11.95             0.47               0.89
2          12.05             0.48               0.88
3          12.15             0.49               0.87
```

One of the three cutoff values can be used.

4. Create two ROC curves that represent the two variables body depth (BD) and rear width (RW) in the same plot. Use the function "roc.test" to test if there is a significant difference in AUC between the two curves.

```
library(MASS) # To access the crab dataset
BD=crabs$BD
Species=crabs$sp
library(pROC)
roc1=roc(Species, BD)
plot(roc1)
RW=crabs$RW
roc2=roc(Species, RW)
lines(roc2,col="red")
legend("bottomright",c("BD","RW"),col=1:2,lty=1,lwd=2)
roc.test(roc1,roc2,paired=TRUE)
DeLong's test for two correlated ROC curves
data:  roc1 and roc2
Z = 3.0898, p-value = 0.002003
alternative hypothesis: true difference in AUC is not
equal to 0
95 percent confidence interval:
 0.02175742 0.09724258
sample estimates:
AUC of roc1   AUC of roc2
  0.7364        0.6769
```

We see that the variable BD has a significantly larger AUC value compared to the variable RW.

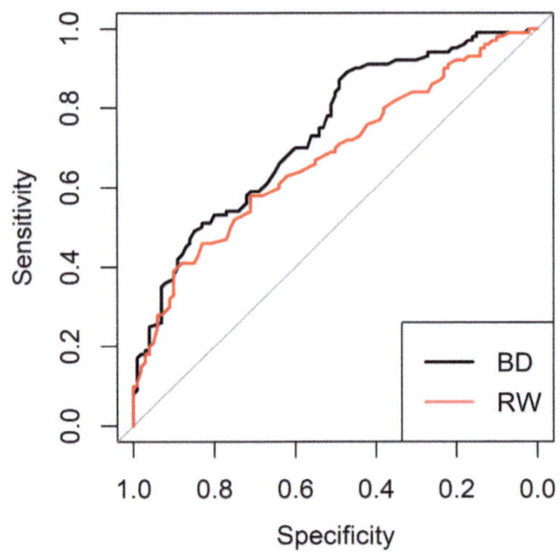

Exercises 10.6

1. Use the hold-out method as a validation method to compute the accuracy of how well the variable body depth (BD) can classify the two-color forms (Blue (B) and Orange (O)). Use the training data (60% of the total data) to compute an appropriate cutoff value based on the ROC curve, using the Youden method. Then, use the test data to see how well this cutoff value can discriminate the two groups. Calculate the accuracy.

```
library(caret)
library(MASS) # To access the crab dataset
set.seed(150) #For reproducibility
ind = createDataPartition(crabs$sp, p = 0.6, list=FALSE)
train = crabs[ind,]
test = crabs[-ind,]
library(pROC)
roc1=roc(train$sp, train$BD)
coords(roc1,"best", best.method="youden",transpose = FALSE)
cutoff=15.65 # Select one of the thresholds
# Blue crabs have generally smaller BD
pred=factor(ifelse(test$BD<cutoff,"B","O"))
(CT=table(pred,test$sp))
  pred  B    O
   B    29   21
   O    11   19
sum(diag(CT))/sum(CT)
0.60
# This also works
confusionMatrix(data=pred,reference=test$sp, positive="O")
```

Note that you might get different values if you have used another seed and/or if you use a different R-version than I used to generate the result (I used version 4.4.2).

2. Use the LOOCV to compute the accuracy of the variable body depth (BD), using all crabs, to classify the two-color forms (Blue (B) and Orange (O)), using the Youden method to determine the cutoff value in every iteration.

```
rm(list=ls()) # Clear environment
library(MASS) # To access the crab dataset
library(pROC)
BD=crabs$BD
Group=crabs$sp
df=data.frame(BD,Group)
n=nrow(df)  # Number of data points
pred=NULL  # Create a vector to save the prediction
for (i in 1:n){
  # Data point with row i will be used as test data
  test=df[i,]
  # Create a new data frame without the data point i
  train=df[-i,]
  roc1=roc(train$Group, train$BD)
  cutoff=coords(roc1,"best", best.method="youden",transpose =
  FALSE)$threshold
  pred[i]=ifelse(test$BD<cutoff,"B","O")
}
(CT=table(pred,Group))
       Group
 pred    B   O
    B   47  13
    O   53  87
sum(diag(CT))/sum(CT)
0.67
```

Answers to the Exercises in Chapter 11

Exercises 11.3

1. Combine the numerical variables in the Crab dataset by using LDA on all data to classify male and female crabs. Create an ROC curve of the discriminant scores. Note that:

```
crabs$sex
M M M  M  …
Levels: F M
```

female crabs are set first, so "female" will be our baseline.

```
rm(list=ls()) # Clear environment
library(MASS) # To access the crab dataset and the lda function
fit = lda(sex ~ FL+RW+CL+CW+BD, data=crabs)
D=as.numeric(predict(fit)$x)
stripchart(D~sex,data=crabs,ylab="Discriminant scores",
vertical = TRUE,xlim=c(0.5,2.5))
abline(h=0,col="red")
library(pROC)
Group=crabs$sex
roc1=roc(Group, D)
data.frame(roc1$thresholds,roc1$sensitivities,
roc1$specificities)
plot(roc1)
roc1
Area under the curve: 0.996
```

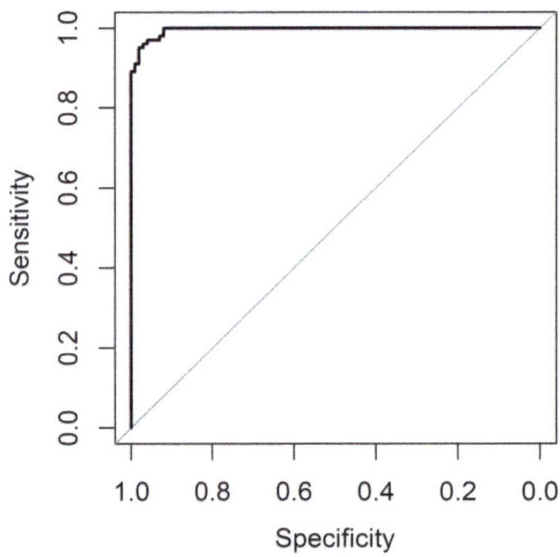

2. Calculate the accuracy, sensitivity, and specificity using the default cutoff value of 0 in the "predict" function. Use the category "female" as the baseline.
   Since the category "female" is our baseline, this will be associated with specificity, whereas the category "male" will be associated with sensitivity (a positive result).

```
library(caret)
pred=predict(fit,crabs[,4:8])$class
confusionMatrix(data=pred,reference=crabs$sex, positive="M")
Prediction  F    M
   F        95   3
   M        5    97
```

```
Accuracy : 0.96
…..
            Sensitivity : 0.9700
            Specificity : 0.9500
# The classification table and accuracy can also be calculated
like this
CT = table(pred, crabs$sex)
CT
pred    F    M
  F    95    3
  M     5   97
sum(diag(CT)/(sum(CT)))
0.96
```

3. Suppose that you find a crab and would like to know the sex of the crab with the following measurements: FL = 8.0, RW = 6.7, CL = 16.2, CW = 18.9, BD = 7.0. Use your LDA model to compute the probability that the crab is a female.

```
new=data.frame(FL=8.0,RW=6.7,CL=16.2,CW=18.9,BD=7.0)
predict(fit,new)
Levels: F M
$posterior
      F            M
1 0.03595855   0.9640415
$x
     LD1
1 0.9565681
```

The probability that the crab is a female is about 3.596%.

4. Build an LDA model based on the Crab dataset to classify male and female crabs. Use the hold-out method to validate your model. Use 70% of the data to train your model and 30% to test your model. Report the accuracy of your model based on the test data.

```
rm(list=ls()) # Clear environment
library(caret)
library(MASS) # To access the crab dataset and the lda function
set.seed(1) #For reproducibility
ind = createDataPartition(crabs$sex, p = 0.7, list=FALSE)
train = crabs[ind,]
test = crabs[-ind,]
fit = lda(sex ~ FL+RW+CL+CW+BD, data=train)
pred=predict(fit, test)$class
tab = table(pred, test$sex)
tab
```

```
pred  F   M
 F   24   1
 M    6  29
sum(diag(tab)/(sum(tab)))
0.8833333
```

Note that the accuracy has been reduced from 0.96 to 0.88 when we use validation. Also, note that you might get different values if you have used another seed and/or if you use a different R-version than I used to generate the result (I used version 4.4.2).

We can also use the "train" function in the caret package:

```
set.seed(1) #For reproducibility
fit = train(sex ~ FL+RW+CL+CW+BD, data=train, method="lda",
        trControl = trainControl(method = "cv"))
pred=predict(fit,test)
confusionMatrix(data=pred,reference=test$sex, positive="M")
0.8833333
```

Exercises 11.5

1. Combine the numerical variables in the Crab dataset by using logistic regression on all data. Create an ROC curve based on the computed probabilities to classify male and female crabs and report the AUC value.

```
rm(list=ls()) # Clear environment
library(MASS) # To access the crab dataset
fit=glm(sex~FL+RW+CL+CW+BD,data=crabs,family=binomial)
Prob=predict(fit,type="response")
stripchart(Prob~sex,data=crabs,ylab="Probabilities",
vertical = TRUE,xlim=c(0.5,2.5))
abline(h=0.5,col="red")
Group=crabs$sex
library(pROC)
roc1=roc(Group, Prob)
plot(roc1)
roc1
Area under the curve: 0.9986
```

Note that, by using logistic regression, we get a bit better prediction than with the LDA since the AUC has increased from 0.996 to 0.9986.

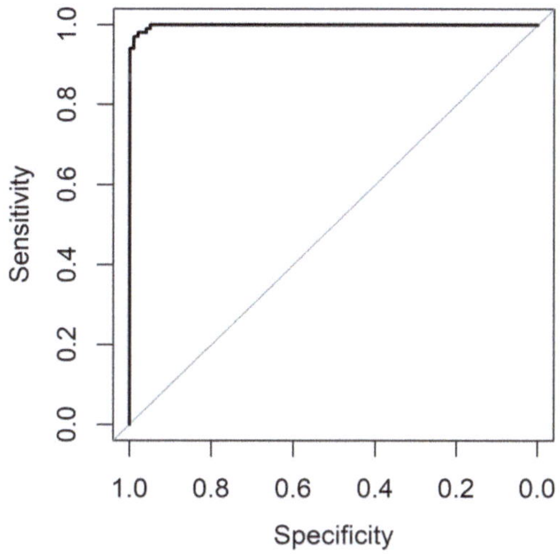

2. Simplify the logistic model by using the "step" function with backward selection. Which variables were included in the simplified model?

```
step(fit,direction="backward")
…..
Step:  AIC=27
sex ~ FL + RW + CL
              Df    Deviance    AIC
<none>              19.003      27.003
- FL          1     24.095      30.095
- CL          1     93.299      99.299
- RW          1     257.286     263.286
```

The variables included in the simplified/reduced model are FL, RW, and CL.

3. Calculate the accuracy of your simplified model versus the full model using a cutoff value of 0.5.
   Full model

```
fit=glm(sex~FL+RW+CL+CW+BD,data=crabs,family=binomial)
pred_prob=predict(fit,type="response")
pred_class=factor(ifelse(pred_prob<0.5,"F","M"))
tab = table(pred_class, crabs$sex)
tab
sum(diag(tab)/(sum(tab)))
0.975
```

   Simplified model

```
fit=glm(sex~FL+RW+CL,data=crabs,family=binomial)
pred_prob=predict(fit,type="response")
pred_class=factor(ifelse(pred_prob<0.5,"F","M"))
tab = table(pred_class, crabs$sex)
```

```
tab
sum(diag(tab)/(sum(tab)))
0.975
```

The full model and the simplified model predict equally well.

4. Suppose that you find a crab and would like to know the sex of the crab with the following measurements: FL = 8.0, RW = 6.7, CL = 16.2, CW = 18.9, BD = 7.0. Use your simplified logistic regression model to compute the probability that the crab is a female.

```
new=data.frame(FL=8.0,RW=6.7,CL=16.2,CW=18.9,BD=7.0)
1-predict(fit,new,type="response")
0.002047452
```

Since we set females as the baseline, the probability that the crab is a male is the one that is computed by the "predict" function. To compute the corresponding probability that it is a female crab, we therefore take one minus the probability for a crab to be a male. The probability that we have a female crab is about 0.2%. Also, since the simplified model only includes FL, RW, and CL, it is enough to use only these measurements.

```
new=data.frame(FL=8.0,RW=6.7,CL=16.2)
1-predict(fit,new,type="response")
0.002047452
```

5. Use the hold-out method to validate your simplified model. Use 70% of the data as your training data and 30% as your test data. Then calculate the accuracy of the model based on the test dataset. Note, as we discussed at the beginning of this chapter, we should perform model selection on a validation data and not on all data as in this example. We will discuss such approach in the next section.

```
set.seed(1) #For reproducibility
ind = createDataPartition(crabs$sex, p = 0.7, list=FALSE)
train = crabs[ind,]
test = crabs[-ind,]
fit = glm(sex~FL+RW+CL,data=train,family=binomial)
pred_prob=predict(fit, test,type="response")
pred_class=ifelse(pred_prob<0.5,"F","M")
pred_class=factor(pred_class)
tab = table(pred_class, test$sex)
tab
 pred_class    F    M
     F         28   0
     M         2    30
sum(diag(tab)/(sum(tab)))
0.9666667
```

Note that you might get different values if you have used another seed and/or if you use a different R-version than I used to generate the result (I used version 4.4.2).
We can also use the "train" function in the caret package:

```
fit = train(sex ~ FL+RW+CL, data=train, method="glm",
family="binomial",
         trControl = trainControl(method = "cv"))
pred=predict(fit,test)
confusionMatrix(data=pred,reference=test$sex, positive="M")
```

Exercises 11.7

1. Use a decision tree to classify female and male crabs of the Crab dataset (you can use all numerical variables as well as the categorical variable species in the dataset to classify). Use all data to create the tree. To avoid overfitting, set the argument minsplit to 80.

```
rm(list=ls()) # Clear environment
library(MASS) # To access the crab dataset
library(rpart)
fit=rpart(sex~FL+RW+CL+CW+BD+sp,data=crabs,
      method="class",minsplit=80,parms = list(split = "gini"))
library(rpart.plot)
rpart.plot(fit,extra=1)
```

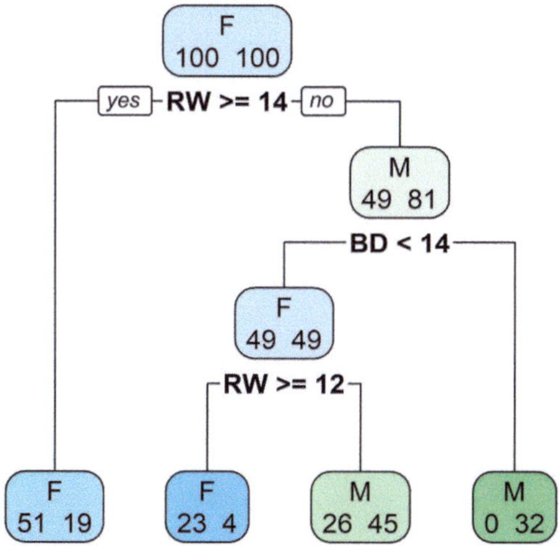

2. Calculate the accuracy of your tree.

```
library(caret)
pred=predict(fit, crabs[,c(1,4:8)], type="class")
confusionMatrix(data=pred,reference=crabs$sex, positive="M")
....
```

```
Accuracy : 0.755
# The classification table and accuracy can also be calculated
like this
tab = table(pred, crabs$sex)
tab
sum(diag(tab)/(sum(tab)))
```

3. Suppose that you find a crab and would like to know the sex of the crab with the following measurements: RW = 6.7, BD = 7.0. Use your tree to compute if the crab is a male or a female. Also, explain in words how the tree makes this prediction.
We need to re-run the "rpart" function to make a prediction based only on the RW and BD:

```
fit=rpart(sex~RW+BD,data=crabs,method="class",minsplit=80,
parms = list(split = "gini"))
new=data.frame(RW=6.7,BD=7.0)
predict(fit,new,type="class")
M
Levels: F M
```

Since the RW is smaller than 14, we first move to the right in the tree. Then we move to the left in the second node because BD is less than 14. Finally, we move to the right because RW is less than 12. The node we end up in is defined as M (male) because the majority of crabs (45 out of 71) in this node are male crabs.
4. Use a decision tree to classify female and male crabs of the Crab dataset (you can use all numerical variables as well as the categorical variable species in the dataset to classify). Use the hold-out method to evaluate your tree. Use 70% of the data to build your tree (to find an appropriate value of the cp parameter) and 30% of the data to test your tree.

```
rm(list=ls()) # Clear environment
library(caret)
library(MASS) # To access the crab dataset
library(rpart)
set.seed(1) #For reproducibility
ind = createDataPartition(crabs$sex, p = 0.7, list=FALSE)
train = crabs[ind,]
test = crabs[-ind,]
fit=rpart(sex~FL+RW+CL+CW+BD+sp,data=train,method="class",
minsplit=1,parms = list(split = "gini"),cp=0)
plotcp(fit)
```

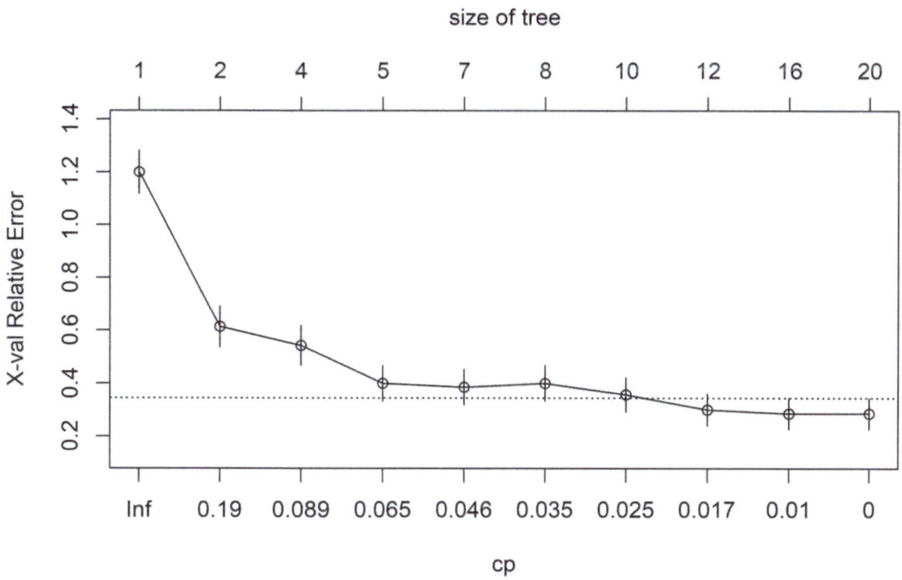

Based on the training data, we select a cp value of 0.017 for our tree. Note that you might get different values if you have used another seed and/or if you use a different R-version than I used to generate the result (I used version 4.4.2).

```
fit=rpart(sex~FL+RW+CL+CW+BD+sp,data=train,method="class",
minsplit=1,parms = list(split = "gini"),cp=0.017)
pred=predict(fit, test, type="class")
tab=table(pred, test$sex)
sum(diag(tab)/(sum(tab)))
0.8
```

To plot the pruned tree, you can run:

```
library(rpart.plot)
rpart.plot(fit,roundint=FALSE,extra=1)
```

We can also use the "train" function in the caret package to tune the hyperparameter based on a 10-fold cross-validation. To train the model, we can, for simplicity, use 41 different cp values that go from 0 to 0.2 with a step size of 0.005, which seems to be a reasonable range according to the figure above.

```
set.seed(1) #For reproducibility
# To try different models with different cp values
cp_grid = data.frame(cp = seq(0,0.2,0.005))
fit = train(sex ~ FL+RW+CL+CW+BD+sp, data=train, method=
"rpart",minsplit=1,parms = list(split = "gini"),trControl =
trainControl(method = "cv"), tuneGrid = cp_grid)
print(fit)
```

```
     cp          Accuracy        Kappa
   0.000        0.7857143     0.5714286
   0.005        0.7857143     0.5714286
   0.010        0.7857143     0.5714286
   0.015        0.7857143     0.5714286
   0.020        0.7857143     0.5714286
   0.025        0.7857143     0.5714286
   0.030        0.7857143     0.5714286
   0.035        0.7642857     0.5285714
   0.040        0.7571429     0.5142857
   0.045        0.7571429     0.5142857
….
```

Based on the 10-fold cross-validation, the “train” function proposed a cp value of 0.03. By using this value:

```
fit=rpart(sex~FL+RW+CL+CW+BD+sp,data=train,method="class",
minsplit=1,parms = list(split = "gini"),cp=0.03)

pred=predict(fit, test, type="class")
tab=table(pred, test$sex)
sum(diag(tab)/(sum(tab)))
0.75
```

we get a bit lower accuracy than if we used the plot to find the optimal value of cp.

Exercises 11.9

1. Create a random forest with 2000 trees to classify female and male crabs of the Crab dataset (you can use all numerical variables as well as the categorical variable species in the dataset to classify). Use all data to create the forest.

```
library(MASS) # To access the Crab dataset
library(randomForest)
set.seed(1) #For reproducibility
RF = randomForest(sex ~ FL+RW+CL+CW+BD+sp,data=crabs,
ntree=2000)
plot(RF)
```

2. Calculate the accuracy of your forest based on the OOB error.

```
tab=RF$confusion
(Accuracy=sum(diag(tab[,-3]))/sum(tab[,-3]))
0.9
1-RF$err.rate[2000,1] #This also works
```

Note that you might get a different accuracy if you have used another seed and/or if you use a different R-version than I used to generate the result (I used version 4.4.2).

3. Suppose that you find a blue crab (sp="B") and would like to know the sex of the crab with the following measurements: FL = 8.0, RW = 6.7, CL = 16.2, CW = 18.9, BD = 7.0. Use your forest to predict if it is a male or a female crab.

```
new=data.frame(FL=8.0,RW=6.7,CL=16.2,CW=18.9,BD=7.0,
sp=factor("B",levels=c("B","O")))
predict(RF,new)
M
Levels: F M
```

4. Use a random forest with 1000 trees to classify female and male crabs of the Crab dataset (you can use all numerical variables as well as the categorical variable species in the dataset to classify). Use the hold-out method to evaluate your forest. Use 70% of the data to build your model and 30% of the data to test your model.

```
rm(list=ls()) # Clear environment
library(caret)
library(MASS) # To access the crab dataset
library(randomForest)
set.seed(123) #For reproducibility
ind = createDataPartition(crabs$sex, p = 0.7, list=FALSE)
train = crabs[ind,]
test = crabs[-ind,]
set.seed(123) #For reproducibility
RF = randomForest(sex ~ FL+RW+CL+CW+BD+sp,data=train,
ntree=1000)
pred=predict(RF,test)
(tab1=table(pred,test$sex))
(accuracy=sum(diag(tab1))/sum(tab1))
0.8833333
```

Note that you might get a different accuracy if you have used another seed and/ or if you use a different R-version than I used to generate the result (I used version 4.4.2).
We can also use the "train" function in the **caret** package:

```
set.seed(123) #For reproducibility
#Tune the mtry parameter
mtry_grid=expand.grid(mtry = c(1,2,3,4,5))
fit = train(sex ~ FL+RW+CL+CW+BD+sp, data=train, method="rf",
ntree=1000,
          trControl = trainControl(method = "cv"),
          tuneGrid = mtry_grid)
print(fit)
...
```

```
Accuracy was used to select the optimal model using the
largest value.
The final value used for the model was mtry = 4
```

The 10-fold cross-validation suggested an optimal value of 4 for the mtry parameter. If we instead use this parameter value to train a random forest:

```
set.seed(123) #For reproducibility
fit = randomForest(sex ~ FL+RW+CL+CW+BD+sp,data=train,
ntree=1000,mtry=4)
pred=predict(fit,test)
tab=table(pred, test$sex)
tab
sum(diag(tab)/(sum(tab)))
0.8666667
```

we get a bit higher accuracy.

5. Use all numeric variables and the variable species (sp) in the Crab dataset to find the most important variable to predict the sex of the crabs.

```
rm(list=ls()) # Clear environment
library(MASS) # To access the crab dataset
library(randomForest)
set.seed(123) #For reproducibility
RF = randomForest(sex ~ FL+RW+CL+CW+BD+sp,data=crabs,
ntree=1000, importance=TRUE)
varImpPlot(RF)
```

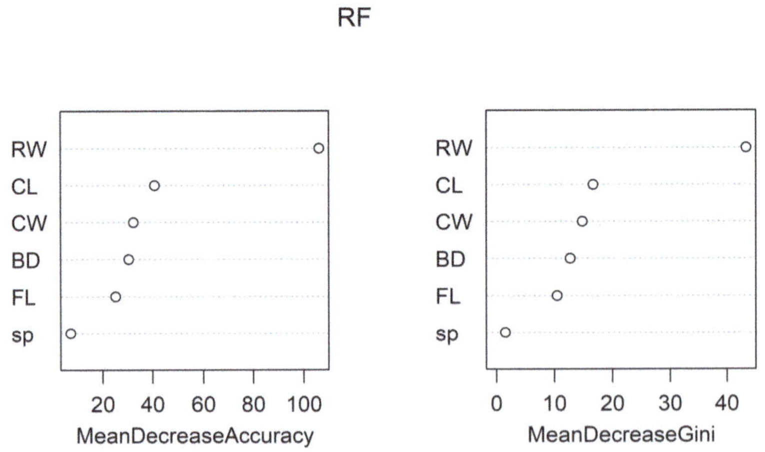

Note that you might get different values in the plot if you have used another seed and/or if you use a different R-version than I used to generate the result (I used version 4.4.2). We see that the variable RW is the most important variable to predict the sex.

Exercises 11.11

1. Suppose that you find a crab and would like to know the sex of the crab with the following measurements: FL = 8.0, RW = 6.7, CL = 16.2, CW = 18.9, BD = 7.0. Use KNN, where you set *k* to 5, to predict if it is a male or female crab based on the numeric variables.

```
rm(list=ls()) # Clear environment
library(MASS) # To access the crab dataset
library(class)
data1=crabs[,c(4:8)]
new=data.frame(FL=8.0,RW=6.7,CL=16.2,CW=18.9,BD=7.0)
knn(data1, new, crabs$sex, k = 5)
[1] M
Levels: F M
```

2. Use KNN to classify female and male crabs of the Crab dataset based on all numeric variables in the dataset. Use the hold-out method to validate your KNN. Use 70% of the data to train your KNN to find an optimal value of *k* and 30% of the data to test your classifier.

```
rm(list=ls()) # Clear environment
library(caret)
library(MASS) # To access the crab dataset
set.seed(3) #For reproducibility
ind = createDataPartition(crabs$sex, p = 0.7, list=FALSE)
train = crabs[ind,]
test = crabs[-ind,]
tune =data.frame(k = seq(1,50,2))
fit = train(sex ~ FL+RW+CL+CW+BD, data=train, method="knn",
         trControl = trainControl(method = "cv"),
         tuneGrid = tune)
print(fit)
…
Accuracy was used to select the optimal model using the
largest value.
The final value used for the model was k = 3.
```

From the hyperparameter tuning, we know that we should set *k* to 3. Let's see how well the KNN predicts the test dataset by using a value of 3 for the parameter *k*:

```
library(class)
data1=train[,c(4:8)] # FL, RW, CL, CW and BD
class1=train$sex # Class membership of training data
pred=knn(data1, test[,c(4:8)], class1, k = 3) # Predict
tab=table(pred, test$sex)
tab
```

```
pred   F    M
  F    26   3
  M    4    27
sum(diag(tab)/(sum(tab)))
0.8833333
```

Note that you might get a different accuracy if you have used another seed and/or if you use a different R-version than I used to generate the result (I used version 4.4.2).

Exercises 11.13

1. Use Naive Bayes to classify female and male crabs, using all numeric variables of the Crab dataset, and calculate its accuracy. Use the default settings in the "naive_bayes" function.

```
library(naivebayes)
model=naive_bayes(sex~FL+RW+CL+CW+BD,crabs)
pred=predict(model)
confusionMatrix(data=pred,reference=crabs$sex, positive="M")
…
Accuracy : 0.88
```

2. Suppose that you find a crab and would like to know the sex of the crab with the following measurements: FL = 8.0, RW = 6.7, CL = 16.2, CW = 18.9, BD = 7.0. Use your NB model to predict if it is a male or female crab based on the numeric variables.

```
new=data.frame(FL=8.0,RW=6.7,CL=16.2,CW=18.9,BD=7.0)
predict(model,new)
[1]  F
Levels: F M
```

3. Use Naive Bayes to classify female and male crabs, using all numeric variables of the Crab dataset. Use the hold-out method to validate your model. Use 70% of the data to build and tune the hyperparameters of your model and 30% of the data to test your model.

```
rm(list=ls()) # Clear environment
library(caret)
library(MASS) # To access the crab dataset
set.seed(10) #For reproducibility
ind = createDataPartition(crabs$sex, p = 0.7, list=FALSE)
train = crabs[ind,]
test = crabs[-ind,]
tune_grid = expand.grid(
  laplace = 0,
  # Try both kernel density estimate and Gaussian distribution
```

```
  usekernel = c(TRUE, FALSE),
  adjust = c(0.5, 1, 2)
)
tune_grid$adjust[tune_grid$usekernel == FALSE] = NA

fit = train(sex ~ FL+RW+CL+CW+BD, data=train,
method="naive_bayes",
        trControl = trainControl(method = "cv"),tuneGrid =
        tune_grid)
print(fit)
…
  usekernel    adjust     Accuracy      Kappa
   FALSE         NA      0.6571429    0.3142857
   TRUE         0.5      0.5571429    0.1142857
   TRUE         1.0      0.6142857    0.2285714
   TRUE         2.0      0.6857143    0.3714286
Tuning parameter 'laplace' was held constant at a value of 0
Accuracy was used to select the optimal model using the
largest value.
The final values used for the model were laplace = 0,
usekernel = TRUE and adjust = 2.
```

From the hyperparameter tuning, we see that a model using a kernel with the parameter "adjust" set to 2 results in the highest cross-validation accuracy. Let's retrain the model with the optimal hyperparameters and evaluate how well it performs on the test dataset.

```
library(naivebayes)
fit=naive_bayes(sex ~ FL+RW+CL+CW+BD,train, usekernel = TRUE,
adjust=2)
pred=predict(fit, test[,4:8])
tab=table(pred, test$sex)
tab
sum(diag(tab))/sum(tab)
0.65
```

Note that you might get a different accuracy if you have used another seed and/or if you use a different R-version than I used to generate the result (I used version 4.4.2).

Naive Bayes results in a very low accuracy (65%), which suggests that this method is clearly not appropriate for this type of data.

Answers to the Exercises in Chapter 12

Exercises 12.2

1. Cluster the 200 crabs based on the numerical variables of the Crab dataset, using average linkage and the Euclidean distance based on standardized data. Show a dendrogram of the clustering.

```
rm(list=ls()) # Clear environment
library(MASS) # To access the crab dataset
data=scale(crabs[,4:8]) # Standardize the numerical variables
h=dist(data, method = "euclidean")
clust=hclust(h,method="average")
plot(clust ,cex=0.3) # Use smaller labels
```

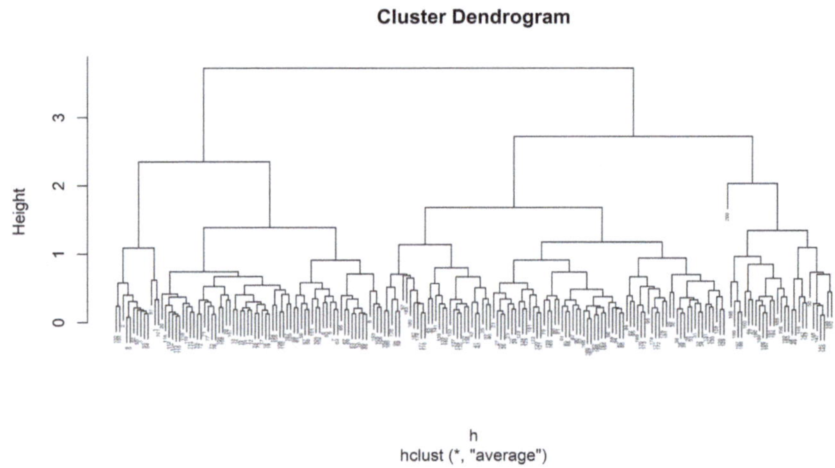

2. Can you identify a crab that is far away from the other crabs?
   Crab number 200 according to the dendrogram above. Export the figure in R to a PDF so that you get a higher resolution of the figure where you can zoom in on the labels.
3. Cut the tree at 1.3. How many clusters do you then obtain? In which cluster can you find crab number 122?

```
abline(h=1.3,col="red") # Place a line in the dendrogram
cutree(clust, h=1.3)
.. 121  122  123  124 .....
     4    4    4    4
# to get the number of clusters and the number of crabs in
each cluster
table(cutree(clust, h=1.3))
 1   2   3   4   5   6   7  8
13  25  37  65  30  17  12  1
```

There are in total eight clusters and crab number 122 can be found in cluster 4.

4. Transpose the dataset so that you instead cluster the standardized numerical variables. Which variables have the most similar profiles across the crabs according to the dendrogram?

```
rm(list=ls()) # Clear environment
library(MASS) # To access the crab dataset
data=t(scale(crabs[,4:8]))
h=dist(data, method = "euclidean")
clust=hclust(h,method="average")
plot(clust)
```

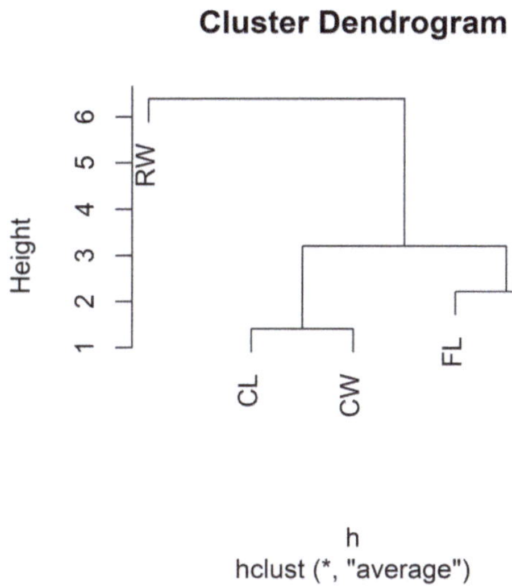

The variables CL and CW have similar profiles across the crabs, whereas the variables FL and BD are similar.

5. Cluster the standardized numerical variables in the Crab dataset. Check which of the linkage functions: average, single, and complete that generates the most robust clusters. Use the Euclidean distance and 1000 bootstraps.

```
library(pvclust)
set.seed(1) #For reproducibility
# Extract and Standardize the numerical variables
data=scale(crabs[,4:8])
fit_aver=pvclust(data, method.hclust="average",
method.dist="euclidean",nboot=1000)
plot(fit_aver)
fit_single=pvclust(data, method.hclust="single",
method.dist="euclidean",nboot=1000)
fit_comp=pvclust(data, method.hclust="complete",
method.dist="euclidean",nboot=1000)
mean(fit_aver$edges$bp)
1
```

```
mean(fit_single$edges$bp)
0.9938185
mean(fit_comp$edges$bp)
1
```

Note that you might get different values if you have used another seed and/or if you use a different R-version than I used to generate the result (I used version 4.4.2).
The complete and average linkage functions resulted in the most robust clusters compared to the single linkage function.

Exercises 12.4

1. Create a heatmap of the standardized numerical variables in the Crab dataset, using the **pheatmap** package. Use complete linkage and the Euclidean distance for the dendrograms. Annotate the rows so that one can see if a crab is a female or male. Tip: export the figure to PDF for a better resolution and set a smaller font size so that you can see the row numbers clearly (fontsize_row = 1.5).

```
library(pheatmap)
library(MASS) # To access the crab dataset
# Standardize the numeric columns
df_scale=as.matrix(scale(crabs[,4:8]))
# Assign row names in the matrix
rownames(df_scale)=rownames(crabs)
library(pheatmap)
pheatmap(df_scale,scale="none",clustering_method="complete",
fontsize_row = 1.5,
         annotation_row = data.frame(Sex=crabs$sex))
```

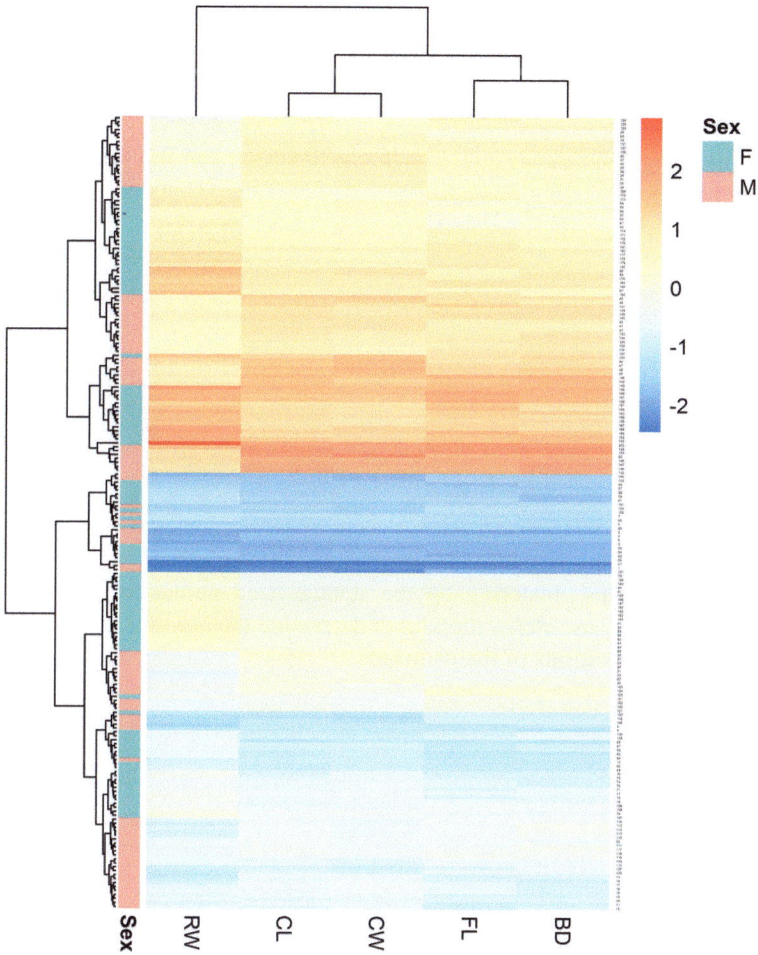

2. Based on the heatmap, can you explain why crab number 200 deviates from the other crabs in the dendrogram?
   It has a relatively large rear width (RW) compared to the other crabs (the dark red band in the RW column).
3. Based on the dendrogram of the crabs, do you think that male and female crabs are well separated?
   No, there is a mixture of male and female crabs in the clusters.
4. There is a distinct cluster of crabs in the middle of the heatmap. What characterizes this cluster?
   This cluster consists of relatively small carbs (the blue bands in the middle).
5. Create a similar heatmap as before but use annotations also for the species of the crabs so that one can identify both the sex and the species. Which type of crabs have the longest rear width (RW) according to the heatmap?
   Orange female crabs have the longest rear width.

```
pheatmap(df_scale,scale="none",clustering_method="complete",
fontsize_row = 1.5,
       annotation_row = data.frame(Sex=crabs$sex,
       Species=crabs$sp))
```

The following code shows how to hide the dendrograms and how to use custom colors for the annotation

```
pheatmap(df_scale,scale="none",clustering_method="complete",
fontsize_row = 1.5,
       annotation_row = data.frame(Sex=crabs$sex,
       Species=crabs$sp),
          treeheight_row = 0, treeheight_col = 0,
          annotation_colors = list(Sex = c("M" = "lightgreen",
          "F" = "red4"),
            Species = c("B" = "navyblue", "O" = "orange"))
)
```

Exercises 12.6

1. Compute K-means clustering on the standardized numerical variables in the Crab dataset. Use the elbow method to determine the optimal value of k. Use 25 random initial positions of the centroids.

```
library(MASS) # To access the crab dataset
Ks=1:20
WCSS=NULL
df=scale(crabs[,4:8])
for (i in Ks) {
  # 25 different random positions
  WCSS[i]=kmeans(df, i, nstart = 25)$tot.withinss
}
plot(Ks, WCSS,type="b", pch = 19, frame=FALSE,
xlab="Number of clusters (k)",
     ylab="Total within cluster sum of squares",xlim=c(0,20))
```

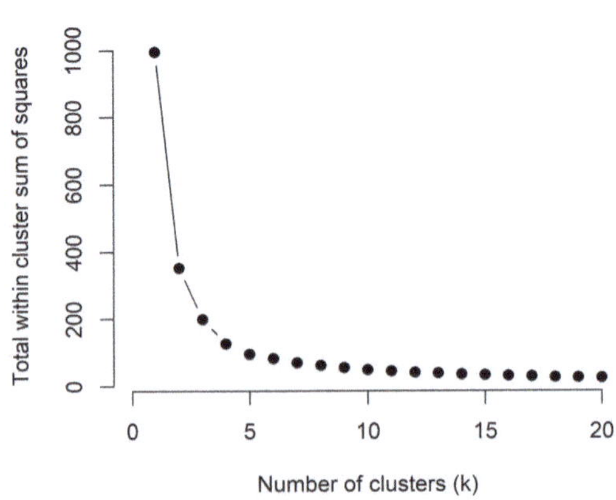

From this plot, it seems like the "elbow" is visible at four clusters, which means that we select four clusters. Note that the random positions of the centroids might result in a slightly different plot every time you run the code.

2. Use K-means clustering to generate four clusters. How many crabs are included in the first cluster (note that the computation involves random processes, which means that you might get different results each time you run your code)?

```
set.seed(1) #For reproducibility
cluster=kmeans(df, 4, nstart = 25 )$cluster
table(cluster)
   cluster
 1   2   3   4
28  71  41  60
```

The first cluster includes 28 crabs. Note that you might get different numbers if you have used another seed and/or if you use a different R-version than I used to generate the result (I used version 4.4.2).

Answers to the Exercises in Chapter 13

Exercises 13.4

1. Use a multiple linear regression model to predict the frontal lobe size (FL) based on the variables RW, CL, CW, and BD from the Crab dataset:
FL~RW+CL+CW+BD
Once you have generated the model, check if your model involves multicollinearity.

```
rm(list=ls()) # Clear environment
library(MASS) # To access the crab dataset
fit=lm(FL~RW+CL+CW+BD,data=crabs)
library(car)
vif(fit)
      RW          CL           CW           BD
6.181286  327.125200   185.836821   52.391501
```

Most of the VIF values are much greater than 5 which indicates that we have problems with multicollinearity.

2. Use instead the **pls** package to compute PCR where you extract only the first principal component. Show the equation with the estimated parameters for this model.

```
library(pls)
library(MASS) # To access the crab dataset
pcr_fit=pcr(FL~RW+CL+CW+BD,ncomp=1,data=crabs)
summary(pcr_fit)
coef(pcr_fit,intercept = TRUE)
```

FL=-0.067+0.062*RW + 0.188*CL + 0.208*CW + 0.089*BD

3. Compute 95% confidence intervals for the parameters in the PCR model based on 1000 bootstrap samples.

```
library(boot)
library(MASS) # To access the crab dataset
set.seed(1) #For reproducibility
bs=function(formula, data, indices){
  bootstrap=data[indices,] # allows boot to select sample
  fit = pcr(formula, data=bootstrap,ncomp=1)
  return(coef(fit,intercept = TRUE))
}
results = boot(data=crabs, statistic=bs, R=1000,
formula=FL~RW+CL+CW+BD)
boot.ci(results, type="perc", index=2)
95%    ( 0.0567,  0.0671 )
boot.ci(results, type="perc", index=3)
95%    ( 0.1821,  0.1942 )
boot.ci(results, type="perc", index=4)
95%    ( 0.2036,  0.2129 )
boot.ci(results, type="perc", index=5)
95%    ( 0.0841,  0.0936 )
```

Note that you might get different values if you have used another seed and/or if you use a different R-version than I used to generate the result (I used version 4.4.2).

4. Use your PCR model to predict the FL size of a crab with the following measurements: RW=6.7, CL=16.1, CW=19.0, BD=7.0.

```
new=data.frame(RW=6.7,CL=16.1,CW=19.0,BD=7.0)
predict(pcr_fit,new)
7.950618
```

5. Use Lasso regression to predict the frontal lobe size (FL) based on the variables RW, CL, CW, and BD in the Crab dataset:
FL~RW+CL+CW+BD
Which variable is suggested by the Lasso model to be unnecessary to predict FL?

```
library(MASS)  # To access the crab dataset
library(glmnet)
# Feature matrix
X = as.matrix(crabs[, c("RW", "CL", "CW", "BD")])
y = crabs$FL           # Response variable
# Find best lambda value
```

```
cv_model = cv.glmnet(X, y, family="gaussian", alpha=1)
lasso_model=glmnet(X, y, family="gaussian", alpha=1,
intercept=TRUE, lambda=cv_model$lambda.min)
coef(lasso_model)
                      s0
(Intercept)     0.69996020
RW              0.16116733
CL              0.08498062
CW              .
BD              0.71997892
```

The variable CW seems to be unnecessary to predict frontal lobe size.

6. Use Lasso regression to predict the sex of the crabs based on the variables sp, FL, RW, CL, CW, and BD in the Crab dataset:
sex~sp+FL+RW+CL+CW+BD
Which variable is suggested by the Lasso model to be unnecessary to predict sex? Note that you need to convert the variable species (sp) to ones and zeros so that the feature matrix only includes numeric data.

```
rm(list=ls())
library(MASS)       # To access the crab dataset
# Extract continuous variables
X1 = as.matrix(crabs[, c("FL", "RW", "CL", "CW", "BD")])
# Convert variable species to numeric 0/1
X2 = ifelse(crabs$sp == "B", 1, 0)
X=cbind(X1,sp=X2)  # Feature matrix
y = crabs$sex             # Response variable
set.seed(1)                # For reproducibility
# Find best value for lambda
cv_model = cv.glmnet(X, y, family="binomial", alpha=1)
lasso_model=glmnet(X, y, family="binomial", alpha=1,
intercept=TRUE, lambda=cv_model$lambda.min)
coef(lasso_model)
                      s0
(Intercept)     11.0176419
FL              -1.1395595
RW              -9.1482211
CL              3.7823981
CW              .
BD              0.2417283
sp             -0.2087569
```

The variable CW seems to be unnecessary to predict sex.

Index

A. Tilevik, *Multivariate Statistics and Machine Learning in R For Beginners*, https://doi.org/10.1007/978-3-032-01851-9

V

W

Z

Functions in R:

A. Tilevik, *Multivariate Statistics and Machine Learning in R For Beginners*, https://doi.org/10.1007/978-3-032-01851-9

Packages in R:

A. Tilevik, *Multivariate Statistics and Machine Learning in R For Beginners*,
https://doi.org/10.1007/978-3-032-01851-9

MIX
Papier aus verantwortungsvollen Quellen
Paper from responsible sources
FSC® C105338

If you have any concerns about our products,
you can contact us on
ProductSafety@springernature.com

In case Publisher is established outside the EU,
the EU authorized representative is:
Springer Nature Customer Service Center GmbH
Europaplatz 3, 69115 Heidelberg, Germany

Printed by Libri Plureos GmbH
in Hamburg, Germany